ORAL DISEASES

An illustrated guide to diagnosis and management
of diseases of the oral mucosa, gingivae, teeth,
salivary glands, bones and joints

ORAL DISEASES

An illustrated guide to diagnosis and management
of diseases of the oral mucosa, gingivae, teeth,
salivary glands, bones and joints

Second Edition

Crispian Scully

MD, PhD, MDS, FDSRCPS, FFDRCSI, FDSRCS, FRCPath
Professor of Oral Medicine, Pathology and Microbiology
Dean, Clinical Director and Director of Studies
Eastman Dental Institute and Hospital for Oral Health Care Sciences
and University College London Hospitals
University of London, UK

Stephen R Flint

MA, PhD, MBBS, FFDRCSI, FDSRCS
Senior Lecturer and Consultant in Oral Medicine
School of Dental Science
Trinity College
Dublin, Ireland

Stephen R Porter

MD, PhD, FDSRCS, FDSRCSE
Head of Department, Senior Lecturer
and Honorary Consultant
Eastman Dental Institute and Hospital for Oral Health Care Sciences
and University College London Hospitals
University of London, UK

MARTIN DUNITZ

© Crispian Scully and Stephen Flint 1989, Martin Dunitz Limited 1996

First published in the United Kingdom in 1989
as *An Atlas of Stomatology*
by Martin Dunitz Limited, The Livery House,
7–9 Pratt Street, London, NW1 OAE

First edition 1989
Second edition 1996

A CIP catalogue record for this title is available
from the British Library.

ISBN: 1–85317–202–2

Publisher's note

This book includes photographs that predate the recommendations
on control of cross-infection: gloves should be worn where appropriate.

Composition by Scribe Design, Gillingham, Kent
Originated, printed and bound in Singapore by Toppan Printing Company (S) Pte Ltd

PREFACE TO THE FIRST EDITION

This atlas gives examples of oral diseases and those lesions in the wide range of systemic disorders that have oral manifestations. It differs from other atlases by the inclusion of a wide range of the more obvious extraoral manifestations and of some disorders of the teeth and hard tissues. It is intended primarily as a pictorial diagnostic aid, both for dentists and physicians, with text that provides a concise synopsis of stomatology. We have added very recent references for most topics, mainly where there are new developments, reviews or points of controversy.

The atlas covers clinical diagnostic features and includes some radiographs, but excludes laboratory tests and does not attempt to discuss management. Neither have we attempted to cover orthodontics, oral surgery or periodontology, as they are dealt with elsewhere.

It is impossible to organize the illustrations in a format that will please all and we have therefore elected to conform fairly closely to the World Health Organization International Classification of Diseases (ICD). This, like any system, cannot suit all needs but it does have the advantage of having received WHO acceptance. We have varied the system where we felt it absolutely necessary.

The illustrations are almost exclusively from our collection in the University Department of Oral Medicine, Surgery and Pathology at Bristol. We are indebted to former and present members of the Department who have contributed to the collection, particularly to the late Professor A I Darling; to Professors J Fletcher and A K Adatia; to Drs S R Porter and J Luker; and to Mr R G Smith. We are also grateful to Professor D K Mason, under whose care some of the patients were seen in Glasgow. A few slides are from other collections: Dr G Laskaris (Athens) has kindly helped with Figures 2.130, 2.131, 2.140, 14.82, 14.83 and 16.58; our colleagues, O Almeida, D Berry, M Griffiths, S Mutlu, F Nally, S Prime, J Ross, J Shepherd and A S Young have also helped with single contributions.

Most of the illustrations have not previously been published. For those that have, we are indebted to Professor R A Cawson as co-author of some publications; to the editors of the *British Dental Journal; Journal of Oral Pathology; Oral Surgery, Oral Medicine and Oral Pathology; Dental Update* and *Hospital update;* and to publishers Churchill Livingstone; Heinemann Medical; Oxford University Press and John Wright for permission to reproduce some of the slides from our collection. We wish to acknowledge any other source whom we may have unwittingly omitted.

We are also grateful to Dr J W Eveson, who joined the Department after this project was started, and who has helped with constructive comments and our further education; to Ni Fathers and Derek Coles, for help with technical aspects related to the illustrations; and to Connie Blake, for typing the manuscript.

CS
SF

PREFACE TO THE SECOND EDITION

The first edition, *An Atlas of Stomatology*, was extremely successful and it became increasingly popular as readers appreciated that it was more than just an atlas, containing also a textual overview of the subject and covering a wider range of oral diseases than most atlases. Since then, the authors have moved to new positions and have had access to a much wider patient base.

This second edition provides one of the most comprehensive illustrated coverages of oral diseases of which we are aware and has been extended and improved to include more data and tables on diagnosis, management and drug use, as well as several new clinical entities. The references have been fully updated.

There is a new chapter on liver disease, and more than 125 new illustrations, covering a range of recently described new entities such as pigmented purpuric stomatitis, superficial mucoceles, idiopathic plasmacytosis, oral lesions induced by cocaine and other drugs, and oral body art. Other conditions appearing for the first time in this edition include a range of lesions seen in AIDS, organ transplants, myiasis, Laband syndrome, larva migrans, giant-cell arteritis, myotonic dystrophy, Munchausen's syndrome, necrotizing fasciitis, toxoplasmosis, lichen sclerosus, adenomatoid hyperplasia, mixed connective tissue disease and lingual thyroid.

The expanded section on diagnosis and management is presented in a clear and easy-to-use format and covers differential diagnoses by symptoms, signs and site, investigations and management of the various conditions covered in the book, the drugs used in the management of oral diseases and the oral and perioral side-effects of drug treatment.

We are grateful to our colleagues who have kindly provided some illustrations; particular thanks are due to Dr A Efeoglu (Istanbul, Turkey), Professor O Almeida (Sao Paulo, Brazil), Mr G Bounds (London, UK), Dr R MacLeod (Edinburgh, UK) and Mr A Babejews (Exeter, UK). We are also grateful to Ms Navdeep Singh (London, UK) for her assistance with tables, to Mr Alan Haddock (King's Lynn, UK) and Mr Alex Redhead (Leeds, UK) for help with references, and to Ms Nicci King and Ms Karen Parr (London, UK) for their help with typing.

Crispian Scully
Stephen R Flint
Stephen R Porter
London and Dublin

CONTENTS

1 DIFFERENTIAL DIAGNOSES AND MANAGEMENT

1.1 DIFFERENTIAL DIAGNOSES BY SYMPTOMS OR SIGNS

Anaesthesia or hypo-aesthesia

Numbness over the chin (numb chin syndrome) may indicate a lesion involving the mental or inferior alveolar nerves or may have more sinister implications.

Traumatic

Mandibular fracture
Direct trauma to trigeminal nerve or branches
Iatrogenic (eg, nerve block anaesthesia or osteotomy)

Idiopathic

Benign trigeminal sensory neuropathy

Neoplasms

Jaw metastases
Intracranial neoplasia
Pharyngeal neoplasia (Trotter's syndrome)
Disseminated malignancy in the absence of identifiable jaw deposits

Systemic non-malignant disease

Connective tissue disorders
Diabetes mellitus
Sarcoidosis
Amyloidosis
Sickle cell disease
Vasculitides

Drugs and poisons

see Section 1.5, page 56

Blisters

(*See* Box 1, page 3)

Skin diseases

Pemphigoid (usually mucous membrane pemphigoid)
Pemphigus (usually pemphigus vulgaris)
Intra-epidermal IgA pustulosis
Dermatitis herpetiformis
Linear IgA disease
Erythema multiforme
Epidermolysis bullosa

Infections

Herpes simplex
Herpes varicella-zoster
Coxsackie viruses

Burns

Angina bullosa haemorrhagica (localized oral purpura)

Drugs

Paraneoplastic disorders

Amyloidosis

False blisters

Cysts
Superficial mucoceles
Abscesses

Burning mouth

Deficiency states

Vitamin B_{12} deficiency
Folate deficiency
Iron deficiency
B complex deficiency

Infections

Candidosis

Others

Erythema migrans (geographic tongue)
Diabetes mellitus
Xerostomia

Psychogenic

Cancerophobia
Depression
Anxiety states
Hypochondriasis

Drugs

Captopril

Box 1 DIFFERENTIATION OF THE MORE IMPORTANT ORAL VESICULOBULLOUS DISORDERS*

	Pemphigus	Mucous membrane pemphigoid	Erythema multiforme	Dermatitis herpetiformis	Linear IgA disease	Localized oral purpura
Incidence	Rare	Uncommon	Uncommon	Rare	Rare	Uncommon
Age mainly affected	Middle age	Late/middle age	Young adults	Middle age	Middle age	Middle age/elderly
Sex mainly affected	F	F	M	M	F	M = F
Geographic factors	Italian, Jewish origin	—	—	—	—	—
Predisposing factors	—	—	Drugs, infections	Gluten-sensitive enteropathy	—	? Steroid inhalers
Oral manifestations	Erosions, blisters rarely persist, Nikolsky sign positive	Blisters (sometimes blood-filled), erosions, Nikolsky sign may be positive	Swollen lips, serosanguinous exudate, large erosions anteriorly, occasional blisters	Blisters, ulcers, erythematous patches	Blisters, ulcers	Blood blisters
Cutaneous manifestations	Large flaccid blisters at some stage	Rare or minor	Target (iris) or other lesions may be present	Pruritic vesicular rash on back and extensor surfaces	Crops of plaques in a characteristic annular or polycyclic pattern on upper trunk, shoulders, limbs, face	—
Histopathology	Acantholysis, intraepithelial bullae	Subepithelial bullae	Subepithelial or intraepithelial bullae	Subepithelial bullae	Subepithelial bullae	Subepithelial bullae
Direct immunostaining	Intercellular IgG in epithelium	Subepithelial/BMZ, C3, IgG	Subepithelial IgG†	Subepithelial IgA	Subepithelial IgA	—
Serology	Antibodies to epithelial intercellular cement in most	Antibodies to epithelial basement membrane in few	—	Antibodies to reticulin or endomysium in some	Antibodies to reticulin and endomysium are rare	—
Other investigations	—	—	—	Biopsy of small intestine	—	Exclude thrombocytopathy

*Lichen planus is rarely bullous; †Non-specific findings; BMZ, basement membrane zone; C3, third component of complement; IgG, immunoglobulin G; IgA, immunoglobulin A.

4

Cacogeusia

Oral disease

Pericoronitis
Chronic periodontitis
Acute necrotizing ulcerative gingivitis
Chronic dental abscesses
Dry socket
Food impaction
Sialadenitis
Neoplasms

Xerostomia

Drugs
Sjögren's syndrome
Sarcoidosis
Irradiation damage

Psychogenic causes

Depression
Anxiety states
Psychoses
Hypochondriasis

Drugs (see also Section 1.5, page 56)

Metronidazole
Disulphiram
Amiodarone
Angiotensin-converting enzyme inhibitors
Allopurinol
Phenylbutazone

Smoking

Starvation

Nasal or pharyngeal disease

Chronic sinusitis
Oroantral fistula
Neoplasm
Nasal foreign body
Pharyngeal disease
Tonsillitis
Neoplasm

Diabetes

Respiratory disease

Bronchiectasis
Neoplasm

Gastrointestinal disease

Pharyngeal pouch
Gastric regurgitation
Liver disease

Central nervous system disease

Temporal lobe tumours
Temporal lobe epilepsy

Renal disease

Uraemia

Discharges

Dental disease

Chronic dental and parodontal abscesses
Dry socket
Cysts
Oroantral fistula
Osteomyelitis
Osteoradionecrosis
Infection by foreign body

Salivary gland disorders

Sialadenitis
Salivary fistulae

Psychogenic (imagined discharges)

Depression
Hypochondriasis
Psychosis

Dry mouth (xerostomia)
(*see also* Section 1.5, page 56)

Drugs with anticholinergic effects

Atropine and analogues (antimuscarinics)
Tricyclic antidepressants
Antihistamines
Antiemetics
Tranquillizers (antipsychotics)

Drugs with sympathomimetic actions

Decongestants
Bronchodilators
Appetite suppressants
Amphetamines

Other drugs

Lithium
Disopyramide
Dideoxyinosine
Diuretics
Interleukin-2
Retinoids

Dehydration

Uncontrolled diabetes mellitus
Diabetes insipidus
Diarrhoea and vomiting
Severe haemorrhage

Psychogenic

Anxiety states
Depression
Hypochondriasis
Bulimia nervosa

Salivary gland disorders

Sjögren's syndrome
Sarcoidosis
Irradiation damage
HIV infection
Bone marrow transplantation/graft-versus-
   host disease
Cystic fibrosis
Ectodermal dysplasia
Amyloidosis

Dysarthria

Oral disease

Painful lesions or loss of mobility of the
   tongue or palate
Cleft palate (including submucous cleft)
Oral neoplasia
Severe scarring

Neurological disorders

Multiple sclerosis
Parkinson's disease
Motor neurone disease
Cerebrovascular accident
Bulbar and pseudo-bulbar palsy
Hypoglossal nerve palsy
Cerebral palsy
Cerebellar disease
Myopathies
Dyskinesias

Drugs (*see also* Section 1.5, page 56)

Phenothiazines
Levodopa
Butyrophenones
Addictive intoxicants, eg, alcohol

Severe xerostomia

Mechanical

Poorly fitting prostheses
Restricted jaw movement

Dysphagia

Oral or pharyngeal disease

Inflammatory, traumatic, surgical or
    neoplastic lesions of tongue, palate or
    pharynx
Xerostomia

Oesophageal disease

Foreign body
Stricture
Neoplasia
Systemic sclerosis
Pharyngeal pouch
Oesophagitis
Extrinsic compressive lesions (eg, mediastinal
    lymphadenopathy)

Psychogenic

Hysteria (globus hystericus)

Neurological disorders

Multiple sclerosis
Cerebrovascular accident
Bulbar and pseudo-bulbar palsy
Parkinson's disease
Syringobulbia/syringomyelia
Achalasia of the cardia
Myopathies (eg, myasthenia gravis)
Lateral medullary syndrome

Facial palsy

Neurological

Bell's palsy
Stroke
Cerebral tumour
Moebius syndrome
Multiple sclerosis
Ramsay-Hunt syndrome
Guillain–Barré syndrome
HIV infection
Trauma to facial nerve or its branches
Diabetes mellitus
Leprosy
Kawasaki disease
Lyme disease
Connective tissue disorders
Botulism

Middle ear disease

Cholesteatoma
Malignancy
Mastoiditis

Parotid lesions

Parotid trauma
Parotid malignancy

Others

Melkersson–Rosenthal syndrome
Sarcoidosis (Heerfordt syndrome)
Reiter's syndrome

Myopathies

Facial swelling

Facial swelling is
commonly inflammatory
in origin, caused by
cutaneous or dental
infections or trauma.

Inflammatory

Oral infections
Cutaneous infections
Insect bites

Traumatic

Post-operative oedema or haematoma
Traumatic oedema or haematoma
Surgical emphysema

Immunological

Allergic angioedema
C_1 esterase inhibitor deficiency

(Contd)

Facial swelling
(Contd)

Endocrine and metabolic

Systemic corticosteroid therapy
Cushing's syndrome and disease
Myxoedema
Acromegaly
Obesity
Nephrotic syndrome

Superior vena cava syndrome

Cysts

Neoplasms

Foreign bodies

Others

Crohn's disease (and orofacial
  granulomatosis)
Sarcoidosis
Melkersson–Rosenthal syndrome
Congenital (eg, lymphangioma)
Lymphoma

Fissured tongue

Fissured tongue is common
and usually
inconsequential, although
erythema migrans is often
associated.

Isolated

With systemic disease

Down's syndrome
Melkersson–Rosenthal syndrome

Halitosis

Oral sepsis

Food impaction
Chronic dental or periodontal sepsis
Acute necrotizing ulcerative gingivitis
Dry socket
Pericoronitis
Xerostomia
Oral ulceration

Oral malignancy

Nasopharyngeal disease

Foreign body
Sinusitis
Tonsillitis
Neoplasm

Volatile foodstuffs

Garlic
Onions
Highly spiced foods

Drugs (*see also* Section 1.5, page 56)

Solvent abuse
Alcohol
Smoking
Chloral hydrate
Nitrites and nitrates
Dimethyl sulphoxide
Disulphiram
Cytotoxic drugs
Phenothiazines
Amphetamines
Paraldehyde

Systemic disease

Acute febrile illness
Respiratory tract infections
Hepatic failure
Renal failure
Diabetic ketoacidosis
Leukaemias

Psychogenic

Neuroses
Psychoses

Hirsutism

Hirsutism is defined as more facial and body hair than is acceptable to a woman living in a particular environment.

ANDROGEN-MEDIATED

Drugs

Androgens
Anabolic steroids
Contraceptive pill

Ovarian

Polycystic ovaries
Ovarian tumours
Insulin resistance

Adrenal

Cushing's syndrome
Congenital adrenal hyperplasia
Androgen-producing tumours

Other

Idiopathic

ANDROGEN-INDEPENDENT

Racial

Pregnancy

Drugs

Minoxidil
Phenytoin
Calcium-channel blockers
Cyclosporin
Corticosteroids
Danazol
Diazoxide

Endocrine

Hypothyroidism
Acromegaly

Hyperpigmentation

See Pigmentation

Loss of taste

Anosmia

Upper respiratory tract infections
Maxillofacial injuries (tearing of olfactory nerves)

Neurological disease

Lesions of chorda tympani
Cerebrovascular disease
Multiple sclerosis
Bell's palsy
Fractured base of skull
Posterior cranial fossa tumours
Cerebral metastases
Trigeminal sensory neuropathy

Psychogenic

Anxiety states
Depression
Psychoses

Drugs (*see also* Section 1.5, page 56)

Penicillamine

Others

Irradiation
Xerostomia
Zinc or copper deficiency

Pain

(See Box 2, page 10)

Local diseases

Diseases of the teeth
Dentine sensitivity
Pulpitis
Periapical periodontitis

Diseases of the periodontium
Lateral (periodontal) abscess
Acute necrotizing ulcerative gingivitis
Pericoronitis
Necrotizing periodontitis

Diseases of the jaws
Dry socket
Fractures
Osteomyelitis
Infected cysts
Malignant neoplasms

Diseases of the maxillary antrum
Acute sinusitis
Malignant neoplasms

Diseases of the salivary glands
Acute sialadentitis
Calculi or other obstruction to duct
Severe Sjögren's syndrome
HIV disease
Malignant neoplasms

Diseases of the temporomandibular joint
Arthritis
Temporomandibular joint dysfunction (facial arthromyalgia)

Vascular disorders
Migraine
Migrainous neuralgia
Giant-cell arteritis

Neurological disorders
Trigeminal neuralgia
Malignant neoplasms involving the trigeminal nerve
Multiple sclerosis
HIV disease
Bell's palsy (rarely)
Herpes zoster (including post-herpetic neuralgia)

Psychogenic pain
Atypical facial pain and other oral symptoms associated with anxiety or depression

Referred pain
Angina, nasopharyngeal, ocular and aural disease
Chest disease (rarely)

Others
Drugs (eg vinca alkaloids)

Box 2   DIFFERENTIATION OF IMPORTANT TYPES OF FACIAL PAIN*

	Idiopathic trigeminal neuralgia	Temporomandibular joint dysfunction	Atypical facial pain	Migraine	Migrainous neuralgia
Age (years)	> 50	Any	30–50	Any	30–50
Sex	F > M	F > M	F > M	F > M	M > F
Site	Unilateral, mandible or maxilla	Unilateral or bilateral mandible, temple	± Bilateral, maxilla	Any	Retro-orbital
Associated features	—	± Anxiety ± Life events ± Depression	± Depression	± Photophobia, ± Nausea, ± Vomiting	± Conjunctival injection, ± Lacrimation ± Nasal congestion
Character	Lancinating	Dull	Dull	Throbbing	Boring
Duration of episode	Brief (seconds)	Hours	Continual	Many hours (usually during day)	Few hours (usually during night, often at same time)
Precipitating factors	± Trigger areas	None	None	± Foods ± Stress	± Alcohol, ± Stress
Relieving factors	Carbamazepine	Analgesics, antidepressants, anxiolytics, others	Antidepressants	Clonidine, ergot derivatives, β-blockers, H_3-blockers	Clonidine, ergot derivatives, β-blockers, H_3-blockers, pizotifen

*Most oral pain is caused by local disease.

Pigmentation

(*see* Box 3, page 11)

GENERALIZED

Racial

Pregnancy

Chloasma

Food/drugs (*see* Section 1.5, page 56)

Endocrinopathies

Addison's disease
Nelson's syndrome
Ectopic ACTH production

Others

Pigmentary incontinence
Albright's syndrome
Haemochromatosis/haemosiderosis
β-thalassaemia
Drugs (eg minocycline, doxorubicin or antimalarials; *see* page 309)
ACTH therapy
Biliary atresia
Permanganate or silver poisoning

LOCALIZED

Ecchymoses
Ephelis
Melanoma
Melanoacanthoma
Melanotic macule
Naevus
Peutz–Jeghers syndrome
Kaposi's sarcoma
Epithelioid angiomatosis
Smoker's melanosis
Acanthosis nigricans
Heavy-metal poisoning (lead, bismuth and arsenic)
Laugier–Hunziker syndrome
von Recklinghausen's neurofibromatosis
Spotty pigmentation, myxoma, endocrine overactivity syndrome
Tattoos (amalgam, lead pencils, ink, dyes, carbon)

Box 3 COMMON BENIGN ISOLATED PIGMENTED LESIONS

Lesion	Main sites	Age affected	Size	Other features
Naevi	Palate	3–4th decade	< 1 cm	Mostly raised and pigmented blue or brown
Melanotic macules	Lips; gingivae	Any	< 1 cm	Macular Mostly in Caucasians Brown or black
Amalgam tattoos	Floor of mouth; mandibular gingivae	Usually after 5 years	< 1 cm	Macular Greyish or black

Purpura

Trauma (including suction)

Platelet and vascular disorders

Thrombocytopenia (especially drugs and leukaemias)
Thrombasthenia
Von Willebrand's disease
Scurvy
Ehlers–Danlos syndrome
Chronic renal failure
'Senile' purpura

Infections

Infectious mononucleosis
Rubella
HIV infection

Localized oral purpura (angina bullosa haemorrhagica)

Amyloidosis

Mixed connective tissue disease

Red areas

Generalized redness

Candidosis
Avitaminosis B complex (rarely)
Irradiation mucositis
Mucosal atrophy (eg avitaminosis B)
Polycythaemia

Localized red patches

Denture-induced stomatitis
Erythroplasia
Purpura
Telangiectases

Angiomas (purple)
Kaposi's sarcoma
Epithelioid angiomatosis
Burns
Lichen planus
Lupus erythematosus
Avitaminosis B_{12}
Sarcoidosis
Psoriasis
Mucoepithelial dysplasia syndrome
Geographic tongue
Drug allergies
Wegener's granulomatosis
Deep mycoses

Sialorrhoea (hypersalivation)

Psychogenic (usually)

Painful lesions in the mouth

Foreign bodies in the mouth

Drugs (*see also* Section 1.5, page 56)
Parasympathomimetics
Buprenorphine
Others

Poor neuromuscular coordination
Parkinson's disease
Facial palsy
Other physical disability

Poisoning
Heavy metals
Mercury
Copper sulphate
Insecticides
Nerve agents

Others
Rabies (rarely)

Telangiectasia

Hereditary haemorrhagic telangiectasia
Chronic liver disease
Scleroderma
Carcinoid

Pregnancy
Oestrogens
Post-irradiation

Trismus

Limited opening of the jaw may have several causes, including the following:

Extra-articular causes
Infection and inflammation near masticatory muscles
Temporomandibular joint dysfunction syndrome (facial arthromyalgia)
Fractured condylar neck
Fibrosis (including scars, systemic sclerosis and submucous fibrosis)
Tetanus
Tetany
Invading neoplasm
Myositis ossificans
Coronoid hypertrophy or fusion to zygomatic arch
Hysteria

Intra-articular causes
Dislocation
Intracapsular fracture
Arthritides
Ankylosis

In contrast, some drugs such as metoclopramide and phenothiazines may cause facial muscle spasm inhibiting the patient from *closing* his or her mouth.

Ulcers

Traumatic

Mechanical (may be artefactual)
Chemical, electrical, thermal, radiation burns

Neoplastic

Carcinoma and other malignant tumours

Recurrent aphthous stomatitis

(including Behçet's syndrome/MAGIC syndrome, Sweet's syndrome and acute febrile illness of childhood)

Systemic disease

Cutaneous disease: Erosive lichen planus, pemphigus vulgaris and others, mucous membrane pemphigoid and bullous pemphigoid, erythema multiforme, dermatitis herpetiformis and linear IgA disease, epidermolysis bullosa, epidermolysis bullosa acquisita, IgA intraepithelial pustular dermatosis, chronic ulcerative stomatitis

Blood or vascular disorders: Anaemia, sideropenia, neutropenias, leukaemias, myelofibrosis, myelodysplasia, multiple myeloma, giant-cell arteritis, periarteritis nodosa

Gastrointestinal: Coeliac disease, Crohn's disease, ulcerative colitis

Connective tissue disease: Lupus erythematosus, Reiter's disease, mixed connective tissue disease, Felty's syndrome

Infective: Herpes simplex, chickenpox, herpes zoster, hand, foot and mouth disease, herpangina, infectious mononucleosis, cytomegalovirus infection, acute necrotizing ulcerative gingivitis, tuberculosis, atypical mycobacterial infections, syphilis, aspergillosis, cryptococcosis, leishmaniasis, tularaemia, lepromatous leprosy, paracoccidioidomycosis, histoplasmosis, coccididioidomycosis, blastomycosis, HIV infection, Gram-negative bacteria

Drugs: Cytotoxics, many others (*see* Section 1.5, page 56)

Others: Wegener's granulomatosis, midline lethal granuloma, Langerhan's cell histiocytoses, angiolymphoid hyperplasia with eosinophilia, necrotizing sialometaplasia, noma

White lesions

Congenital

White sponge naevus
Dyskeratosis congenita
Pachyonychia congenita

Acquired

Inflammatory

Infective: Candidosis, hairy leukoplakia, syphilitic leukoplakia, Koplik's spots, papillomas

Non-infective: Lichen planus, lichen sclerosis, lupus erythematosus, pyostomatitis vegetans, xanthomatosis, dermatomyositis

Neoplastic and possibly pre-neoplastic

Keratoses (leukoplakias)
Carcinoma

Others

Drug burns
Grafts

The lips

Angular stomatitis (cheilitis, cheilosis)

Candidosis (denture-induced stomatitis or
  other types)
Staphylococcal, streptococcal or mixed infections
Ariboflavinosis (rarely), iron, folate or B_{12}
  deficiency
Crohn's disease and orofacial granulomatosis
Anaemia
Acrodermatitis enteropathica
HIV infection

Bleeding

Trauma
Cracked lips
Erythema multiforme
Angiomas
Underlying haemorrhagic disease aggravates
  tendency to bleed

Blisters

Herpes labialis
Burns
Herpes zoster
Erythema multiforme
Pemphigus vulgaris
Epidermolysis bullosa
Mucoceles
Impetigo
Allergic cheilitis

Desquamation and crusting

Dehydration
Exposure to hot dry winds
Acute febrile illness
Chemical or allergic cheilitis
Mouth-breathing
Actinic cheilitis
Candidal cheilitis
Erythema multiforme
Psychogenic (self-induced)
Drugs

Swellings

There is a wide individual and racial
variation in the size of the lips

Diffuse swellings

Oedema (trauma or infection or insect bite)
Angioedema: allergic or C_1 esterase inhibitor
  deficiency
Crohn's disease and orofacial granulomatosis
Cheilitis granulomatosa
Cheilitis glandularis

Melkersson–Rosenthal syndrome
Lymphangioma
Haemangioma
Macrocheilia
Ascher's syndrome

Localized swellings

Mucoceles
Chancre
Salivary adenoma
Squamous cell carcinoma
Basal cell carcinoma
Other tumours
Keratoacanthoma
Cysts
Abscesses
Insect bites
Haematomas
Tuberculosis
Leprosy
Rhinoscleroma
Anthrax
Trichiniasis

Ulceration

Infective

Herpes labialis
Herpes zoster
Syphilis
Leishmaniasis
Mycoses
Impetigo

Tumours

Squamous cell carcinoma
Basal cell carcinoma
Keratoacanthoma

Burns

Mucocutaneous disease

Lupus erythematosus
Pemphigus
Pemphigoid
Trauma

White lesions

Keratoses
Carcinoma
Lichen planus
Lupus erythematosus
Fordyce spots
Actinic keratosis
Scars

The gingivae

Red areas

Redness is usually a sign of chronic gingivitis or periodontitis, but is then restricted to the gingival margins. Other red lesions which may affect the gingiva include:

Congenital

Mucoepithelial dysplasia syndrome
Hereditary haemorrhagic telangiectasia

Acquired

Trauma: physical, chemical, radiation, thermal

Drugs: eg chlorhexidine, cinnamonaldehyde

Infections: candidosis, *Geotrichum candidum*

Desquamative gingivitis: lichen planus, mucous membrane pemphigoid, pemphigus vulgaris, dermatitis herpetiformis, linear IgA disease, lupus erythematosus, pyostomatitis vegetans, psoriasis

Epithelioid angiomatosis

Wegener's granulomatosis

Sarcoidosis

Dermatomyositis

Primary biliary cirrhosis

Leukaemia(s)

Premalignancy (eg erythroplasia)

Malignancy — Kaposi's sarcoma

Plasma cell gingivitis

Bleeding

Periodontal disease

Chronic gingivitis
Chronic periodontitis
Acute ulcerative gingivitis
HIV gingivitis
HIV periodontitis

(Contd)

Haemorrhagic disease

Primary platelet disorders
Lymphoproliferative disorders
Myelodysplastic disorders
Myelofibrosis
Myeloproliferative disorders
Idiopathic thrombocytopenic purpura
Hereditary haemorrhagic telangiectasia
Ehlers–Danlos syndrome
Scurvy
Angiomas

Drugs

Anticoagulants
Non-steroidal anti-inflammatory drugs
Cytotoxics
Sodium valproate

Clotting defects

Hepatobiliary disease
Haemophilias
Von Willebrand's disease

Gingival swelling

Generalized and congenital

Gingival fibromatosis
Jones' syndrome
Murray–Puretic–Drescher syndrome
Mucolipidosis (I-cell disease)
Rutherfurd syndrome
Zimmermann–Laband syndrome
Cross syndrome
Ramon syndrome
Gingival fibromatosis with growth hormone deficiency (Byars–Jurkiewicz syndrome)
Mucopolysaccharidosis 1-H
Fucosidosis
Aspartylglucosaminuria
Leprechaunism (Donohue syndrome)
Pfeiffer syndrome
Amyloidosis
Lipoid proteinosis
Infantile systemic hyalinosis

The gingivae

(Contd)

Generalized and acquired

Acute myeloid leukaemia
Preleukaemic leukaemia
Aplastic anaemia
Drugs (*see also* Section 1.5, page 56)
   Phenytoin
   Cyclosporin
   Calcium-channel blockers
      Nifedipine
      Diltiazem
      Nitrendipine
      Felodipine
      Verapamil
      Amlodipine
   Others
      Sodium valproate (rare)
      Tranexamic acid (rare)
Vitamin C deficiency

Localized and congenital

Fabry's syndrome (angiokeratoma corporis
   diffusum universale)
Cowden's syndrome (multiple hamartoma
   and neoplasia syndrome)
Tuberous sclerosis
Focal dermal hypoplasia
Sturge–Weber angiomatosis
Congenital gingival granular cell tumour

Localized and acquired

Heck's disease
Lymphomas
Langerhan's cell tumours
Multiple myeloma
Plasmacytomas
Other primary and secondary neoplasms, eg
   papillomas, squamous cell carcinoma,
   Kaposi's sarcoma
Wegener's granulomatosis
Pregnancy epulis
Fibroepithelial epulis
Giant cell epulis
Sarcoidosis
Crohn's disease and related disorders
Epithelioid angiomatosis

Ulcers

Ulcers that affect predominantly the gingivae
are usually traumatic, acute ulcerative
gingivitis or occasionally results of
immunodeficiency, especially acute
leukaemia, neutropenias or HIV disease. The
gingivae can, however, be affected by most
other causes of mouth ulcers (*see* page 13).

Enhanced periodontal destruction

Primary immunodeficiencies

Reduced neutrophil number
   Cyclic neutropenia
   Benign familial neutropenias
   Other
Defective neutrophil function
   Hyperimmunoglobulinaemia E
   Chronic granulomatous disease
   Kartagener's syndrome
   Chediak–Higashi syndrome
   Acatalasia
Other immunodeficiencies
   Fanconi's anaemia
   Down's syndrome
   Severe combined immunodeficiency (SCID)

Other congenital disorders

Papillon–Lefèvre syndrome
Hypophosphatasia
Ehlers–Danlos syndrome type VIII
Acro-osteolysis (Hajdu–Cheney syndrome)
Type 1b glycogen storage disease
Oxalosis
Dyskeratosis benigna intraepithelialis
   mucosae et cutis hereditara

Secondary immunodeficiencies

Malnutrition
HIV disease
Pregnancy
Diabetes mellitus
Crohn's disease
Leukaemias

Other acquired causes

Vitamin C deficiency
Tobacco use

The palate

Lumps

Developmental

Unerupted teeth
Torus palatinus
Cysts

Inflammatory

Abscesses
Cysts
Papillary hyperplasia
Necrotizing sialometaplasia
Adenomatoid hyperplasia
Sarcoidosis
Franklin's heavy chain disease

Neoplasms

Oral or antral carcinoma
Salivary tumours
Fibrous overgrowths
Kaposi's sarcoma
Papillomas
Lymphomas
Others

Redness

Redness restricted to the denture-bearing area of the palate is almost invariably denture-induced stomatitis (candidosis), although erythematous candidosis of HIV disease can commonly occur as a red patch of the palate. Other red lesions may be erythroplasia, Kaposi's sarcoma or other lesions (*see* page 11).

The tongue

Swellings or lumps

Localized

Congenital: Lingual thyroid, haemangioma, lymphangioma, lingual choristoma

Inflammatory: Infection, abscess, median rhomboid glossitis, granuloma, foliate papillitis, insect bite

Traumatic: Oedema, haematoma

Neoplastic: Fibrous lump, papilloma, neurofibroma, carcinoma, sarcoma, granular cell tumour (granular cell myoblastoma)

Others: Foreign body, cysts

Diffuse

Congenital: Down's syndrome, cretinism, mucopolysaccharidoses, lymphangioma, haemangioma

Inflammatory: Infection, insect bite, Ludwig's angina

Traumatic: Oedema, haematoma

Others: Multiple endocrine adenomatosis type III; angioedema; amyloidosis; cyst; acromegaly; muscular (Beckwith–Wiedeman syndrome); deposits (glycogen storage disease, I cell disease, mucopolysaccharidoses)

Sore tongue

With obvious localized lesions

Any cause of oral ulceration (*see* page 13)
Geographic tongue
Median rhomboid glossitis
Foliate papillitis

Glossitis (generalized redness and depapillation)

Anaemias
Candidosis
Avitaminosis B
Post-irradiation

With no identifiable physical abnormality

Anaemia/sideropenia
Depression or cancerophobia
Glossodynia
Diabetes
Hypothyroidism

The major salivary glands

Swellings

Inflammatory

Mumps
Recurrent parotitis
Sjögren's syndrome
Ascending sialadenitis
Recurrent sialadenitis
Sarcoidosis
Actinomycosis

Neoplasms

Others

Duct obstruction
Sialosis
Mikulicz disease (lymphoepithelial lesion and
  syndrome)
Amyloidosis
HIV disease

Drug-associated (*see also* Section 1.5, page 56)

Chlorhexidine
Phenylbutazone
Iodine compounds
Thiouracil
Catecholamines
Sulphonamides
Phenothiazines
Methyldopa

Salivary gland pain

Inflammatory

Mumps
Stones or other causes of obstruction
Sjögren's syndrome
Acute sialadenitis
Recurrent sialadenitis

Neoplastic

Salivary gland malignant tumours

Drug-associated (*see also* Section 1.5, page 56)

Antihypertensive drugs
Cytotoxic drugs
Vinca alkaloids

The neck

Swellings in the neck

Cervical lymph nodes

Inflammatory: Lymphadenitis (nasopharyngeal,
antral, dental, tonsillar, aural, facial or scalp
infections), glandular fever syndromes (EBV,
CMV, Brucella, *Toxoplasma*, HIV), tuberculosis
or other mycobacterial infections, other
infections (rubella, cat scratch, syphilis)

Neoplasms: Secondary carcinoma (oral,
nasopharyngeal or thyroid primary),
lymphoma, leukaemia

Others: Connective tissue disease, drugs (eg,
phenytoin), mucocutaneous lymph node
syndrome, sarcoidosis

Salivary glands

Mumps
Tumours
Sjögren's syndrome
Sarcoidosis
Sialadenitis
Sialosis

Side of the neck

Actinomycosis
Branchial cyst
Parapharyngeal cellulitis
Pharyngeal pouch
Cystic hygroma
Carotid body tumours or aneurysms

Muscle or other soft tissue neoplasm

Focal myositis
Myositis ossificans
Proliferative myositis
Nodular pseudosarcomatous fasciitis

Midline of the neck

Submental lymphadenopathy
Thyroglossal cyst
Ectopic thyroid
Thyroid tumours or goitre
'Plunging' ranula
Ludwig's angina
Dermoid cyst
Other skin lesions

Oral complaints frequently associated with psychogenic factors*

*Organic causes should first be excluded.

Dry mouth
Sore or burning mouth
Bad or disturbed taste
Atypical facial pain
Atypical odontalgia
Supposed anaesthesias and dysaesthesias

Temporomandibular joint dysfunction
Non-existent discharges
Gripping dentures
Vomiting or nausea caused by dentures
Supposed sialorrhoea
Non-existent lumps or spots

1.3 GUIDE TO THE DIAGNOSIS AND MANAGEMENT OF ORAL DISEASES

Condition	Typical main clinical features	Diagnosis
Abscess (dental)	Pain ± swelling	Clinical mainly
Acanthosis nigricans	Hyperpigmented confluent papillomas mainly in groin/axillae	Clinical plus biopsy
Acquired immune deficiency syndrome (AIDS)	Opportunistic infections (especially fungal and viral), Kaposi's sarcoma, lymphomas, encephalopathy	Confirmed by HIV antibodies
Acromegaly	Increasing prognathism and hand size, headaches, tunnel vision, lethargy, weight gain	Enlarging pituitary fossa Increased growth hormone
Actinomycosis	Purplish indurated swelling(s) over mandible or neck	Clinical plus microbiology 'Sulphur granules'
Acute bacterial sialadenitis	Painful salivary swellings ± fever and/or trismus	Clinical plus bacteriology
Acute necrotizing ulcerative gingivitis	Interdental papillary ulceration and bleeding, halitosis, pain	Clinical mainly
Addison's disease	Weakness, lassitude, loss of weight, hyperpigmentation	Clinical plus low blood pressure, hyponatraemia, hyperkalaemia, reduced cortisol and increased ACTH
Adenoid cystic carcinoma	Firm salivary swelling	Clinical plus investigations
Agammaglobulinaemia	Recurrent pyogenic infections, especially respiratory and cutaneous	Reduced immunoglobulins
Albright's syndrome	Fibrous dysplasia, precocious puberty, hyperpigmentation, endocrine disease	Clinical plus investigations
Alveolar osteitis (dry socket)	Empty painful extraction socket, halitosis	Clinical
Amalgam tattoo	Grey to black pigmented area(s) usually over the mandible	Clinical
Ameloblastoma	Slow growing swelling, usually in mandible	Clinical plus investigations
Angioedema [see also hereditary angioedema]	Facial swelling	Clinical
Angular cheilitis	See Cheilitis	
Aphthae	Recurrent oral ulcers only	Clinical

Investigations	Management
Radiography ± vitality test	Drain either by incision if pointing, or through tooth. Analgesics ± antimicrobials
Biopsy, gastroscopy, barium studies Exclude diabetes mellitus	Treat underlying cause
HIV antibodies CD4 lymphocyte count	Reverse transcriptase inhibitors [AZT, DDI, DDC]. Prophylaxis/treatment of infections
Lateral skull radiography, growth hormone assays, visual fields, CT/MRI	Treatment of pituitary adenoma
Pus for microscopy and culture	Antimicrobial: penicillin for 4 weeks+
Pus for culture and sensitivity	Antimicrobial: flucloxacillin
Smear may help Consider excluding HIV	Antimicrobial: penicillin or metronidazole. Oral hygiene improvement. Mechanical debridement
Blood pressure, electrolytes, 24 hr cortisol Synacthen test	Corticosteroids
Biopsy and radiography	Surgery
Serum immunoglobulins	Immunoglobulin replacement Antimicrobials
Radiography ± bone biopsy	± Surgery ± calcitonin
Radiography to exclude fracture or foreign body	Debridement, obtundent dressing ± antimicrobial
± Radiography	Reassurance. Biopsy if any doubt
Radiography *and* biopsy	Surgery
C1 esterase inhibitor, IgE, C3 and C4 levels	Antihistamines/corticosteroids
Full blood picture. Exclude underlying systemic disease	Corticosteroids topically

Condition	Typical main clinical features	Diagnosis
Atypical facial pain	Persistent dull ache typically in one maxilla in a female	Clinical
Bell's palsy	Lower motor neurone facial palsy only	Clinical
Behçet's syndrome	Recurrent oral and genital ulceration, other systemic features	Clinical
Black hairy tongue	Black hairy tongue	Clinical
Bourneville–Pringle disease	Papules or nodules around nose/mouth, subungual fibromas, ash leaf patches	Clinical plus cerebral radio-opacities
Bruton's syndrome	*See* Agammaglobulinaemia	
Bulima nervosa	Recurrent self-induced vomiting	Clinical
Burning mouth syndrome	*See* Glossodynia	
Calculus, salivary	Recurrent salivary swelling ± pain at mealtimes	Clinical ± investigations
Cancrum oris	Chronic ulceration	Clinical ± investigations
Candidosis	White or red persistent lesions	Clinical ± investigations
Carcinoma	Ulcer, lump or red or white lesion	Clinical plus investigations
Central papillary atrophy	*See* Median rhomboid glossitis	
Chancre	Single, painless indurated ulcer usually on lip or tongue	Syphilis serology
Cheek-chewing	Shredded or keratotic lesions around occlusal line and/or on lower labial mucosa	Clinical
Cheilitis, actinic	Soreness and/or keratosis on lower lip Sun exposure	Clinical
angular	Soreness of commissures	Clinical
Cherubism	Slowly enlarging swellings over mandible or maxillae	Clinical plus investigations
Child abuse syndrome	Various injuries inconsistent with history	Clinical ± radiography

Investigations	Management
Clinical and radiographic exclusion of organic disease	Reassurance, tricyclic antidepressants, 5HT antagonists
Consider excluding middle ear lesion, Lyme disease, cerebellopontine angle tumour	Corticosteroids systemically. Protect cornea with pad
Full blood picture, white cell count and differential	Colchicine, thalidomide or azathioprine may be indicated
—	Reassurance. Brush tongue ± tretinoin
Skull radiography. Biopsy skin lesions	Anticonvulsants
Full blood picture, electrolytes	Reassurance. Psychiatric care Restoration of dental erosions
Radiography/sialography	Surgery ± lithotripsy
Consider biopsy Consider immune defect	Debridement. Antimicrobial Improve nutrition
Smear plus culture Consider immune defect	Antifungal
Biopsy. Chest radiography	Surgery ± radiotherapy
Syphilis serology ± biopsy	Antimicrobial: penicillin
—	Avoid habit
—	Avoid exposure. Bland UV protecting creams. ± Laser excision
Haematological screen Denture assessment	Denture modification/replacement Oral and denture hygiene Antifungal: miconazole
Radiography + biopsy	Reassurance
Photographs + radiography	Protect child from further abuse

24

Condition	Typical main clinical features	Diagnosis
Chronic granulomatous disease	Recurrent pyogenic infections, cervical lymphadenopathy	Clinical plus investigations
Chronic mucocutaneous candidosis	Persistent mucocutaneous candidosis	Clinical plus investigations
Cicatricial pemphigoid	*See* Mucous membrane pemphigoid	
Cleidocranial dysplasia	Patent fontanelles, clavicles can approximate	Clinical plus radiographs
Coeliac disease	Loose stool, malabsorption, loss of weight/failure to thrive	Clinical plus jejunal villous atrophy
Condyloma acuminata	Warts (condylomas)	Clinical
CREST syndrome	Raynaud's phenomenon, changing facial appearance. Mucosal telangiectases ± Sjögren's syndrome	Clinical plus investigations
Crohn's disease	Loose stool, malabsorption, abdominal pain ± orofacial granulomatosis	Clinical plus investigations
Cyclic neutropenia	Recurrent pyogenic infections	Clinical plus neutropenia
Denture-induced hyperplasia	Hyperplasia close to denture flange	Clinical
Denture-induced stomatitis	Erythema in denture-bearing area	Clinical
Dermatitis herpetiformis	Pruritic rash	Clinical plus investigations Small bowel biopsy
Dermatomyositis	Proximal limb and trunk weakness plus heliotrope rash	Clinical plus investigations
Dermoid cyst	Submental swelling	Clinical plus investigations
Desquamative gingivitis	Erythematous desquamating gingivae	Clinical plus biopsy
Diabetes mellitus	Polyuria, polydipsia	Hyperglycaemia
Discoid lupus erythematosus	*See* Lupus	
Dry mouth	*See* Sjögren's syndrome	
Dry socket	*See* Alveolar osteitis	

Investigations	Management
Assay neutrophil phagocytosis and killing of bacteria	Antimicrobial Bone marrow transplantation
Assay T cell function. Biopsy + fungal culture	Antifungals
Radiography of skull and clavicles	Remove supernumary teeth/cysts
Gliadin, reticulin or endomysial antibodies + small bowel biopsy	Gluten-free diet
Biopsy	Surgery
Clinical + anti-centromere antibodies + radiographs	Immunosuppressives
Barium meal and follow-through	Sulphasalazine or corticosteroids
Serial neutrophil counts	Antimicrobial, colony-stimulating factor
—	Ease denture flange; excise hyperplasia
Fungal culture	Leave denture out at night stored in antifungal
Lesional biopsy + small bowel biopsy + gliadin antibodies	Gluten-free diet Dapsone or sulphapyridine
Serum creatine kinase and aldolase Electromyography Skin/muscle biopsy	Systemic corticosteroids and acetyl salicyclic acid
Radiography	Surgery
Biopsy ± immunofluorescence	Topical corticosteroids, improve oral hygiene
Blood sugar (fasting) Glucose tolerance test	Diet or insulin ± oral hypoglycaemic agent

Condition	Typical main clinical features	Diagnosis
Ectodermal dysplasia	Dry thin hair, dry skin, fever, hypodontia	Clinical
Ephelis	*See* Freckles	
Epidermolysis bullosa	Blisters at sites of trauma	Clinical plus histology
Epiloia	*See* Bourneville–Pringle disease	
Epulis		
congenital	Firm nodule on gingiva	Clinical
fibrous	Firm nodule on gingiva	Clinical
fissuratum	Firm leaflike swellings	Clinical
giant cell	Purplish swelling in premolar area	Clinical plus investigations
in pregnancy	Soft swelling typically on anterior gingivae	Clinical
Erythema		
migrans	Desquamating patches on tongue	Clinical
multiforme	Oral ulcers, swollen lips. Target lesions	Clinical
nodosum	Tender red lumps on shins	Clinical plus investigations
Erythroplakia [erythroplasia]	Red velvety patch	Clinical plus histology
Facial arthromyalgia	TMJ pain, click, limitation of movement	Clinical
Familial fibrous dysplasia	*See* Cherubism	
Familial white folded gingivostomatitis	White persistent lesions in mouth, rectum, vagina	Clinical plus family history
Felty's syndrome	Rheumatoid arthritis, splenomegaly, neutropenia	Clinical plus investigations
Fibroepithelial polyp	Firm pink polyp	Clinical
Fibroma, leaf	*See* Fibroepithelial polyp	
Fibromatosis, gingival	Firm pink gingival swellings	Clinical
Fibrous dysplasia	Bony swelling	Clinical plus investigations
Fibrous lump	*See* Fibroepithelial polyp	
Foliate papillitis	Painful swollen foliate papilla	Clinical
Fordyce spots	Yellowish granules in buccal mucosae or lips	Clinical
Fragilitas ossium	Spontaneous fractures, blue sclera	Clinical plus investigations

Investigations	Management
Radiography for hypodontia	Restorative dentistry
Biopsy	Protect against trauma Vitamin E ± phenytoin
—	Excise if no resolution
—	Excise
—	Change denture. Excise
Exclude hyperparathyroidism	Surgery
Pregnancy test	Leave or excise
—	Reassurance
—	Corticosteroids, acyclovir if herpes-induced
Biopsy ± serum for immune complexes	Treat underlying cause
Biopsy	Excise
Radiography ± arthroscopy	Reassurance, occlusal splint, anxiolytics or antidepressants
± Biopsy	Reassurance
Full blood picture, rheumatoid factor, erythrocyte sedimentation rate	Salicylates
—	Excision
—	Excision
Radiographs and biopsy	Excision or await resolution
—	Reassurance
—	Reassurance
Radiography	Orthopaedic care

Condition	Typical main clinical features	Diagnosis
Freckles [ephelides]	Brown macules	Clinical
Frey's syndrome	Gustatory sweating	Clinical
Gardner's syndrome	Osteomas, desmoid tumours, colonic polyps	Clinical plus investigations
Geographic tongue	*See* Erythema migrans	
German measles	Macular rash, fever, occipital lymphadenopathy	Clinical
Glandular fever	Fever, sore throat, generalized lymphadenopathy	Serology for definitive diagnosis

Glossitis
  atrophic
  benign migratory
  in iron deficiency
  median rhomboid
  Moeller's in vitamin
    B12 deficiency
	
	Depapillated tongue
	See Erythema migrans
	Depapillated tongue
	See Central papillary atrophy
	Depapillated tongue
		
		Clinical plus investigations
		
		Clinical plus investigations
		
		Clinical plus investigations

Glossodynia	Burning normal tongue	Clinical plus investigations
Gorlin–Goltz syndrome (Gorlin's syndrome)	Odontogenic keratocysts, basal cell naevi, skeletal anomalies	Clinical plus investigations
Haemangioma	Blush or reddish swelling	Clinical ± aspiration
Haemophilia	Haemarthroses, ecchymoses, severe bleeding after trauma	Clinical plus investigations
Hairy leukoplakia	White lesions on tongue	Clinical
Halitosis	Oral malodour	Clinical
Hand, foot and mouth disease	Oral ulcers, mild fever, vesicles on hands and/or feet	Clinical
Heck's disease	Oral papules	Clinical
Heerfordt's syndrome	Uveitis, parotitis, fever, facial palsy	Clinical plus investigations
Hereditary angioedema	Recurrent facial swellings	Clinical plus investigations
Hereditary haemorrhagic telangiectasia	Telangiectasia on lips, mouth, hands	Clinical

Investigations	Management
—	Reassurance
Starch-iodine test	Glycopyrrolate
Radiography of jaws, colonoscopy	Excision of colonic polyps
—	Symptomatic
White cell count and differential, Paul Bunnel test, consider HIV and other viral serology	Symptomatic, corticosteroids systemically if airway threatened
Full blood picture, haematinic assay	Treat underlying cause
Full blood picture, serum ferritin	Treat underlying cause
Full blood picture, serum B12	Treat underlying cause
Full blood picture, haematinic assay, fasting blood glucose	Treat underlying cause where possible ± antidepressants
Radiography skull, jaws, chest	Remove cysts. ± Etretinate
Empties on pressure	Leave or cryoprobe, laser or sclerosant
Haemostasis assays	Cover surgery with factor replacement ± antifibrinolytics
HIV serology ± biopsy	Leave
Oral/ENT examination and radiography	Treat underlying cause
—	Symptomatic
—	Observe or remove
Chest radiography. Biopsy, serum angiotensin-converting enzyme, calcium levels	Corticosteroids
C1 esterase inhibitor, C3 and C4 assays	Danazol or stanazolol
Full blood picture and haemoglobin	Laser or cryoprobe to bleeding telangiectases

Condition	Typical main clinical features	Diagnosis
Herpangina	Oral ulcers, mild fever	Clinical
Herpetic stomatitis	Oral ulcers, gingivitis, fever	Clinical
Herpes labialis	Vesicles, pustules, scabs at mucocutaneous junction	Clinical
Herpes zoster	*See* Shingles	
Histiocytosis (Langerhan's cell)	Osteolytic lesions	Clinical plus investigations
Histoplasmosis	Cough, fever and weight loss	Histology
Hodgkin's lymphoma	Chronic lymph node swelling ± fever	Histology
Horner's syndrome	Bilateral pupil constriction, ptosis	Clinical
Human immunodeficiency virus (HIV)	*See* AIDS	
Human papillomavirus infections	Warty lesions	Clinical
Hyperparathyroidism	Renal calculi, polyuria, abdominal pain Brown tumour in jaws	Investigations
Hypo-adrenocorticism	*See* Addison's disease	
Hypohidrotic ectodermal dysplasia	*See* Ectodermal dysplasia	
Hypoparathyroidism, congenital	Tetany, cataracts, enamel hypoplasia	Investigations (may be part of polyendocrinopathy syndrome)
Hypophosphatasia	Anorexia, bone pain, weakness	Clinical plus investigations
Idiopathic midfacial granuloma syndrome	Ulceration	Histology
Impetigo	Facial rash, blisters, often golden yellow	Microbiology
Infectious mononucleosis	*See* Glandular fever	
Kaposi's sarcoma	Purplish macules or nodules	Histology
Kawasaki disease	Lymphadenopathy, conjunctivitis, dry lips, strawberry tongue, desquamation, cardiomyopathy/myocarditis	Clinical mainly

Investigations	Management
—	Symptomatic
Sometimes smear or serology	Symptomatic ± acyclovir
—	Acyclovir
Biopsy Skeletal survey	Depends on type; from no treatment to chemotherapy and irradiation
Biopsy + chest radiography	Fluconazole
Biopsy ± lymphangiogram ± MRI	Radiotherapy / chemotherapy
—	Reassure. Identify cause
—	Excise or intralesional interferon
Jaw + skeletal radiography, plasma calcium, phosphate and parathyroid hormone, bone scan	Remove parathyroid adenoma
Plasma parathormone, calcium phosphate levels	Calcium, vitamin D
Plasma calcium phosphate and alkaline phosphatase levels	Calcium, vitamin D
Biopsy, anti-neutrophil cytoplasmic antibody (ANCA)	Chemotherapy
Culture and sensitivity	Antimicrobial: penicillin
Biopsy. HIV serology	Chemotherapy or radiotherapy
Full blood picture, erythrocyte sedimentation rate, electrocardiogram	Symptomatic

Condition	Typical main clinical features	Diagnosis
Keratoconjunctivitis sicca	*See* Sjögren's syndrome	

Keratosis
  frictional
  smoker's
  verrucous
  sublingual
	White lesion
	White lesion in palate
	Raised or warty white lesion
	White lesion in floor of mouth and ventrum of tongue
		Clinical
		Clinical
		Clinical and histology
		Clinical and histology

Langerhan's cell histiocytoses	*See* Histiocytosis	
Leishmaniasis	Mucocutaneous ulceration, lymphadenopathy	Clinical and histology
Leprosy	Hypo- or hyperpigmented patches, lymphadenopathy, neuropathy	Clinical and histology
Letterer–Siwe disease	*See* Histiocytosis	
Leukaemia	Anaemia, bleeding tendency, infections, lymphadenopathy	Blood picture, biopsy
Leukopenia	Recurrent infections	Blood picture, biopsy
Leukoplakia	*See* Keratosis and *see* Hairy leukoplakia	
Lichen planus	Mucosal white lesions. Polygonal purple pruritic papules on skin	Clinical and histology
Lichenoid lesions: drug-induced	Mucosal white lesions. Polygonal purple pruritic papules on skin	Clinical and histology
Linear IgA disease	Mucosal vesicles or desquamative gingivitis	Clinical and histology
Localized oral purpura	Blood blisters only in mouth	Clinical
Ludwig's angina	Tender brawny submandibular swelling, fever	Clinical
Lupus erythematosus	Arthralgia, fever, rash, lymphadenopathy, lichenoid mucosal lesions	Clinical plus investigations
Lyme disease	Acute arthritis – mainly knee, rash ± facial palsy	Clinical plus serology
Lymphadenitis acute	Tender swollen lymph nodes	Clinical plus investigations
chronic	Chronically enlarged lymph nodes	Clinical plus investigations

Investigations	Management
—	Try to eliminate cause
—	Try to eliminate cause
Biopsy	Excise if dysplastic, stop tobacco use
Biopsy	Excise if dysplastic, stop tobacco use
Biopsy	Pentamidine or stibogluconate
Biopsy	Dapsone or clofazimine
Full blood picture + film, bone marrow biopsy	Chemotherapy
Full blood picture, bone marrow biopsy	Antimicrobial
Biopsy ± immunofluorescence	Corticosteroids topically, stop tobacco use
Biopsy	Corticosteroids topically, stop taking drug
Biopsy ± immunofluorescence	Dapsone ± sulphapyridine
Platelet count, biopsy may be needed to differentiate from pemphigoid	Reassurance ± deflate blisters
Pus for culture and sensitivity	Drainage, antimicrobials: penicillin in high dose
Antibodies to double-strand DNA	Corticosteroids, antimalarials
Serology	Antimicrobials
Temperature, examine drainage area White cell count and differential	Depends on cause
Temperature, examine drainage area White cell count and differential chest radiograph. Consider biopsy ± HIV testing	Depends on cause

Condition	Typical main clinical features	Diagnosis
Lymphangioma	Swelling but empties on pressure	Clinical
Lymphoma	Wide spectrum. Swollen lymph nodes, fever, weight loss	Clinical plus histology
Lymphosarcoma	*See* Lymphomas	
McCune–Albright syndrome	*See* Albright's syndrome	
Maffucci's syndrome	Enchondromatosis plus cavernous haemangiomas	Clinical plus investigations
MAGIC syndrome	*See* Behçet's syndrome	
Masseteric hypertrophy	Masseter enlarged on both or occasionally one side	Clinical
Measles	Fever, lymphadenopathy, conjunctivitis, rhinitis, maculopapular rash	Clinical
Median rhomboid glossitis	Rhomboidal red or nodular and depapillated or white, in midline of dorsum of tongue, just anterior to circumvallate papillae	Clinical and microbiology
Melanoma	Usually hyperpigmented papule in palate	Clinical plus histology
Melanotic macules	Hyperpigmented macule	Clinical
Melkersson–Rosenthal syndrome	Facial swelling, fissured tongue, facial palsy	Clinical plus investigations
Migrainous neuralgia	Nocturnal unilateral retro-ocular pain	Clinical
Molluscum contagiosum	Umbilicated papules	Clinical
Morsicatio buccarum	*See* Cheek chewing	
Mucoceles	Fluctuant swelling with clear or bluish contents	Clinical
Mucoepidermoid tumour	Firm salivary swelling	Clinical plus investigations
Mucormycosis	Sinus pain and discharge plus fever and palatal ulceration	Clinical plus investigations
Mucous membrane pemphigoid	Blisters, mainly in mouth occasionally on conjunctivae, genitals or skin. Scarring	Clinical and histology
Multiple basal cell naevus syndrome	*See* Gorlin–Goltz syndrome	

Investigations	Management
—	Leave or surgery, cryotherapy, laser therapy or sclerosant
Biopsy. Radiography	Chemotherapy ± radiotherapy
Radiography	Reassurance
—	Symptomatic Rarely surgery ± botulinum toxin
—	Symptomatic Avoid aspirin
Smear of lesion	Antifungals if *Candida* present Stop smoking
Biopsy (wide excision)	Surgery
—	Reassurance
Exclude Crohn's disease and sarcoidosis	Reassurance ± salazopyrine ± dapsone ± intralesional steroids
—	H_3 blockers, analgesics
Consider HIV infection	Pierce with orangewood stick
—	Surgery or cryotherapy
Biopsy ± radiography	Surgery
Biopsy. Radiography. Full blood picture. Exclude diabetes	Surgery. Antifungals
Biopsy + immunostaining	Topical corticosteroids

Condition	Typical main clinical features	Diagnosis
Multiple myeloma	Bone pain, anaemia, nausea, infections, amyloidosis	Clinical plus investigations
Mumps	Fever, painful swollen salivary gland(s) but no pustular discharge from duct	Clinical mainly
Mycosis fungoides	Variable rash	Clinical plus investigations
Myelodysplastic syndrome	Ulcers, anaemia, neutropenia, thrombocytopenia	Clinical plus investigations
Necrotizing sialometaplasia	Ulceration in palate	Clinical ± investigations
Neurofibromatosis	Neurofibromas and skin pigmentation	Clinical usually
Noma	*See* Cancrum oris	
North American blastomycosis	Chronic oral ulceration, pulmonary involvement	Clinical plus investigations
Oral dysaesthesia	*See* Burning mouth	
Oral submucous fibrosis	Firm fibrous bands in cheek and/or palate History of chilli use	Clinical
Orf	Umbilicated nodule	Clinical and history
Orofacial granulomatosis	Facial swelling, mucosa cobblestoned, ulcers, angular stomatitis (*See also* Crohn's disease)	Clinical plus investigations
Osler–Rendu–Weber syndrome	*See* Hereditary haemorrhagic telangiectasia	
Osteogenesis imperfecta	*See* Fragilitis ossium	
Osteomyelitis	Pain, swelling, fever	Clinical plus investigations
Osteopetrosis	Anaemia, cranial neuropathies, hepatosplenomegaly	Clinical plus investigations
Osteoradionecrosis	*See* Osteomyelitis	
Osteosarcoma	Pain, swelling	Clinical plus investigations
Paget's disease	Pain, craniofacial neuropathies, cardiac failure	Clinical plus investigations
Pain dysfunction syndrome	*See* Facial arthromyalgia	
Papillary hyperplasia	Small papillae in palate	Clinical

Investigations	Management
Radiography. Serum and urine electrophoresis. Bone marrow biopsy	Radiography and chemotherapy
Serology may be helpful	Symptomatic
Biopsy. Full blood picture Bone marrow biopsy	Topical chemotherapy ± radiotherapy
Full blood picture. Bone marrow biopsy	Chemotherapy
Biopsy may be indicated	Self-healing
Radiography and biopsy may help	Excise symptomatic tumours
Biopsy ± chest radiography	Antifungals: fluconazole, ketoconazole or amphotericin
—	Avoid chillis and pan. Corticosteroids intralesionally
Electron microscopy ± biopsy	Spontaneous resolution
Exclude Crohn's disease/sarcoidosis Biopsy ± allergy testing	Avoid allergens. Reassurance Corticosteroids intralesionally
Radiography. Pus for culture and sensitivity	Drainage. Antimicrobials
Radiography. Biopsy	Bone marrow transplant
Radiography. Biopsy	Surgery ± chemotherapy
Radiography, serum alkaline phosphatase, urinary hydroxyproline	Diphosphonates, acetylsalicyclic acid, calcitonin
—	Surgery or leave alone

Condition	Typical main clinical features	Diagnosis
Paracoccidioidomycosis	Chronic oral ulceration, pulmonary involvement. Time in Latin America	Clinical plus investigations
Parodontal abscess	Painful swelling alongside a periodontally involved tooth	Clinical
Pemphigoid	*See* Mucous membrane pemphigoid	
Pemphigus	Skin vesicles + bullae. Mouth ulcers	Clinical plus histology
Periadentitis mucosa necrotica recurrens (Sutton's ulcers)	*See* Aphthae	
Periarteritis nodosa	*See* Polyarteritis nodosa	
Pericoronitis	Painful swelling of operculum of partially erupted tooth ± trismus ± fever	Clinical
Periodontitis (acute apical)	Pain, tenderness on touching tooth	Clinical plus investigations
Perleche	*See* Cheilitis, angular	
Phycomycosis	*See* Mucormycosis	
Pleomorphic salivary ademona	Firm salivary swelling	Clinical plus investigations
Polyarteritis nodosa	Fever, weakness, arthralgia, myalgia, abdominal pain, hypertension	Clinical plus raised ESR Histology
Polycythaemia rubra vera	Headache, thromboses, haemorrhage, splenomegaly	Clinical plus investigations
Polyps – fibroepithelial	*See* Fibroepithelial polyp	
Pulpitis	Toothache	Clinical plus investigations
Pyogenic arthritis	Pain, fever, limited jaw movement, swelling	Clinical mainly
Pyogenic granuloma	Swelling, usually on lip, tongue or gum	Clinical
Pyostomatitis vegetans	Irregular oral ulcers and pustules	Clinical plus investigations
Ranula	*See* Mucocele	
Recurrent aphthous stomatitis	*See* Aphthae	

Investigations	Management
Biopsy ± chest radiography	Antifungals: fluconazole, ketoconazole or amphotericin
Radiography, culture pus	Drain. Antimicrobial: penicillin
Biopsy. Serology Immunostaining	Corticosteroids systemically Consider azathioprine or gold
Radiography	Debridement ± antimicrobial Reduce occlusion. Consider extracting offending tooth
Radiography ± vitality test	Open tooth for drainage and relieve occlusion (or extract), analgesics ± antimicrobial
Biopsy ± radiography	Surgery
Full blood picture, erythrocyte sedimentation rate. Biopsy	Systemic corticosteroids
Haemoglobin, full blood picture, marrow biopsy	Phlebotomy ± chemotherapy
Radiography ± vitality test	Open tooth (or extract). Extirpate pulp. Analgesics
Radiography, culture joint aspirate	Antimicrobial, analgesics
Biopsy [excision]	Excise
Biopsy. Exclude Crohn's disease and ulcerative colitis	Treat underlying condition

Condition	Typical main clinical features	Diagnosis
Recurrent parotitis	Recurrent painful parotid swelling	Clinical
Reiter's syndrome	Arthritis, conjunctivitis, mucocutaneous lesions, urethritis	Clinical mainly
Rheumatoid arthritis	Painful swollen small joints ± deformities Associated with Sjögren's syndrome	Clinical plus investigations Check for xerostomia
Rickets	Skeletal deformities, retarded growth, fractures	Clinical plus investigations
Rubella	*See* German measles	
Rubeola	*See* Measles	
Sarcoidosis	Various – especially hilar lymphadenopathy and rashes	Clinical plus investigations
Scleroderma	Tightening facial and other skin Associated with Sjögren's syndrome	Clinical and serology
Scrotal tongue	Fissured tongue	Clinical
Scurvy	Purplish chronically swollen gingivae	Clinical
Shingles	Painful facial rash and oral ulcers if affecting maxillary or mandibular division of trigeminal nerve	Clinical
Sialolithiasis	*See* Calculus, salivary	
Sialorrhoea	Excess salivation	Clinical
Sialosis	Painless persistent bilateral salivary gland swelling	Clinical plus investigations
Sinusitis (acute)	Pain especially on moving head	Clinical plus radiography
Sjögren's syndrome	Autoimmune exocrinopathy. Dry eyes, dry mouth and often a connective tissue disease	Clinical plus investigations
Smoker's keratosis	*See* Keratosis	
South American blastomycosis	*See* Paracoccidioidomycosis	

Investigations	Management
Sialography. Exclude Sjögren's syndrome	Consider duct dilatation. Antimicrobials
Full blood picture, erythrocyte sedimentation rate. Radiography	Tetracycline. Non-steroidal anti-inflammatory drugs
Rheumatoid factor, full blood picture Radiography	Salicylates. Non-steroidal anti-inflammatory drugs
Blood calcium, phosphate, alkaline phosphatase. Radiography. Renal function tests	Vitamin D. Calcitonin
Chest radiograph + serum angiotensin-converting enzyme	Corticosteroids systemically
Serology SCl-70 antibody	Supportive
—	Reassurance
White blood cell count Vitamin C levels	Vitamin C
Consider underlying immune defect	Analgesics, ± acyclovir, ± protect cornea
Salivary flow rate	Avoid anticholinesterases, otherwise reassurance or consider atropinics
Exclude alcoholism, diabetes, bulimia, sarcoidosis, Sjögren's syndrome, liver disease	Remove underlying cause
Radiography	Decongestants, analgesics and antimicrobial
Serology — SS-A (Ro) and SS-B (La) antibodies. Consider labial gland biopsy ± salivary flow rate ± sialography ± scan	Artificial tears and saliva. Preventive dentistry

Condition	Typical main clinical features	Diagnosis
Staphylococcus aureus lymphadenitis	Painful swollen lymph node(s) ± fever	Clinical mainly
Stevens–Johnson syndrome	*See* Erythema multiforme	
Streptococcal tonsillitis	Sore throat. Tonsillar exudate	Clinical mainly
Stroke	Hemiplegia usually ± facial palsy	Clinical
Subluxation-temporo-mandibular joint	Limited jaw movement ± pain, condyle palpably displaced	Clinical
Surgical emphysema	Swelling which crackles on palpation	Clinical
Tori	Asymptomatic bony lumps	Clinical
Toxoplasmosis	Lymphadenopathy ± chorioretinitis	Clinical plus investigations
Trigeminal neuralgia	Severe lancinating pain often associated with trigger zone	Clinical mainly
Tuberculosis	Cough, cervical, lymphadenopathy, weight loss, oral ulceration	Clinical plus investigations
White sponge naevus	*See* Familial white folded gingivostomatitis	
Zygomycosis	*See* Mucormycosis	

Investigations	Management
Pus for culture and sensitivity	Antimicrobials
Throat swab	Antimicrobials
—	Physiotherapy
—	Reduce. Consider Dawtry operation
—	Reassurance. Antimicrobials
—	Reassurance. Surgery if interfering with denture wear
Serology	Sulphonamide + pyrimethamine
Skull base CT	Avoid trigger zone. Carbamazepine ± phenytoin, baclofen or clonazepam
Chest radiograph Sputum microscopy and culture Biopsy	Antimicrobials: rifampicin, isoniazid, ethambutol, streptomycin

1.4 GUIDE TO DRUGS USED IN THE MANAGEMENT OF ORAL DISEASES

Always check doses, possible interactions and adverse effects before using a drug. While every attempt has been made to include accurate data, the authors and publishers accept no liability for Tables 1 to 15.

Table 1 ANALGESICS (INCLUDING OPIOIDS)

Drug	Comments	Route	Adult dose
Aspirin	Mild analgesic: NSAID Causes gastric irritation Interferes with haemostasis Contraindicated in bleeding disorders, asthma, children, late pregnancy, peptic ulcers, renal disease, aspirin allergy	Oral	300–600 mg up to 6 times a day after meals; maximum 4 g daily (use soluble or dispersible or enteric-coated aspirin)
Mefenamic acid	Mild analgesic: NSAID May be contraindicated in asthma, gastro-intestinal, liver and renal disease and pregnancy May cause diarrhoea or haemolytic anaemia	Oral	250–500 mg up to 3 times a day
Diflunisal	Analgesic for mild to moderate pain: NSAID Long action: twice a day dose only Effective against bone and joint pain Contraindicated in renal and liver disease, peptic ulcer, pregnancy, allergies	Oral	250–500 mg twice a day
Paracetamol	Mild analgesic: not usually termed an NSAID Hepatotoxic in overdose or prolonged use Contraindicated in liver or renal disease	Oral	500–1000 mg up to 6 times a day
Codeine phosphate*	Analgesic for moderate pain Contraindicated in liver disease and late pregnancy Avoid alcohol May cause sedation and constipation Reduces cough reflex	Oral	10–60 mg up to 6 times a day (or 30 mg IM)
Dextropropoxyphene*	Analgesic for moderate pain Risk of respiratory depression in overdose, especially if taken with alcohol May cause dependence Occasional hepatotoxicity No more effective than paracetamol or aspirin alone	Oral	65 mg up to 4 times a day
Diclofenac	Analgesic for moderate pain: NSAID Contraindicated in peptic ulcer, aspirin sensitivity and pregnancy Caution in elderly, renal, liver or cardiac disease	Oral or IM	25–75 mg up to twice daily
Dihydrocodeine tartrate*	Analgesic for moderate pain May cause nausea, drowsiness and constipation Contraindicated in children, asthma, hypothyroidism and renal disease May increase post-operative dental pain	Oral	30 mg up to 4 times a day (or 50 mg IM)

Table 1 (Contd)

Drug	Comments	Route	Adult dose
Nefopam	Analgesic for moderate pain May cause nausea, dry mouth or urine retention Contraindicated in epilepsy	Oral	60 mg up to 3 times a day
Pentazocine*	Analgesic for moderate pain May produce dependence, hallucinations or provoke withdrawal symptoms in narcotic addicts Contraindicated in pregnancy, children, hypertension, respiratory depression, head injuries or raised intracranial pressure There is a low risk of dependence	Oral	50 mg up to 4 times a day (or 30 mg IM or IV)
Buprenorphine*	Potent analgesic More potent than pentazocine and longer action than morphine No hallucinations May cause salivation, sweating, dizziness and vomiting Respiratory depression in overdose Can cause dependence Contraindicated in pregnancy, children, with MAOIs, liver or respiratory disease	Sub-lingual	0.2–0.4 mg up to 4 times a day (or 0.3 mg IM)
Meptazinol*	Potent analgesic Claimed to have low incidence of respiratory depression Side-effects as buprenorphine	IM or IV	75–100 mg up to 6 times a day
Phenazocine*	Analgesic for severe pain May cause nausea	Oral or sub-lingual	5 mg up to 4 times a day
Pethidine*	Potent analgesic Less potent than morphine Contraindicated with MAOI Risk of dependence	SC or IM	25–100 mg up to 4 times a day
Morphine*	Potent analgesic Often causes nausea and vomiting Reduces cough reflex, causes pupil constriction	SC or IM or oral	5–10 mg as required
Diamorphine*	Potent analgesic More potent than pethidine and morphine but more dependence	SC or IM or oral	2.5 mg by injection; 5–10 mg orally

*Opioids; NSAID, non-steroidal anti-inflammatory drug; IM, intramuscular; IV, intravenous; SC, subcutaneous; MAOI, monoamine oxidase inhibitor

Table 2 ANTIFUNGALS FOR THE TREATMENT OF ORAL CANDIDOSIS

Drug	Dose	Comments
Amphotericin	10–100 mg 6-hourly	Dissolve in mouth slowly Active topically Negligible absorption from gastro-intestinal tract
Nystatin	500 000 unit lozenge, 100 000 unit pastille, or 100 000 unit per ml of suspension 6-hourly	Dissolve in mouth slowly Active topically Negligible absorption from gastro-intestinal tract
Miconazole	250 mg tablet 6-hourly or 25 mg/ml gel used as 5 ml 6-hourly	Dissolve in mouth slowly Active topically Also has antibacterial activity Negligible absorption from gastro-intestinal tract Theoretically best antifungal to treat angular cheilitis
Ketoconazole	200–400 mg once daily with meal	Absorbed from gastro-intestinal tract Useful in intractable candidosis Contra-indicated in pregnancy and liver disease May cause nausea, rashes, pruritus and liver damage Enhances nephrotoxicity of cyclosporin
Fluconazole	50–100 mg once daily	Absorbed from gastro-intestinal tract Less toxic than ketoconazole Contraindicated in pregnancy, infants and renal disease May cause nausea and abdominal pain

Table 3 ANTIVIRAL THERAPY OF ORAL HERPETIC INFECTIONS

Virus	Disease	Otherwise healthy patient	Immunocompromised patient
Herpes simplex	Primary herpetic gingivostomatitis	Consider oral acyclovir[a,b] 100–200 mg, five times daily as suspension or tablets	Acyclovir 250 mg/m^2 IV[b] every 8 hours
	Recurrent herpetic infection, eg herpes labialis	5% acyclovir cream	Consider systemic acyclovir[b] as above depending on risk to patient of infection
Herpes varicella-zoster	Chickenpox	—	As above
	Zoster (shingles)	Consider oral acyclovir[a] 800 mg, five times daily	

[a]In neonate, treat as if immunocompromised.
[b]Systemic acyclovir: caution in renal disease and pregnancy; occasional increase in liver enzymes and urea, rashes.

Table 4 ANTIBACTERIALS

Drug	Comments*	Route	Dose
PENICILLINS	Most oral bacterial infections respond well to drainage ± penicillin Oral phenoxymethyl penicillin is usually effective and cheap Amoxycillin is often used and is usually effective, but almost four times as expensive		
Amoxycillin	Orally effective (absorption better than ampicillin) Broad-spectrum penicillin derivative *Staphylococcus aureus* often resistant Not resistant to penicillinase Contraindicated in penicillin hypersensitivity Rashes in infectious mononucleosis, cytomegalovirus infection, lymphoid leukaemia, allopurinol. May cause diarrhoea	Oral, IM or IV	250–500 mg 8-hourly
Augmentin (Co-amoxiclav)	Mixture of amoxycillin and potassium clavulanate Inhibits some penicillinases and therefore active against *Staphylococcus aureus* Inhibits some lactamases and is therefore active against some Gram-negative and penicillin-resistant bacteria Contraindicated in penicillin hypersensitivity Beware of hepatobiliary events	Oral	125/250 mg 8-hourly
Ampicillin	Less oral absorption than amoxycillin, otherwise as for amoxycillin (There are many analogues but these have few, if any, advantages) Contraindicated in penicillin hypersensitivity	Oral, IM or IV	250–500 mg 6-hourly
Benzylpenicillin	Not orally active Most effective penicillin where organism sensitive Not resistant to penicillinase Contraindicated in penicillin hypersensitivity Large doses may cause K$^+$ to fall and Na$^+$ to rise	Oral or IM	300–600 mg 6-hourly
Flucloxacillin	Orally active penicillin derivative Effective against most, but not all, penicillin-resistant staphylococci Contraindicated in penicillin hypersensitivity	Oral or IM	250 mg 6-hourly
Phenoxymethyl penicillin (Penicillin V)	Orally active Best taken on empty stomach Not resistant to penicillinase Contraindicated in penicillin hypersensitivity	Oral	250–500 mg 6-hourly
Procaine penicillin	Depot penicillin Not resistant to penicillinase Contraindicated in penicillin hypersensitivity Rarely psychotic reaction	IM	300 000 units every 12 hours
Benethamine penicillin (Triplopen)	Depot penicillin Contains benzyl (300 mg), procaine (250 mg) and benethamine (475 mg) penicillins Not resistant to penicillinase Contraindicated in penicillin hypersensitivity	IM	1 vial every 2–3 days *Contd*

IM, intramuscular; IV, intravenous; K$^+$, potassium; Na$^+$, sodium.
*It should be noted that some antibacterials impair the activity of oral contraceptives.

Table 4 (Contd)

Drug	Comments*	Route	Dose
SULPHONAMIDES	Main indications are in prophylaxis of post-traumatic meningitis but meningococci increasingly resistant Co-trimoxazole may be used to treat sinusitis Contraindicated in pregnancy and in renal disease In other patients, adequate hydration must be ensured to prevent the (rare) occurrence of crystalluria Other adverse reactions include erythema multiforme, rashes and blood dyscrasias		
Co-trimoxazole	Combination of trimethoprim and sulphamethoxazole Orally active Broad spectrum Occasional rashes or blood dyscrasias Contraindicated in pregnancy, liver disease May increase the effect of protein-bound drugs	Oral or IM	960 mg twice daily or 3–4.5 ml IM twice daily
TETRACYCLINES	Broad-spectrum antibacterial but of the many preparations there is little to choose between them However, doxycycline is useful since a single dose is adequate, and minocycline is effective against meningococci; both are safer for patients with renal failure than most of the tetracyclines, which are nephrotoxic Tetracyclines cause discoloration of developing teeth and have absorption impaired by iron, antacids, milk, etc Use of tetracyclines may predispose to candidosis, and to nausea and gastro-intestinal disturbance Orally active Broad spectrum Contraindicated in pregnancy and children at least up to 8 years Reduced dose indicated in renal failure, liver disease, elderly Frequent mild gastro-intestinal effects	Oral	250–500 mg 6-hourly
Doxycycline	Orally active Broad spectrum Single daily dose Contraindicated in pregnancy and children up to at least 8 years Safer than tetracycline in renal failure (excreted in faeces) Reduce dose in liver disease and elderly Mild gastro-intestinal effects	Oral	100 mg once daily
Minocycline	Orally active Broad spectrum: active against meningococci Safer than tetracycline in renal disease (excreted in faeces) May cause dizziness and vertigo Absorption not reduced by milk Contraindicated in pregnancy and children up to at least 8 years May also cause oral pigmentation in adults	Oral	100 mg twice daily
VANCOMYCIN	Reserved for serious infections Extravenous extravasation causes necrosis and phlebitis May cause nausea, rashes, tinnitus, deafness Rapid injection may cause 'red neck' syndrome Contraindicated in renal disease, deafness Very expensive	Oral or IV	500 mg 6-hourly for pseudomembranous colitis. 1 g IV by slow injection for prophylaxis of endocarditis

IM, intramuscular; IV, intravenous.
*It should be noted that some antibacterials impair the activity of oral contraceptives.

Table 5 OTHER ANTIBACTERIAL AGENTS USED OCCASIONALLY

Drug	Comments*	Route	Adult dose
CEPHALOSPORINS AND CEPHAMYCINS	Broad spectrum, expensive and bactericidal antibiotics with few absolute indications for use in dentistry, although they may be effective against *Staphylococcus aureus* They produce false-positive results for glycosuria with 'Clinitest' Hypersensitivity is the main side-effect Some cause a bleeding tendency Some are nephrotoxic Cefuroxime is less affected by penicillinases than other cephalosporins and is currently the preferred drug of the many available		
Cefotaxime and ceftazidime	Not orally active Broad spectrum; third generation cephalosporins Contraindicated if history of anaphylaxis to penicillin Expensive	IM or IV	1 g 12-hourly
Cefuroxime	Not orally active Broad spectrum; second generation cephalosporin Contraindicated if history of anaphylaxis to penicillin	IM or IV	250–750 mg 8-hourly
Ceftriaxone	Orally active; third generation cephalosporin Longer action than most cephalosporins Contraindicated in liver disease or history of anaphylaxis to penicillin	IM or IV	1 g daily as single dose
ERYTHROMYCIN	Similar antibacterial spectrum to penicillin and is therefore used in penicillin-allergic patients Active against most staphylococci, *Mycoplasma* and *Legionnella*, but not always against oral *Bacteroides* Do not use erythromycin estolate, which may cause liver disease		
Erythromycin stearate	Orally active Useful in those hypersensitive to penicillin Effective against most staphylococci and streptococci May cause nausea Rapid development of resistance Reduced dose indicated in liver disease Can increase cyclosporin absorption and toxicity	Oral	250–500 mg 6-hourly
Erythromycin lactobionate	Used where parenteral erythromycin indicated Give not as a bolus but by infusion Comments as above	IV	2 g daily
GENTAMICIN	Reserved for serious infections Can cause vestibular and renal damage, especially if given with frusemide Contraindicated in pregnancy and myasthenia gravis Reduce dose in renal disease	IM or IV	Up to 5 mg/kg daily *Contd*

IM, intramuscular; IV, intravenous. *It should be noted that some antibacterials impair the activity of oral contraceptives.

Table 5 (Contd)

Drug	Comments*	Route	Adult dose
METRONIDAZOLE	Orally active Effective against anaerobes Use only for 7 days (or peripheral neuropathy may develop, particularly in liver-disease patients) Avoid alcohol (disulfiram-type reaction) May increase warfarin effect May cause tiredness IV preparation available but expensive Suppositories effective Contraindicated in pregnancy	Oral or IV	200–400 mg 8-hourly (take with meals)
RIFAMPICIN	Reserved mainly for treatment of tuberculosis Safe and effective but resistance rapidly occurs Body secretions turn red May interfere with oral contraception Occasional rashes, jaundice or blood dyscrasias	Oral or IV	0.6–1.2 g daily in 2–4 divided doses

IM, intramuscular; IV, intravenous. *It should be noted that some antibacterials impair the activity of oral contraceptives.

Table 6 SOME TOPICAL CORTICOSTEROIDS (many more potent preparations are available)

Drug	Dose 6-hourly	Comments
Hydrocortisone hemisuccinate pellets	2.5 mg	Dissolve in mouth close to lesions Use at early stage
Triamcinolone acetonide in carmellose gelatin paste	Apply thin layer	Adheres best to dry mucosa Affords mechanical protection Of little value on tongue or palate
Betamethasone phosphate tablets	0.5 mg as a mouth wash	More potent than preparations above but may produce adrenal suppression
Beclomethasone dipropionate (inhaler)	Spray on lesion, 50–200 µg	More potent than preparations above but may produce adrenal suppression

Table 7 SOME INTRALESIONAL CORTICOSTEROIDS

Drug	Dose	Comments
Prednisolone sodium phosphate	Up to 24 mg	Short acting
Methylprednisolone acetate	4–80 mg every 1 to 5 weeks	Also available with lignocaine
Triamcinolone acetonide	2–3 mg every 1 to 2 weeks	—
Triamcinolone hexacetonide	Up to 5 mg every 3 to 4 weeks	—

Table 8 SOME INTRA-ARTICULAR CORTICOSTEROIDS*

Drug	Dose	Comments
Dexamethasone sodium phosphate	0.4–5 mg at intervals of 3 to 21 days	More expensive than hydrocortisone acetate
Hydrocortisone acetate	5–50 mg	Usual preparation used

*Also used are those listed in Table 7 under intralesional corticosteroids.

Table 9 SYSTEMIC IMMUNOMODULATORY DRUGS

Drug	Comments	Adult dose
Prednisolone	May be indicated systemically for pemphigus and Bell's palsy, and occasionally other disorders	Initially 40–80 mg orally each day in divided doses, reducing as soon as possible to 10 mg daily Give enteric-coated prednisolone with meals
Dexamethasone	May be used to reduce post-surgical oedema after minor oral surgery	5 mg IV with premedication followed by 0.5–1.0 mg daily for 5 days, orally if possible
Betamethasone	May be useful to reduce post-surgical oedema after minor oral surgery	1 mg orally the night before operation 1 mg orally with premedication 1 mg orally every 6 hours for 2 days post-operatively
Methylprednisolone	May be useful to reduce post-surgical oedema after major surgery	Methylprednisolone succinate 1 g IV at operation, 500 mg on evening of operation followed by 125 mg IV every 6 hours for 24 hours. Then methylprednisolone acetate orally 80 mg every 12 hours for 24 hours
Azathioprine	Steroid-sparing for immuno-suppression Myelosuppressive and hepatotoxic, and long-term may predispose to neoplasms Contraindicated in pregnancy	Orally 2–2.5 mg/kg daily
Dapsone	May be used in some dermatoses Occasional neuropathy, headache, anaemia, rashes Contraindicated in glucose-6-phosphate dehydrogenase deficiency, pregnancy, anaemia, cardiorespiratory disease	Orally up to 1–2 mg/kg daily
Colchicine	May be used in severe oral ulceration Occasional nausea, abdominal pain, or blood dyscrasia Contraindicated in pregnancy, renal or gastro-intestinal disease	Orally up to 500 µg 4 times daily *Contd*

IV, intravenous.

52

Table 9 (Contd)

Drug	Comments	Adult dose
Thalidomide	May be used in severe oral ulceration Peripheral neuropathy in prolonged use Contraindicated in pregnancy	Orally 50–200 mg preferably on alternate days

Table 10 SOME SEDATIVES AND TRANQUILLIZERS

Drug	Comments	Preparations	Route	Adult dose
Chlorpromazine	Major tranquillizer May cause dyskinesia, photosensitivity, eye defects. and jaundice Contraindicated in epilepsy IM use causes pain and may cause postural hypotension	25 mg tablet 25 mg/ml syrup 50 mg/2 ml injection	Oral or IM	25 mg 8-hourly
Chlordiazepoxide	Anxiolytic Reduce dose in elderly	5 mg or 10 mg	Oral	5–10 mg 8-hourly
Diazepam	Anxiolytic Reduce dose in elderly	2 mg, 5 mg or 10 mg	Oral, IM or IV	2–30 mg daily in divided doses
Thioridazine	Major tranquillizer Phenothiazine with fewer adverse effects than chlorpromazine Rare retinopathy	10 mg or 25 mg	Oral	10–50 mg 8-hourly
Propranolol	Useful anxiolytic which does not cause amnesia, but reduces tremor and palpitations Contraindicated in asthma, cardiac failure, pregnancy	10 mg or 40 mg	Oral	80–100 mg daily
Haloperidol	Major tranquillizer Useful in elderly	500 µg	Oral	500 µg 12-hourly

IM, intramuscular; IV, intravenous.

Table 11 SOME OTHER DRUGS USED IN THE MANAGEMENT OF ORAL DISEASES

Drug	Comments	Route	Adult dose
Etretinate	Vitamin A analogue which may be used in treatment of erosive lichen planus Effect begins after 2 to 3 weeks Treat for 6 to 9 months, followed by similar rest period Most patients develop dry, cracked lips May cause epistaxis, pruritus, alopecia Contraindicated in pregnancy/liver disease	Oral	0.5–1.0 mg/kg daily in two divided doses
Carbamazepine	Prophylactic for trigeminal neuralgia — not analgesic Occasional dizziness, diplopia and blood dyscrasia, usually with a rash and usually in the first 3 months of treatment Potentiated by cimetidine, dextropropoxyphene and isoniazid Potentiates lithium Interferes with oral contraceptives	Oral	Initially 100 mg once or twice daily. Many patients need about 200 mg 8-hourly. Do not exceed 1800 mg daily

Table 12 SOME ANTIDEPRESSANTS

Drug	Comments	Route	Adult dose
Amitriptyline	Tricyclic Antidepressant effect may not be seen until up to 30 days after start Sedative effect also When treatment established, use single dose at night	Oral	25–75 mg daily in divided dose
Dothiepin	Tricyclic Anxiolytic effect also useful in atypical facial pain When treatment established, use single dose at night	Oral	25 mg three times a day or 75 mg at night
Clomipramine	Tricyclic Equally effective as amitriptyline but less sedative effect Useful in phobia or obsessional states	Oral	10–100 mg daily in divided doses
Fluoxetine	Selective serotonin re-uptake inhibitor Less sedative or cardiotoxic than tricyclics Contraindicated in cardiovascular, hepatic or renal disease, pregnancy, diabetes and epilepsy	Oral	20 mg daily
Flupenthixol	Not a tricyclic or MAOI Fewer side-effects Contraindicated in cardiovascular, hepatic or renal disease, Parkinsonism or overexcitable/over-active patients	Oral	1–3 mg in the morning

MAOI, monoamine oxidase inhibitor

Table 13 ANTIDEPRESSANTS: INTERACTIONS AND CAUTIONS

Tricyclics and tetracyclics	Monoamine oxidase inhibitors (MAOIs)
USE WITH CAUTION IN: Cardiovascular disease Epilepsy Liver disease Diabetes Hypertension Glaucoma Mania Urinary retention Prostatic hypertrophy	**USE WITH CAUTION IN:** Cardiovascular disease Epilepsy Liver disease Phaeochromocytoma
MAY INTERACT WITH: Barbiturates MAOIs Antihypertensives General anaesthetics	**MAY INTERACT WITH:** Barbiturates Some sympathomimetic amines Tricyclics Narcotics Antihypertensives Foods such as some meat or yeast extracts, cheese, wine

Note: Neither group significantly interact with lignocaine, prilocaine or doses of adrenaline found in dental local analgesic solutions. Either group may worsen xerostomia.

Table 14 SOME HYPNOTICS

Drug	Comments	Preparations	Route	Adult dose
Chlormethiazole	Contraindicated in liver disease Useful in elderly May cause dependence	192 mg capsule 250 mg/5 ml syrup	Oral	500 mg
Diazepam	Useful hypnotic Reduce dose in elderly May cause dependence	5 mg or 10 mg	Oral	5–10 mg
Dichloralphenazone	Derivative of chloral hydrate Contraindicated in porphyria, with oral anticoagulants Useful in elderly	650 mg	Oral	1300 mg
Nitrazepam	No more useful than diazepam Avoid in elderly May cause dependence Hangover effect	5 mg	Oral	5–10 mg
Temazepam	Useful in elderly May cause dependence Less hangover effect than nitrazepam	10 mg	Oral	10–20 mg

Table 15 ANTIFIBRINOLYTIC AGENTS

Drug	Comments	Route	Adult dose
ε-amino caproic acid	Useful in some bleeding tendencies May cause nausea, diarrhoea, dizziness, myalgia Contraindicated in pregnancy, history of thromboembolism, renal disease	Oral	3 g, 4–6 times daily
Tranexamic acid	As above, but tranexamic acid is usually the preferred drug	Oral, IV	1–1.5 g, 6 or 12 hourly Slow injection 1 g 8-hourly

IV, intravenous.

1.5 GUIDE TO THE ORAL AND PERIORAL SIDE-EFFECTS OF DRUG TREATMENT

Most oral and perioral side-effects to drug treatment are rare but the more common causes are indicated in **bold** in the following section. For further details the reader is referred to the British National Formulary.

ANGIOEDEMA

Acetylsalicylic acid
Angiotensin-converting enzyme (ACE) inhibitors
Asparaginase
Barbiturates
Captopril
Carbamazepine
Cephalosporin derivatives
Clonidine
Co-trimoxazole
Disulphite sodium
Enalapril
Epoetin alpha
Ibuprofen
Indomethacin
Iodine contrast media
Ketoconazole
Local anaesthetics
Miconazole
Naproxen
Nitrofurantoin
Penicillamine
Penicillin derivatives
Pyrazolone derivatives
Quinine
Streptomycin
Sulphonamide derivatives
Thiouracil derivatives

BURNING MOUTH

Captopril

CANDIDOSIS

Broad-spectrum antibiotics
Corticosteroids
Drugs causing xerostomia
Immunosuppressants

CERVICAL LYMPH-NODE ENLARGEMENT

Phenytoin
Phenylbutazone
Primidone

DERMATITIS HERPETIFORMIS-LIKE REACTIONS

Acetylsalicylic acid
Amitriptyline
Diclofenac
Flurbiprofen
Indomethacin
Phenobarbitone
Sulphonamides

CHEILITIS

Actinomycin
Busulphan
Cytotoxics
Ethyl alcohol
Isoniazid
Lithium salts
Menthol
Penicillamine
Phenothiazines
Retinoids
Selegiline

ERYTHEMA MULTIFORME (INC. STEVENS-JOHNSON SYNDROME)

Acetylsalicylic acid
Allopurinol
Amlodipine
Arsenic
Atropine
Barbiturates
Carbamazepine
Chloral hydrate
Chloramphenicol
Chlorpropamide
Clindamycin
Co-trimoxazole
Codeine
Diclofenac
Diflunisal
Digitalis glycosides
Diltiazem
Ethyl alcohol
Fluconazole
Fluorouracil
Griseofulvin
Hydantoin
Hydrochlorothiazide
Indapamide
Measles/mumps/rubella vaccine
Meclofenamic acid

Mercury
Mesterolone
Nifedipine
Omeprazole
Oxyphenbutazone
Penicillin derivatives
Phenolphthalein
Phenothiazine derivatives
Phenylbutazone
Phenytoin
Piroxicam
Progesterone
Pyrazolone derivatives
Quinine
Radiotherapy
Retinol
Rifampicin
Streptomycin
Sulindac
Sulphasalazine
Sulphonamides
Sulphonylurea derivatives
Tenoxicam
Tetracyclines
Theophylline
Tocainide
Trimethadione
Vancomycin
Verapamil
Zidovudine

EPIDERMOLYSIS BULLOSAE-LIKE ERUPTIONS

Frusemide
Penicillamine
Sulphonamides

FACIAL OEDEMA

Cinoxacin
Corticosteroids
Cyclosporin
Trilostane

FACIAL FLUSHING

Adenosine
Alprostadil
Buserilin

Calcitonin
Calcium channel blockers
Carboprost
Chlorpropamide
Clomiphene
Co-dergocrine
Danazol
L-Dopa
Flumazenil
Formestane
Loxapine
Morphine
Nicotinic acid
Oxpentifylline
Pentamidine
Protirelin
Quinine
Rifampicin
Ritodrine
Sermorelin
Tamoxifen
Thymoxamine
Thyroxine
Trilostane

FACIAL HIRSUTISM

Cyclosporin
Cyproterone
Formestane
Medroxyprogesterone
Nandrolone
Norethisterone
Oxymetholone
Phenytoin
Testosterone
Tibolone

FACIAL PAIN

Phenothiazines
Stilbamidine
Vinca alkaloids

FACIAL PALSY

Botulinum A toxin

GINGIVAL HYPERPLASIA

Amlodipine
Cyclosporin A
Diltiazem
Diphenoxylate
Ethosuximide
Felodipine
Interferon-alpha
Lacidipine
Mephenytoin
Nifedipine
Nitrendipine
Norethisterone + mestranol
Norethynodrel + mestranol
Phenytoin
Valproic acid
Verapamil

GLOSSITIS

Captopril
Chloramphenicol
Cytotoxics
Enalapril
Ergot alkaloids
Flunisolide
Gold
Griseofulvin
Isoniazid
Methyldopa
Metronidazole
Phenelzine
Phenothiazine derivatives
Streptomycin
Sulindac
Tetracycline
Tricyclic antidepressants
Zidovudine

HALITOSIS

Dimethyl sulphoxide
Disulfiram
Isosorbide dinitrate

HYPERSALIVATION

Anticholinesterases
Buprenorphine
Clonazepam
Clozapine

Copper sulphate
Ethionamide
Iodides
Ketamine
Mercurials
Nicardipine
Niridazole
Remoxipride

INVOLUNTARY FACIAL MOVEMENTS

Butyrophenones
Carbamazepine
L-dopa
Lithium
Metirosine
Methyldopa
Metoclopramide
Phenothiazines
Phenytoin
Tetrabenazine
Tricyclic antidepressants
Trifluoperazine

LABIAL CRUSTING

Etretinate

LICHENOID REACTIONS

Allopurinol
Antimalarials
β-Adrenergic blockers
Barbiturates
BCG vaccine
Captopril
Chloral hydrate
Chlorpropamide
Cholera vaccine
Colchicine
Dapsone
Griseofulvin
Hepatitis B vaccine
Interferon-alpha
Mercury
Metformin
Methyldopa
NSAIDs

Contd

Oral contraceptives
Para-aminosalicylate
Penicillamine
Penicillin derivatives
Phenylbutazone
Phenytoin
Piroxicam
Prazosin
Procainamide
Propylthiouracil
Quinine
Rifampicin
Sulphonamides
Tocainide
Tetracyclines

MUCOUS MEMBRANE DISCOLORATION

Blue:
Amiodarone
Antimalarials
Bismuth overdose
Mepacrine
Minocycline
Phenazopyridine
Quinidine
Silver
Sulphasalazine

Brown (hypermelanosis):
Aminophenazone
Betel nut
Busulphan
Clofazimine
Contraceptives
Cyclophosphamide
Diethylstilbestrol
Doxorubicin
Doxycycline
Fluorouracil
Heroin
Hormone-replacement therapy
Ketoconazole
Menthol
Methaqualone
Minocycline
Phenolphthalein
Propranolol
Zidovudine

Black:
Amiodiaquine

Betel nut
Methyldopa

Green:
Copper

Grey:
Amiodiaquine
Chloroquine
Fluoxetine
Hydroxychloroquinine
Lead
Silver
Tin/zinc

PEMPHIGUS VULGARIS

Ampicillin
Arsenic
Benzylpenicillin
Captopril
Cephadroxil
Cephalexin
Gold
Interferon-beta
Interleukin-2
Oxyphenbutazone
Penicillamine
Phenobarbitol
Phenylbutazone
Piroxicam
Probenecid
Procaine penicillin
Rifampicin

PEMPHIGOID-LIKE REACTIONS

Amoxycillin
Azapropazone
Clonidine
Frusemide
Ibuprofen
Isoniazid
Mefenamic acid
Nadolol
Penicillin V
Penicillamine
Phenacetin
Psoralens
Practolol
Salicylic acid derivatives
Suphasalazine

Sulphonamides

SALIVA COLOURED RED

Rifabutin
Rifampicin

SALIVARY GLAND PAIN

Bethanidine
Bretylium
Clonidine
Cytotoxics
Guanethidine
Methyldopa

SALIVARY GLAND SWELLING

Anti-thyroid agents
Chlorhexidine
Cimetidine
Clonidine
Ganglion-blocking agents
Insulin
Interferon
Iodides
Isoprenaline
Methyldopa
Nicardipine
Nifedipine
Nitrofurantoin
Oxyphenbutazone
Phenothiazines
Phenylbutazone
Ritodrine
Sulphonamides

SCALDED MOUTH SENSATION

Captopril

SJÖGREN'S SYNDROME

Hydralazine
Levamisole
Practolol
Procainamide
Sucralfate

TASTE DISTURBANCE

Anti-thyroids
Aurothiomalate
Aztreonam

Baclofen
Biguanides
Calcitonin
Captopril
Carbimazole
Cefacetril
Cilazapril
Clarithromycin
Enalapril
Ethionamide
Etidronate
Fosinopril
Gold
Griseofulvin
Guanoclor
Imipenem
Lincomycin
Lisinopril
Lithium
Metformin
Metronidazole
Nedocromil
Niridazole
Oxyfedrine
Penicillamine
Pentamidine
Perindopril
Phenindione
Propafenone
Prothionamide
Quinapril
Ramipril
Terbinafine
Thiouracil
Trandolapril
Zopiclone

TOOTH DISCOLORATION

Betel nut
Chlorhexidine
Fluoride
Iron
Mercury
Nitrofurantoin
Tetracyclines
Vitamin E

TRIGEMINAL PARAESTHESIA

Acetazolamide
Colistin

Ergotamine
Hydralazine
Isoniazid
Labetalol
Methysergide
Monoamine oxidase inhibitors
Nalidixic acid
Nitrofurantoin
Phenytoin
Propofol
Propranolol
Stilbamidine
Streptomycin
Sulphonylureas
Sulthiame
Tricyclic antidepressants
Trilostane

ULCERATION

Acetylsalicylic acid
Allopurinol
Aurothiomalate
Aztreonam
Carbamazepine
Cocaine
Cytotoxics
Diclofenac
Dideoxycytidine
Emepromium
Flunisolide
Gold
Indomethacin
Interleukin-2
Isoprenaline
Ketorolac
Molgramostim
Naproxen
Pancreatin
Penicillamine
Phenindione
Phenylbutazone
Phenytoin
Potassium chloride
Proguanil
Sulindac
Vancomycin

XEROSTOMIA

Alfuzosin
Amoxapine

Amiloride
Amitriptyline
Amphetamines
Antihistamines
Atropinics
Benzhexol
Benztropine
Biperiden
Buspirone
Chlormezanone
Chlorpromazine
Clomipramine
Clonidine
Cyclizine
Desipramine
Dexamphetamine
Diazepam
Dicyclomine
Dideoxyinosine
Disopyramide
Dothiepin
Doxepin
Ephedrine
Fenfluramine
Fluoxetine
Ganglion-blocking agents
Hyoscine
Imipramine
Indoramine
Interleukin-2
Iprindole
Isocarboxazid
Ketorolac
Ketotifen
L-Dopa
Lithium
Lofepramine
Lofexidine
Maprotiline
Mepenzolate
Methyldopa
Mianserine
Monoamine oxidase inhibitors
Morphine
Nabilone
Nefopam
Nortriptyline
Opiates
Orphenadrine
Oxitropium
Paraxetine

Contd

Phenelzine
Phenothiazine
Pipenzolate
Pirenzipine
Poldine
Pratropium

Procyclidine
Propafenone
Propantheline
Selegiline
Sertraline
Sucralfate

Tranylcypromine
Trazodone
Triamterene
Trimipramine
Tricyclic antidepressants
Viloxazine

2 INFECTIOUS AND PARASITIC DISEASES

TUBERCULOSIS

Tuberculosis is usually caused by *Mycobacterium tuberculosis*, although atypical mycobacteria may be implicated particularly in immunocompromised patients. Oral lesions of tuberculosis are rare. The most common is a painless, irregular ulcer of the dorsum of the tongue, secondary to pulmonary tuberculosis (**Figure 2.1**). Typically the edge of the ulcer is undermined. Tuberculosis can be spread by the respiratory route.

The most common form of skin tuberculosis is lupus vulgaris. Lesions appear most frequently on the head and neck (**Figure 2.2**), rarely intraorally. Lupus vulgaris begins as multiple red lesions, from their appearance called 'apple-jelly nodules'. The lesions ulcerate and scar (**Figure 2.3**).

Tuberculous cervical lymphadenitis (**Figure 2.4**) is uncommon but may be seen particularly in Asian patients and may be caused by *Mycobacterium tuberculosis* or *M. bovis*. The site of entry of the organism is usually the tonsils and, in some cases, *M. scrofulaceum*, *M. avium-intracellulare* or *M. kansasii* may be implicated. Tuberculous lymphadenitis caseates and discharges through multiple fistulae (scrofula), with scars on healing (**Figure 2.5**).

Haematogenous spread of tuberculosis is usually to vertebrae or long bones — rarely to the jaw (**Figure 2.6**).

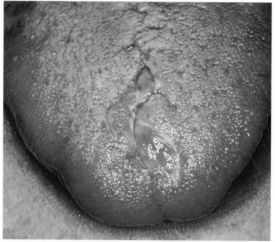

2.1

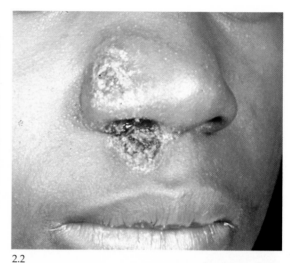

2.2

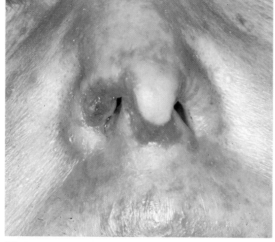

2.3

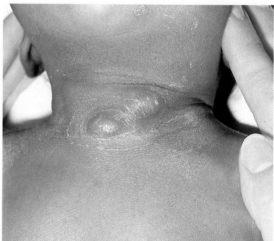

2.4

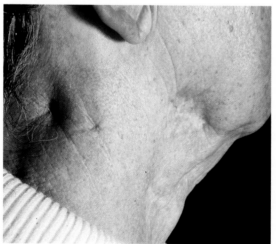

2.5

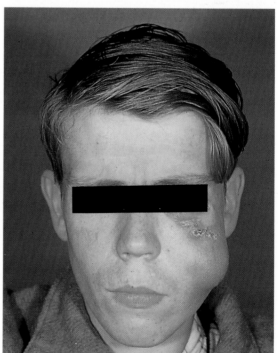

2.6

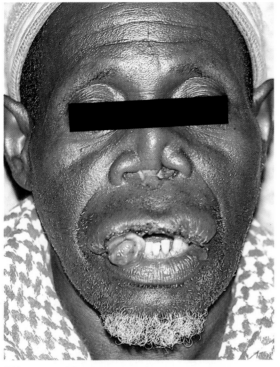

2.7

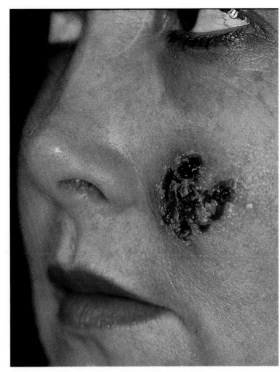

2.8

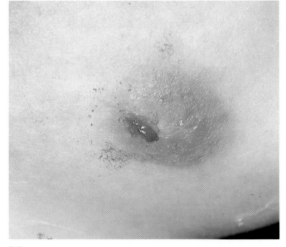

2.9

LEPROSY

Lepromatous leprosy, caused by *Mycobacterium leprae*, can produce widespread lesions, sometimes involving the mouth. Nodules can involve the lips or gingiva and elsewhere (**Figure 2.7**). The palate may necrose. The classic neural form of leprosy causes thickening of the greater auricular nerve and there may be cranial nerve lesions.

ANTHRAX

Cutaneous anthrax presents as a black eschar at the site of inoculation (malignant pustule) (**Figure 2.8**).

ACTINOMYCOSIS

Cervicofacial actinomycosis is more common than thoracic or abdominal actinomycosis. *Actinomyces israelii* is a common oral commensal but rarely causes disease. Trauma, such as jaw fracture or tooth extraction, appears to initiate infection, which usually presents on the skin of the upper neck, typically just below or over the angle of the mandible (**Figure 2.9**). The lesion appears as a purplish firm swelling that enlarges and may eventually discharge through multiple sinuses, although this classical presentation is now uncommon. Rare cases affect bone or salivary glands.

UVULITIS

Uvulitis is a rare, potentially serious, infection. *Haemophilus influenzae* type b, may cause uvulitis in isolation or associated with epiglottitis and/or bacteraemia. Group A streptococci may also cause uvulitis. The uvula is often more oedematous than shown here (**Figure 2.10**) and the airway may be threatened. There may be palatal petechiae.

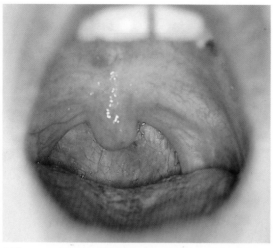

2.10

VACCINIA

Auto-inoculation of vaccinia virus from a vaccination site can produce single or multiple vaccinial lesions, with central scab and pronounced erythema and oedema (**Figure 2.11**).

Although vaccinia was extremely rare, it could affect the tongue or lip (**Figure 2.12**). Occasionally, in young children especially, vaccinial lesions were disseminated widely by auto-inoculation. Vaccination is no longer necessary, since smallpox has been eradicated.

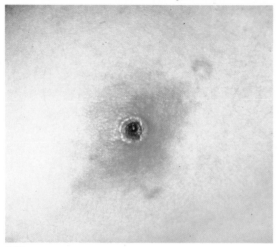

2.11

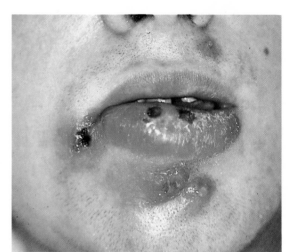

2.12

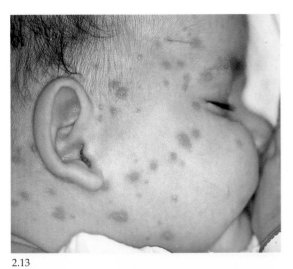

2.13

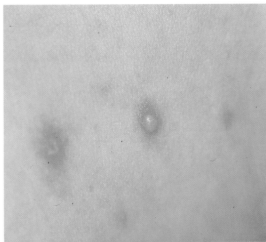

2.14

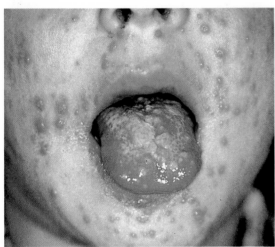

2.15

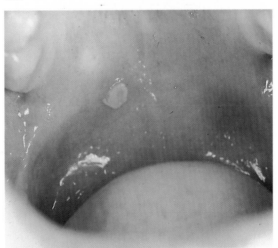

2.16

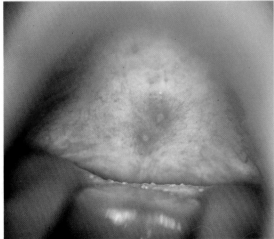

2.17

VARICELLA
(*Chickenpox*)

Varicella is a highly contagious infection caused by the varicella-zoster virus (VZV). After an incubation period of 2–3 weeks, a variably dense rash appears, concentrated mainly on the trunk and head and neck (**Figure 2.13**).

The typical rash goes through macular, papular, vesicular and pustular stages before crusting (**Figure 2.14**). The rash crops in waves over 2–4 days, so that lesions at different stages are typically seen (**Figure 2.15**).

The oral mucosa is commonly involved but there may be isolated lesions only. Vesicles appear, especially in the palate, and then rupture (**Figure 2.16**). Ruptured oral vesicles produce painful round or ovoid ulcers with an inflammatory halo (**Figure 2.17**).

HERPES ZOSTER
(*Shingles*)

Herpes zoster is caused by reactivation of VZV latent in dorsal root ganglia and, rarely, by reinfection. Zoster typically affects the elderly and those with cellular immune defects, especially HIV infection, and causes pain and a rash restricted to a dermatome (the mandibular division of the trigeminal nerve, in **Figure 2.18**). Healing is usually uneventful, but there may be bone necrosis, tooth loss or hypoplasia of developing teeth.

Ipsilateral oral ulceration in the distribution of the mandibular division of the trigeminal nerve is seen in **Figure 2.19** (same patient as **Figure 2.18**). Mandibular and maxillary zoster may simulate toothache — the pain may precede the rash.

Zoster of the maxillary division of the trigeminal nerve causes a rash and periorbital oedema but the eye is not involved (**Figure 2.20**). The rash of zoster resembles that of varicella and occasionally pocks are seen beyond the affected dermatome (note lesions on forehead). Occasionally, oral lesions appear in the absence of a rash. Ipsilateral oral ulceration in maxillary zoster involves the palate (**Figure 2.21**) and vestibule.

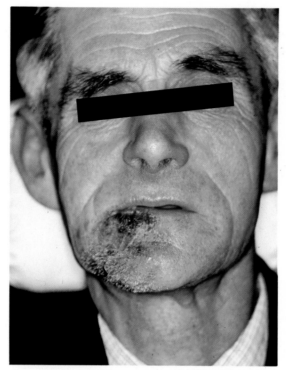

2.18

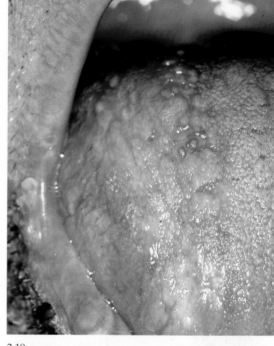

2.19

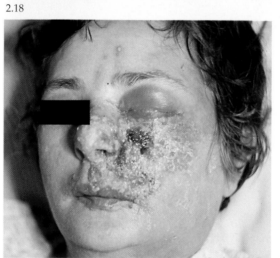

2.20

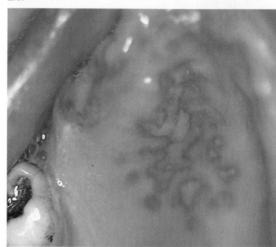

2.21

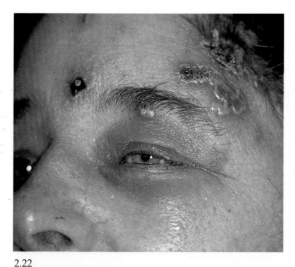

2.22

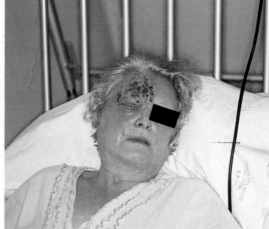

2.23

Zoster of the ophthalmic division of the trigeminal nerve (**Figure 2.22**) does threaten sight, with the possibility of corneal ulceration, or panophthalmitis. Ophthalmic zoster also produces chemosis and periorbital oedema which may become bilateral (**Figure 2.23**). Involvement of the central nervous system is common when zoster affects cranial nerves, and meningeal signs and symptoms are frequent.

Zoster more typically affects thoracic dermatomes (**Figure 2.24**). It has a bimodal distribution affecting a group of young adults who appear perfectly healthy otherwise, and also the elderly.

Occasionally, cervical dermatomes are affected (**Figure 2.25**).

(Contd)

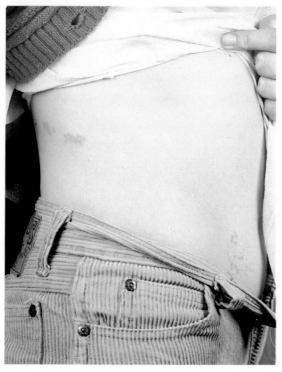

2.24

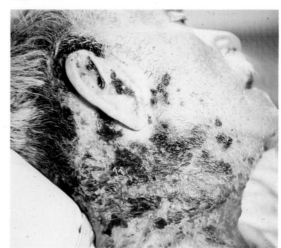

2.25

HERPES ZOSTER
(Contd)

There is an increased prevalence of zoster in persons with immunocompromised cellular immunity, including those with HIV infection (*see* **Figure 2.78**), malignancy, and following bone marrow transplants. This patient, with Hodgkin's lymphoma, has sciatic zoster (**Figure 2.26**). Radiotherapy and chemotherapy also reactivate VZV.

Zoster may leave sequelae such as scarring (here, **Figure 2.27**, from mandibular zoster), sometimes with pigmentation, and post-herpetic neuralgia. Tissue destruction and severe post-herpetic neuralgia are more common in those who are immunocompromised. Infection of zoster lesions with *Staphylococcus aureus* can lead to a form of impetigo with delayed healing, greater scarring of the zoster lesions and dissemination of the bacterial lesions.

ZOSTER
(Ramsay-Hunt syndrome)

Although zoster almost invariably affects sensory nerves, motor nerves may be involved occasionally. In Ramsay-Hunt syndrome, zoster of the geniculate ganglion of the facial nerve can cause ipsilateral lower motor neurone facial palsy (**Figure 2.28**) with ipsilateral pharyngeal ulceration.

A rash may be seen in the external ear, in the distribution of a sensory branch of the facial nerve (**Figure 2.29**).

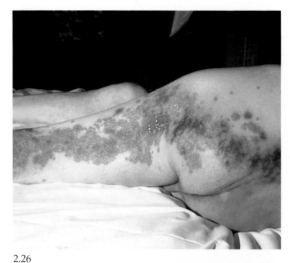

2.26

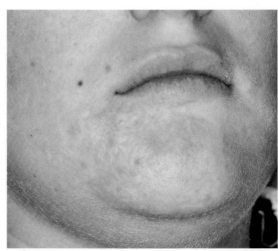

2.27

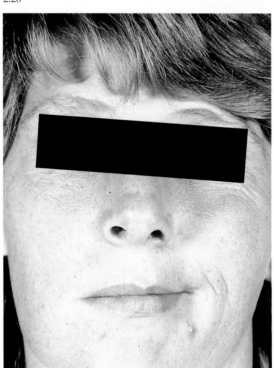

2.28

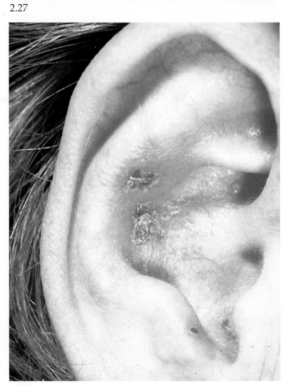

2.29

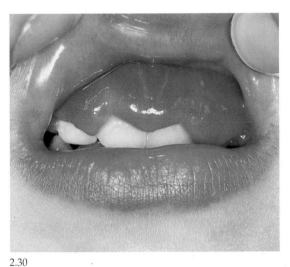

2.30

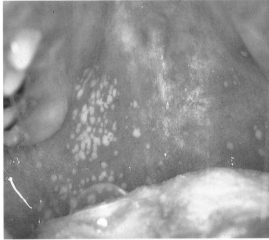

2.31

HERPES SIMPLEX INFECTIONS

After an incubation period of approximately 6–7 days, gingival oedema, erythema and ulceration (**Figure 2.30**) are prominent features of primary infection with herpes simplex virus (HSV), usually caused by HSV-1. Widespread vesicles break down to leave pin-point ulcers that enlarge and fuse to produce irregular painful oral ulcers (**Figure 2.31**).

Typically a childhood infection between ages 2–4 years, an increasing number of adults are now affected and HSV-2 is sometimes implicated in orofacial infection (**Figure 2.32**).

Affected patients, especially adults, can be severely ill, with malaise, fever and cervical lymph node enlargement. The tongue is often coated (**Figure 2.33**) and there is halitosis. Rarely, acute ulcerative gingivitis follows. Additionally, the saliva is heavily infected with HSV which may cause lip and skin lesions (**Figures 2.34** and **2.35**) and is a source for cross-infection.

Rare complications of HSV infection include encephalitis and mononeuropathies.

(Contd)

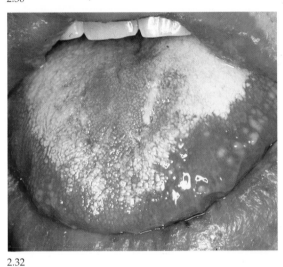

2.32

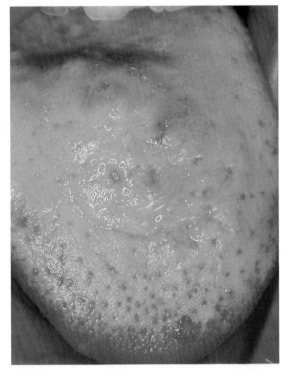

2.33

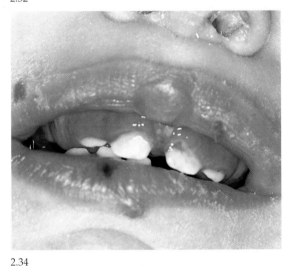

2.34

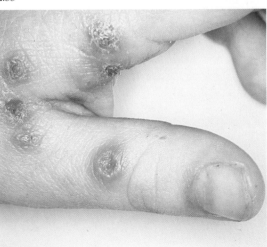

2.35

HERPES SIMPLEX INFECTIONS
(Contd)

Primary infection of the finger by HSV can cause a painful whitlow (**Figure 2.36**). This is an occupational hazard for non-immune dental, medical or paramedical personnel if they do not wear protective gloves.

RECURRENT HERPES SIMPLEX INFECTION

Reactivation of HSV latent in the trigeminal ganglion — for example, by fever, sunlight, trauma or immunosuppression — can produce herpes labialis (**Figure 2.37**). It presents as macules that rapidly become papular and vesicular, typically at the mucocutaneous junction of the lip. Lesions then become pustular, scab and heal without scarring (**Figures 2.38** and **2.39**).

Some 6–14 per cent of the population have recurrent HSV infections. Any mucocutaneous site can be affected, including the anterior nares (**Figure 2.40**). Occasionally infection can recur at sites other than mucocutaneous junctions and can simulate zoster (**Figure 2.41**). Similarly, impetigo can mimic (or complicate) herpes labialis.

(Contd)

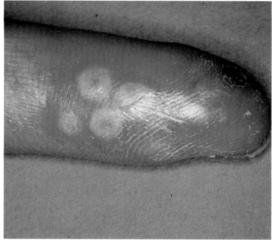

2.36

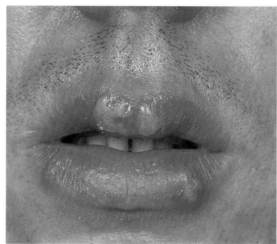

2.37

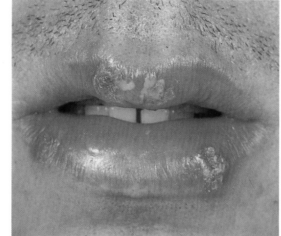

2.38

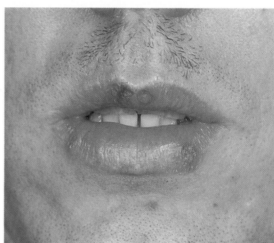

2.39

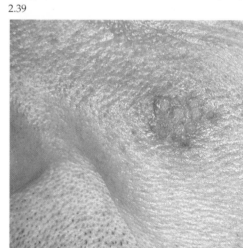

2.40

2.41

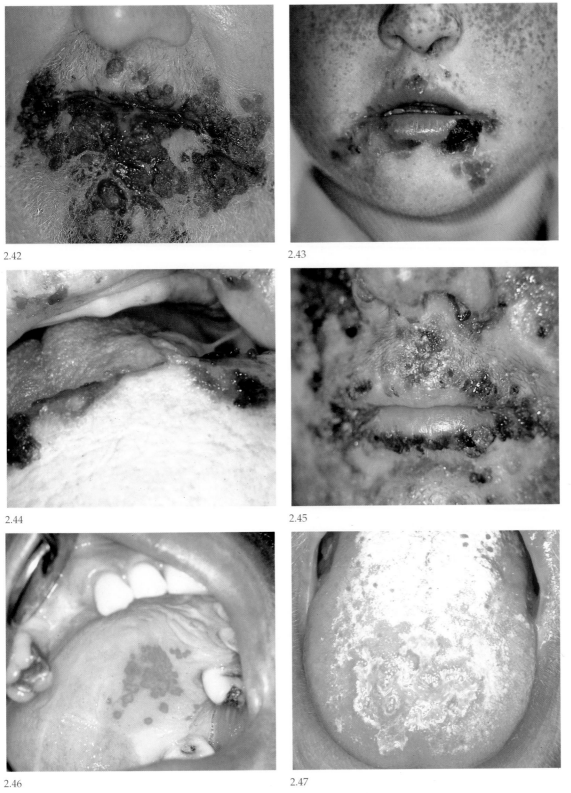

2.42

2.43

2.44

2.45

2.46

2.47

The lesions of herpes labialis eventually heal after crusting. Widespread lesions can affect debilitated patients, such as this man recovering from pneumonia (**Figure 2.42**).

Patients with T-cell immune defects are predisposed to recurrent herpes (**Figure 2.43**).

Haemorrhage into lesions produces a deceptive appearance in a leukaemic or other patient with thrombocytopenia (**Figure 2.44**).

ECZEMA HERPETICUM

Eczema, other diseases of the skin, and the use of topical corticosteroids predispose to disseminated herpetic lesions (eczema herpeticum, Kaposi's varicelliform eruption, **Figure 2.45**). Skin lesions in otherwise healthy patients are rare but a macular, vesicular or purpuric rash may be seen.

RECURRENT INTRAORAL HERPES

Herpes simplex infection due to reactivation of latent HSV is rare intraorally, but may follow the trauma of a local anaesthetic injection (**Figure 2.46**) or may be seen in immunocompromised patients. Recurrent intraoral herpes in normal patients tends to affect the tongue, hard palate or gingiva and heals within 1–2 weeks.

Immunocompromised patients may develop chronic, often dendritic, ulcers from HSV reactivation. Clinical diagnosis tends to underestimate the frequency of these lesions. So-called 'geometric herpetic stomatitis' may be seen in HIV disease or leukaemia (**Figure 2.47**).

MEASLES
(*Rubeola*)

Measles is an acute contagious infection with a paramyxovirus. The incubation of 7–10 days is followed by fever, rhinitis, cough, conjunctivitis (coryza) and then a red maculopapular rash (**Figure 2.48**). The rash appears initially on the forehead and behind the ears, and spreads over the whole body (**Figure 2.49**). It is less immediately obvious in a dark-skinned patient (**Figure 2.50**).

Mucosal lesions include conjunctivitis (**Figure 2.51**) and Koplik's spots — small, whitish, necrotic lesions, said to resemble grains of salt (**Figure 2.52**). These spots are found in the buccal mucosa and occasionally also in the conjunctiva or genitalia. They precede the rash by 1–2 days and are pathognomonic.

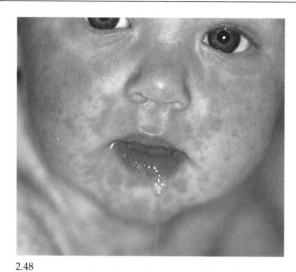

2.48

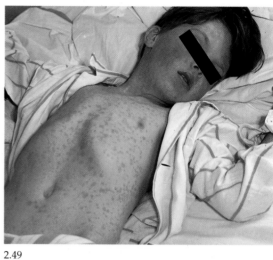

2.49

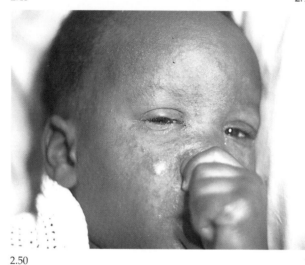

2.50

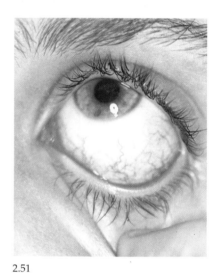

2.51

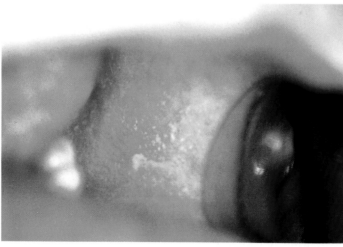

2.52

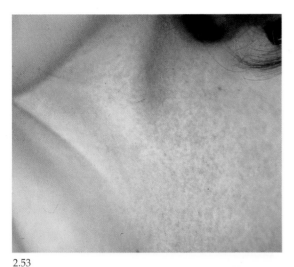

2.53

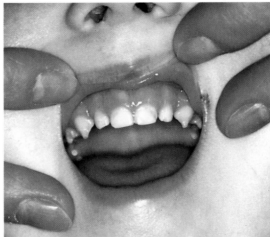

2.54

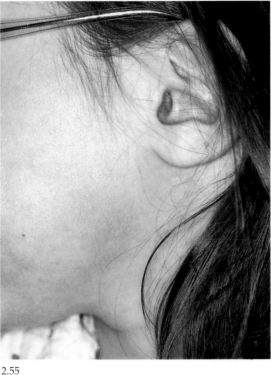

2.55

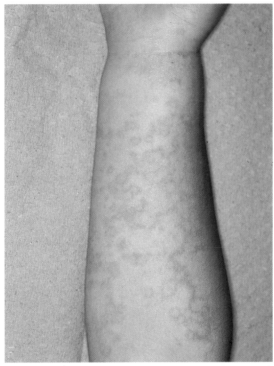

2.56

RUBELLA
(German measles)

Rubella is a togavirus infection with an incubation period of 2–3 weeks, followed by mild fever, mild conjunctivitis, a diffuse maculopapular rash (**Figure 2.53**) and lymphadenopathy. Some enteroviruses, especially echovirus type 9, may cause a similar rash. There are no specific oral manifestations but there may be oral petechiae, known as Forcheimer's spots.

Maternal infection during the first trimester of pregnancy may lead to congenital rubella, causing mental handicap, deafness, blindness and cardiac defects, depending on the timing of the intrauterine infection. Congenital rubella may cause hypoplasia of the deciduous dentition (**Figure 2.54**). Similar defects may be found in other intrauterine infections, such as toxoplasmosis, cytomegalovirus, herpes simplex and Coxsackie B.

PARVOVIRUS INFECTION

Parvovirus is a DNA virus that may cause an acute febrile illness (fifth disease or erythema infectiosum), with rash that produces a 'slapped cheek' appearance on the face (**Figure 2.55**).

Pharyngitis, conjunctivitis, lymph node enlargement, splenomegaly and polyarthritis may occasionally be seen, especially in adults. The exanthem typically evolves into a reticular configuration (**Figure 2.56**).

Parvovirus infection may occasionally precipitate aplastic crises, especially in those with sickle-cell anaemia.

74

HIV DISEASE

Infection with human immunodeficiency viruses (HIV) may cause an initial glandular fever-like illness, but may be asymptomatic. The incubation period (i.e. the time from infection to AIDS) may extend over ten or more years. **Oral candidosis**, especially thrush, is seen in over 90 per cent of HIV-infected patients (**Figure 2.57**). It is the most common oral feature of HIV disease and may be a predictor of other opportunistic infections and of oesophageal thrush. Extensive and chronic oral candidosis in HIV disease (**Figure 2.58**) may become resistant to fluconazole.

Other types of oral candidosis may be seen, including angular stomatitis (**Figure 2.59**). In healthy persons this is usually a local infection, emanating from a reservoir of *Candida* beneath an upper denture. Erythematous candidosis is another common feature seen especially in the palate (**Figure 2.60**). It may produce a thumb-print type pattern in the palate (**Figure 2.61**), and the red lesions of candidosis (**Figure 2.62**) may be overlooked by the uninitiated.

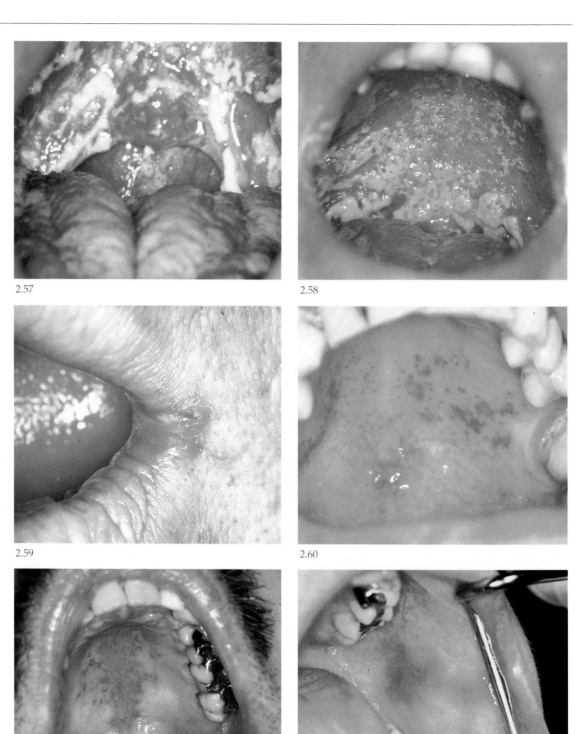

2.57

2.58

2.59

2.60

2.61

2.62

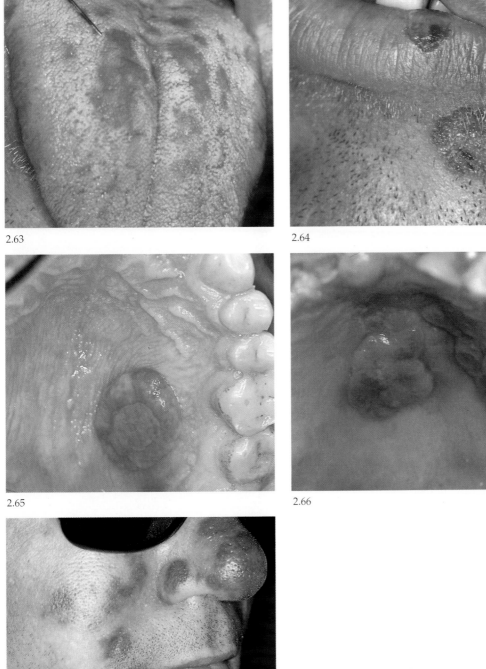

2.63

2.64

2.65

2.66

2.67

Erythematous candidosis on the tongue may be multifocal (**Figure 2.63**), or may simulate median rhomboid glossitis. Unusual infections or combinations of lesions may be seen in HIV disease, such as candidosis plus herpes labialis (**Figure 2.64**).

Kaposi's sarcoma is a late feature of infection with HIV, especially in male homosexuals with AIDS, but may be seen occasionally in other groups of immunocompromised patients (**Figure 2.65**). It may be caused by a novel herpesvirus. Oral lesions are macules or nodules, red to purple in colour, and most common in the palate. Multiple Kaposi's sarcomas are common (**Figure 2.66**).

Epithelioid angiomatosis, a bacterial infection, is the main differential diagnosis. Kaposi's sarcoma is not uncommon extraorally, especially on the nose (**Figure 2.67**).

(Contd)

HIV DISEASE
(Contd)

Hairy leukoplakia of the tongue is a common feature of HIV disease (**Figure 2.68**). This lesion is not known to be premalignant, but may be a predictor of bad prognosis. Flat white lesions may be seen on the tongue in about one-third of cases (**Figure 2.69**). Mild hairy leukoplakia may be overlooked by the tyro (**Figure 2.70**) and hairy leukoplakia is typically more corrugated than it is hairy (**Figure 2.71**).

Hairy leukoplakia is usually bilateral on the lateral margins and the ventrum of the tongue (**Figure 2.72**) and can simulate candidosis (**Figure 2.73**). It is usually associated with Epstein–Barr virus and may resolve with antivirals such as acyclovir.

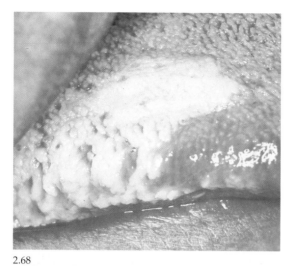

2.68

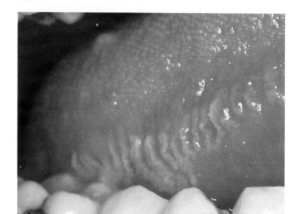

2.70

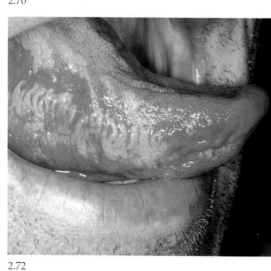

2.72

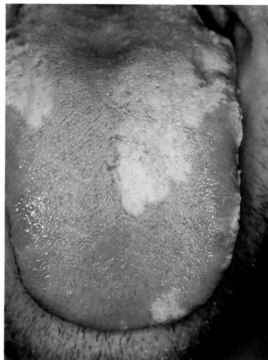

2.69

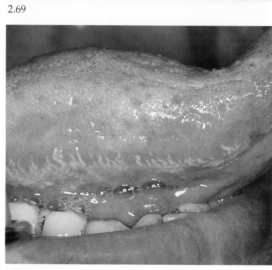

2.71

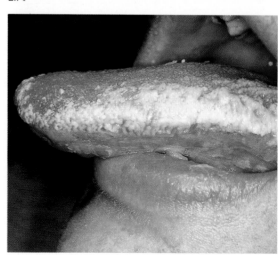

2.73

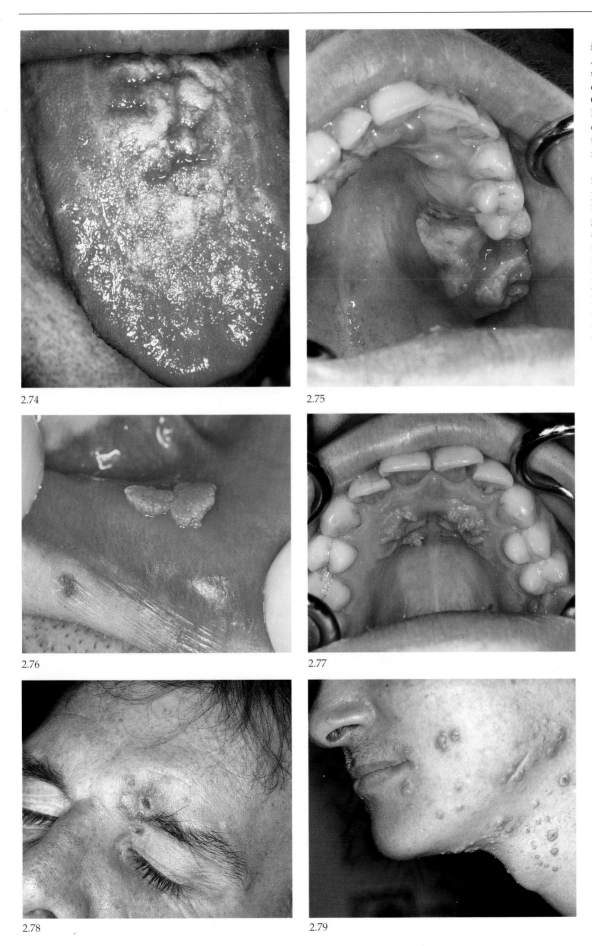

2.74

2.75

2.76

2.77

2.78

2.79

Recurrent herpes simplex infection may be intraoral in AIDS, often as a dendritic ulcer in the midline dorsum of the tongue (Figure 2.74). Chronic herpetic lesions in HIV disease (Figure 2.75) can occasionally become resistant to acyclovir, in which cases foscarnet may be required.

Other viral infections, including human papillomavirus (HPV) infections and, in particular, genital warts (condyloma acuminata) may also be seen in the mouth (Figure 2.76). It is interesting to note that the patient in Figure 2.76 additionally has a healing lesion of herpes labialis; multiple lesions are not uncommon in HIV disease. Types of papillomavirus which are uncommonly associated with oral lesions can cause oral lesions in HIV-infected persons (Figure 2.77) and VZV infection may supervene in AIDS (Figure 2.78). Molluscum contagiosum may complicate HIV disease (Figure 2.79).

(Contd)

HIV DISEASE
(Contd)

Ulcerative gingivitis (**Figure 2.80**) and destructive periodontitis may be features of HIV infection. The ulcerative or necrotizing gingivitis may be widespread and chronic (**Figure 2.81**), although localized necrotic periodontal lesions may arise (**Figure 2.82**). Periodontal necrosis may result not only from periodontitis, but also from viral or fungal infections, or Kaposi's sarcoma (**Figure 2.83**). Localized destructive periodontal lesions are not uncommon (**Figure 2.84**) and alveolar sequestration may follow (**Figure 2.85**).

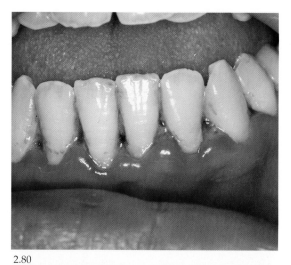

2.80

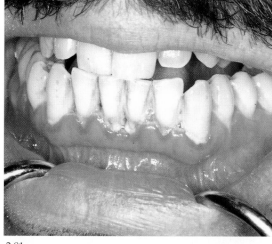

2.81

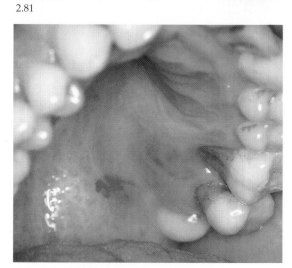

2.82

2.83

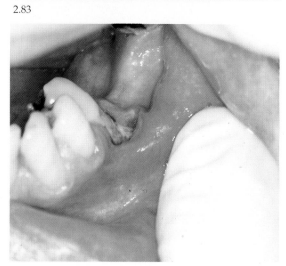

2.84

2.85

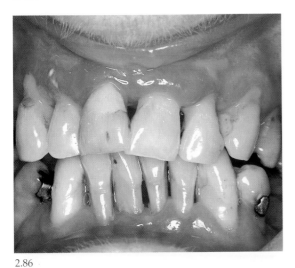

2.86

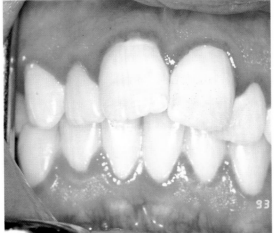

2.87

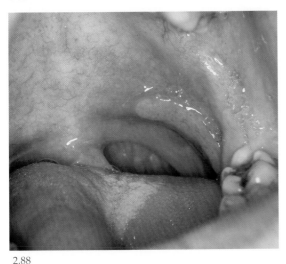

2.88

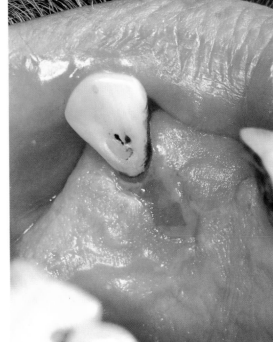

2.89

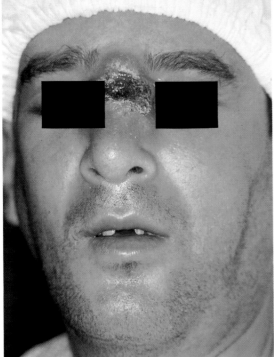

2.90

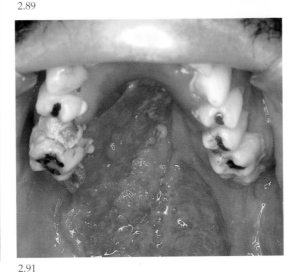

2.91

Occasionally, widespread rapidly destructive periodontitis may be seen (**Figure 2.86**). Finally, linear gingival erythema is sometimes seen in HIV disease (**Figure 2.87**), but necrotic lesions are more sinister.

Aphthous-type ulcers, especially of the major type (**Figure 2.88**) may appear in HIV disease. Mouth ulcers are also occasionally caused by opportunistic pathogens such as herpes viruses, cytomegalovirus (CMV), mycobacteria and rarely by *Histoplasma* or *Cryptococcus*.

In HIV disease, chronic oral ulcers associated with CMV infection are typically seen when the infection is disseminated (**Figure 2.89**).

Oral or cutaneous lesions of histoplasmosis are uncommon in many areas of the world, although histoplasmosis is an increasingly common systemic mycosis in AIDS patients. *Histoplasma capsulatum*, the causal organism, is found particularly in north eastern and central USA. It is found especially in bird and bat faeces and in the endemic areas, is a soil saprophyte. In these areas, over 70% of all adults appear to be infected, typically subclinically.

Clinical presentations include acute and chronic pulmonary, cutaneous, and disseminated histoplasmosis, the latter of which can affect the reticuloendothelial system, lungs, kidneys and gastrointestinal tract and is typically seen in HIV infection (**Figure 2.90**) and in other immunocompromised persons.

Oral lesions of *Histoplasma capsulatum* infection have recently been recorded in persons with pulmonary or disseminated histoplasmosis. The oral lesions are usually ulcerative or nodular (**Figure 2.91**), have been found on the tongue, palate, buccal mucosa or gingiva, and rarely have invaded the jaws.

(Contd)

80

HIV DISEASE
(Contd)

Other oral and perioral lesions in HIV infection include cervical lymph node enlargement, lymphomas (typically non-Hodgkin's lymphomas seen in the oropharynx or fauces (**Figure 2.92**)), salivary gland swelling (**Figure 2.93**) which may cause xerostomia (**Figure 2.94**), petechiae, cranial neuropathies and parotitis — possibly caused by CMV. Lichenoid lesions may be seen in the buccal mucosa (**Figure 2.95** — note that the palatal lesions in this patient are candidosis).

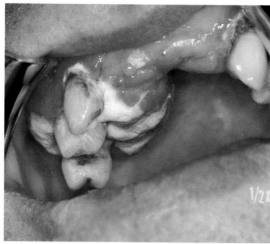

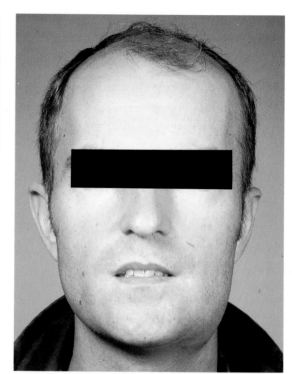

2.92

2.93

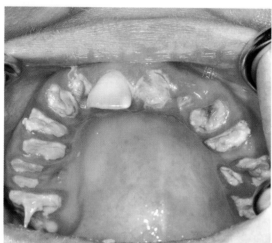

2.94

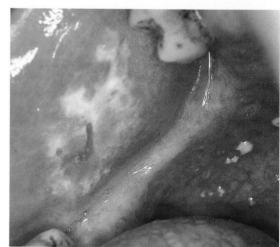

2.95

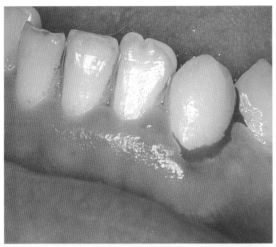

2.96

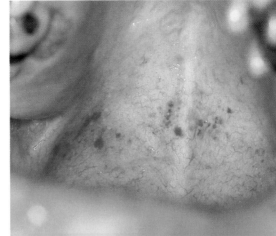

2.97

Spontaneous oral bleeding is sometimes seen in HIV infection (**Figure 2.96**). This may result from the thrombocytopenia which can also cause petechiae (**Figure 2.97**). Oral hyper-pigmentation may also be seen and this may arise from several causes, especially as a drug side-effect (e.g. clofazimine or zidovudine) or as a consequence of adrenocortical damage (**Figure 2.98**). Necrotizing stomatitis (**Figure 2.99**) can be a complication, and syphilis may present atypically (**Figure 2.100**). Finally, osteomyelitis and other severe oral infections may supervene in AIDS (**Figure 2.101**) and intrauterine infection with HIV may rarely cause facial dysmorphogenesis and a fetal AIDS syndrome.

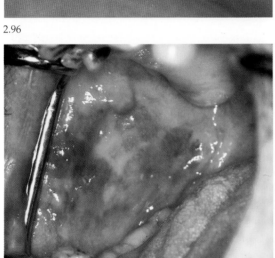

2.98

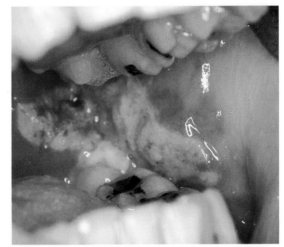

2.99

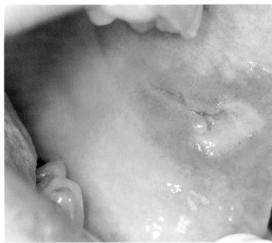

2.100

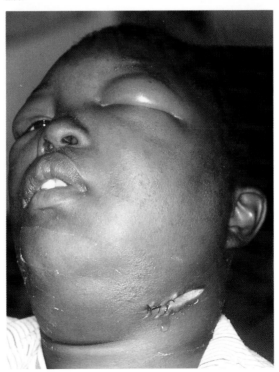

2.101

MUMPS

Mumps is an acute viral infection that predominantly affects the major salivary glands. The parotid glands are usually affected and there is tender swelling with trismus. This may be unilateral (**Figure 2.102**), but is more frequently bilateral. The usual causal agent is a paramyxovirus but some Coxsackie, echo-, and other viruses occasionally cause similar features.

The incubation period of 2–3 weeks is followed by fever, malaise and sialadenitis, which can affect not only the parotids but also the submandibular glands (**Figure 2.103**). Pancreatitis, oöphoritis and orchitis are less common features.

The most obvious intraoral feature of mumps is swelling and redness at the duct orifice of the affected gland (papillitis) (**Figure 2.104**).

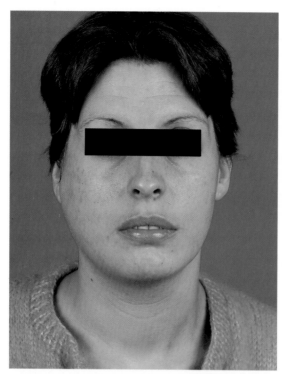

2.102

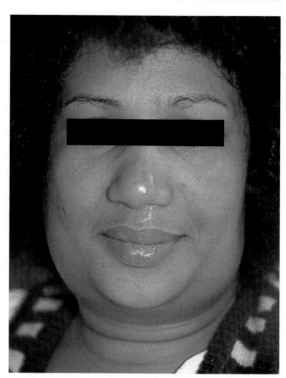

2.103

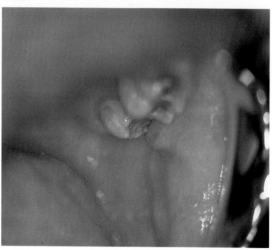

2.104

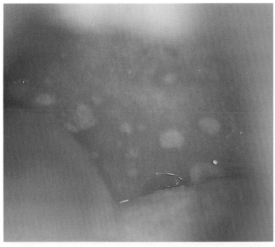

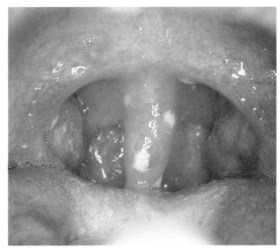

HERPANGINA

Herpangina, a Coxsackie virus infection, presents with fever, malaise, headache, and a sore throat caused by an ulcerating vesicular eruption in the oropharynx (**Figure 2.105**).

The vesicles rupture to leave painful, shallow, round ulcers, mainly on the fauces and soft palate (**Figure 2.106**). Ulcers heal spontaneously in 7–10 days.

Herpangina is usually caused by Coxsackie viruses A1–A6, A8, A10, A12 or A22, but similar syndromes can be caused by other viruses, especially Coxsackie B and echoviruses (**Figure 2.107**).

Herpangina Zahorsky, caused by Coxsackie virus A4, particularly affects infants and small children. Most herpangina is seen in schoolchildren and their contacts.

Lesions resembling Koplik's spots may be seen in echovirus 9 infections, along with a rash and aseptic meningitis. Faucial ulcers, sometimes with a rash and aseptic meningitis, are characteristics of echovirus 16 infection.

2.105

2.106

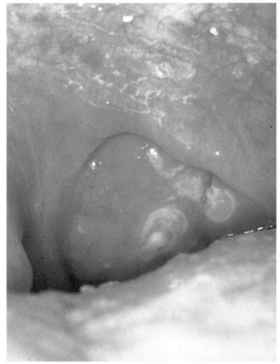

2.107

HAND, FOOT AND MOUTH DISEASE (*Vesicular stomatitis with exanthem*)

This Coxsackie virus infection produces small painful vesicles surrounded by an inflammatory halo especially on the dorsum and lateral aspect of the fingers and toes (**Figures 2.108** and **2.109**). The infection has an incubation period of up to a week. Coxsackie virus A16 is usually implicated, but A5, A7, A9 and A10 or viruses of the B9 group or other enteroviruses may be responsible.

A rash is not always present or may affect more proximal parts of the limbs or buttocks. The vesicles usually heal spontaneously in about 1 week. Reports of other systemic manifestations such as encephalitis are very rare, except in enterovirus 71 infection.

The oral lesions in this condition are non-specific, usually affecting the tongue or buccal mucosa. Ulcers are shallow, painful and very small, surrounded by an inflammatory halo (**Figure 2.110**).

LYMPHONODULAR PHARYNGITIS

Lymphonodular pharyngitis is an acute Coxsackie virus infection associated with strain A10. Similar to herpangina, lymphonodular pharyngitis presents with fever and multiple small (2–5 mm) yellowish papules on the soft palate and oropharynx (**Figure 2.111**).

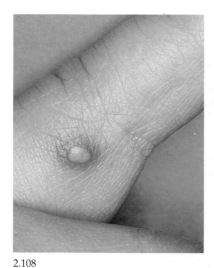

2.108

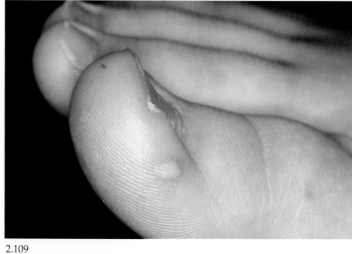

2.109

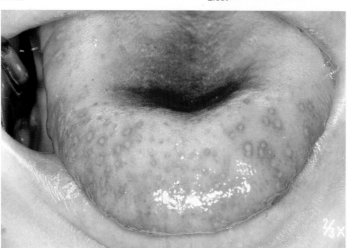

2.110

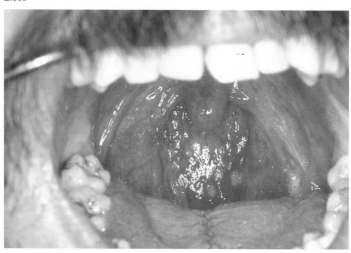

2.111

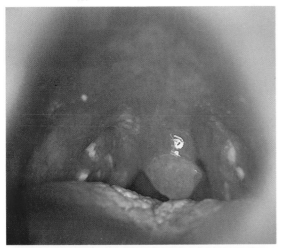

2.112

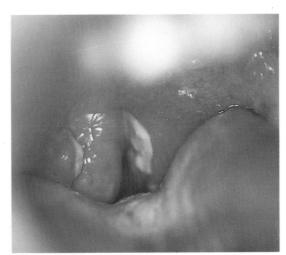

2.113

INFECTIOUS MONONUCLEOSIS
(Paul–Bunnell positive glandular fever)

Infectious mononucleosis (IM) is caused by Epstein–Barr virus (EBV). More common in teenagers and young adults, the incubation of 30–50 days is followed by fever, sore throat and lymph node enlargement. Mouth ulcers may be seen together with faucial oedema and tonsillar exudate (**Figure 2.112**: the white lesion on the soft palate is candidosis).

The faucial oedema and a thick yellow to white tonsillar exudate are typical of IM (**Figure 2.113**) although diphtheria may also produce a tonsillar pseudomembrane. There can be severe dysphagia and on rare occasions the faucial oedema can obstruct the airway (**Figure 2.114**).

Palatal petechiae, especially at the junction of the hard and soft palate, are almost pathognomonic of IM, but can be seen in other infections such as HIV (**Figure 2.115**).

A rare presentation of IM is an isolated lower motor neurone facial palsy.

(Contd)

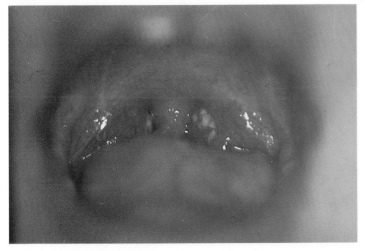

2.114

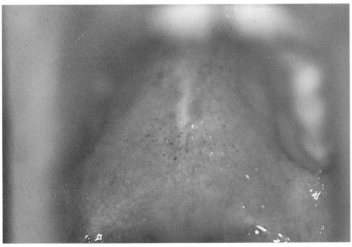

2.115

INFECTIOUS MONONUCLEOSIS
(Contd)

A glandular fever type of illness in young adults is still usually caused by IM. Generalized lymph node enlargement is present and the degree of cervical lymphadenopathy can be seen in **Figure 2.116**.

A feature that may suggest IM is the occurrence of a rash if the patient is given ampicillin or amoxycillin (this may also be seen in lymphoid leukaemias) (**Figure 2.117**). A few patients develop a maculopapular rash even if they are not taking synthetic penicillins. The rash is often morbilliform and does not represent penicillin allergy (**Figure 2.118**).

EBV may also cause persistent malaise, and has associations with Duncan's disease (X-linked lymphoproliferative syndrome), hairy leukoplakia (*see* page 76), and Burkitt's lymphoma and other neoplasms (*see* page 113).

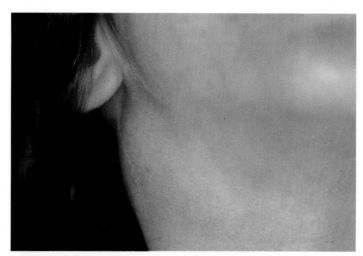

2.116

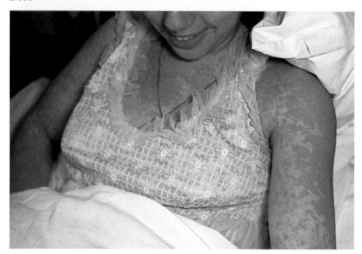

2.117

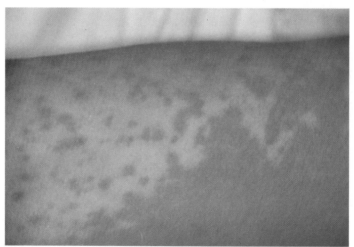

2.118

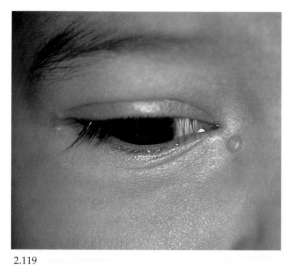

2.119

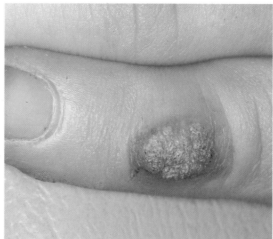

2.120

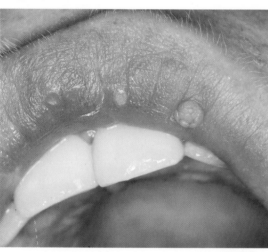

2.121

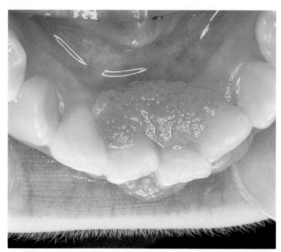

2.122

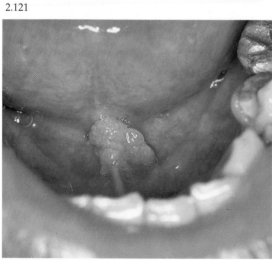

2.123

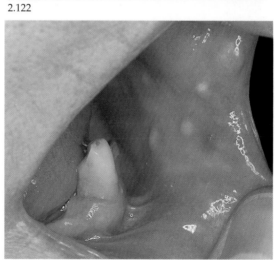

2.124

MOLLUSCUM CONTAGIOSUM

Molluscum contagiosum is a pox virus infection producing characteristic umbilicated non-tender papules, typically on the skin of male children (**Figure 2.119**; *see also* **Figure 2.79**). Oral lesions are very rare.

HUMAN PAPILLOMAVIRUS INFECTIONS

Human papillomavirus infections (HPV) cause verruca vulgaris (common wart) (**Figure 2.120**), condyloma acuminatum (genital wart) and papilloma.

Infection of the oral regions by contact spread can lead to warts, especially on the lips or tongue (**Figure 2.121**).

Papillomas are most common on the palate or gingiva. The cauliflower-like appearance is obvious but indistinguishable from a wart (**Figure 2.122**).

Condyloma acuminatum (genital wart) is caused by HPV. It usually results from orogenital or oroanal contact and appears as a cauliflower-like lump, mainly in the anterior mouth (**Figure 2.123**). The lesions are increasingly common, especially in sexually-active patients and as a complication of HIV disease (*see* **Figures 2.76** and **2.77**).

Focal epithelial hyperplasia (Heck's disease) is an HPV-13 or HPV-32 infection most frequent in Eskimos and North American Indians. Multiple painless, sessile, soft papules, generally whitish in colour, are found, usually in the buccal or lower labial mucosa (**Figure 2.124**).

CONGENITAL SYPHILIS

Congenital syphilis is rare. *Treponema pallidum*, the causal bacterium of this sexually-transmitted disease, crosses the placenta only after the fifth month and can then produce dental defects, typically Hutchinson's incisors (**Figure 2.125**). The teeth have a barrel-shape, often with a notched incisal edge. The molars may be hypoplastic (Moon's molars or mulberry molars (**Figures 2.126** and **2.127**). Dysplastic permanent incisors, along with nerve deafness and interstitial keratitis, are combined in Hutchinson's triad.

Other stigmata include scarring at the commissures (rhagades or Parrot's furrows), high-arched palate and a saddle-shaped nose (**Figure 2.128**). Frontal and parietal bossing (nodular focal osteoperiostitis of the frontal and parietal bones called Parrot's nodes) may be seen, and mental handicap is common (**Figure 2.129**).

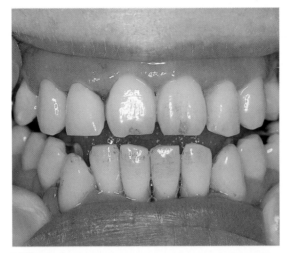

2.125

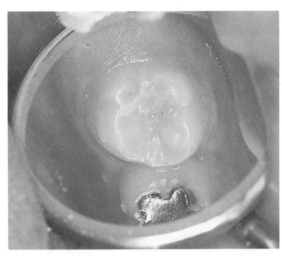

2.126

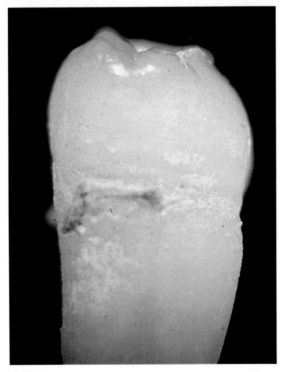

2.127

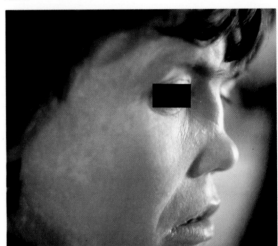

2.128

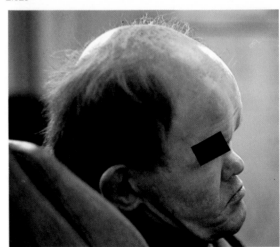

2.129

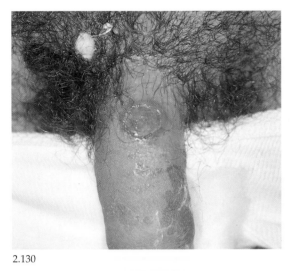

2.130

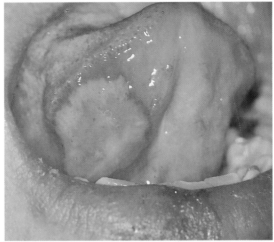

2.131

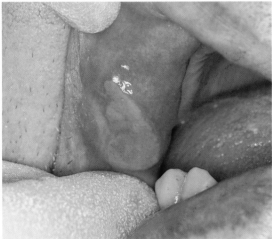

2.132

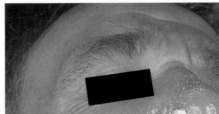
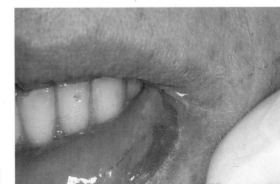

2.133

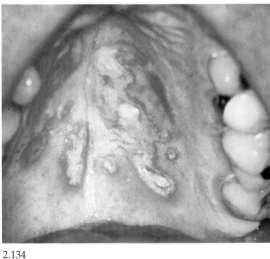

2.134

2.135

PRIMARY SYPHILIS

The incubation period of acquired syphilis is 10–90 days and the primary lesion (chancre) is usually seen in the anogenital region (**Figure 2.130**).

Oral chancres (hard or Hunterian chancre) begin as a papule which becomes a painless lump then a hard-based ulcer with regional lymph node enlargement (**Figures 2.131** and **2.132**). The chancre, which is usually on the lip, tongue or palate, heals in a few weeks but the patient remains infected and infectious

Occasionally, chancres appear on the nose or elsewhere (**Figure 2.133**).

SECONDARY SYPHILIS

Some 6–8 weeks after primary infection, the patient develops non-specific general symptoms, such as fever and malaise, with generalized lymph node enlargement. Rashes are common — typically a macular rash on the palms and soles — but are extremely variable. Papular rashes (papular syphilides) and maculopapular rashes may be seen. Flat, painless, oval or round patches (mucous patches) or ulcers (snailtrack ulcers) may appear in the mouth (**Figure 2.134**), or on the genital mucosae. Atypical lesions may be seen in HIV disease (*see* **Figure 2.100**).

Lesions at the commissure (split papules) are not uncommon in secondary syphilis (**Figure 2.135**). Oral lesions are highly infectious.

TERTIARY SYPHILIS

Tertiary or late, syphilis appears 4–8 years after infection and may cause mucocutaneous, cardiovascular and/or neurological disease (involvement of the cardiovascular or nervous system has been called quaternary syphilis). Meningovascular syphilis, general paresis and tabes dorsalis are the main syndromes of neurosyphilis. Bilateral ptosis (**Figure 2.136**) causes the typical compensatory wrinkled brow.

Another feature of tertiary syphilis is gumma, a painless nodule that undergoes necrosis, forming a punched-out ulcer that eventually heals with scarring. The site of predilection in the mouth is the hard palate, but lesions may affect the tongue or other sites (**Figure 2.137**). Any organ may be affected.

Atrophy of the papillae of the dorsum of the tongue produces, with endarteritis, an atrophic glossitis which leads to leukoplakia with a high premalignant potential (**Figure 2.138**).

Syphilitic osteitis is a rare complication of this stage of the disease (**Figure 2.139**).

LEISHMANIASIS (*Mucocutaneous leishmaniasis: espundia*)

The protozoa *Leishmania brasiliensis* is found mainly in South America. A sandfly bite transmits infection and this usually heals although, in some, there is later metastasis to the mucocutaneous junctions of the mouth or nose (**Figure 2.140**). The palate is frequently affected and ulcerates. Leishmaniasis may also be found around the Mediterranean (*L. donovani* or *L. tropica*). Chronic ulcers or swellings may be seen on the lips or face.

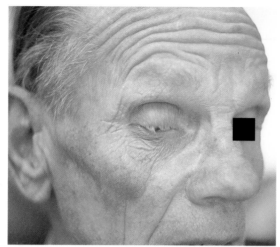

2.136

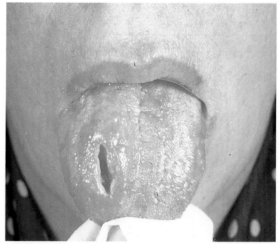

2.137

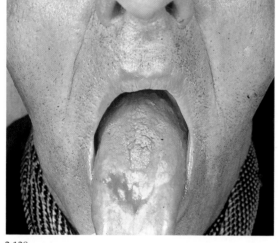

2.138

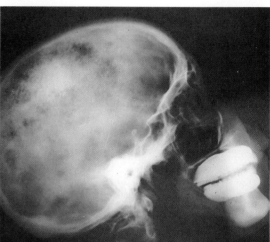

2.139

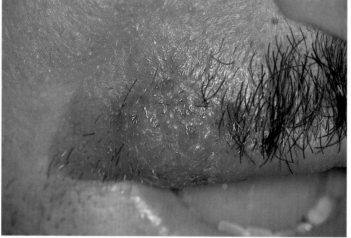

2.140

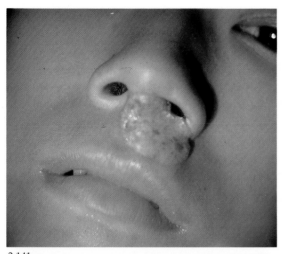

2.141

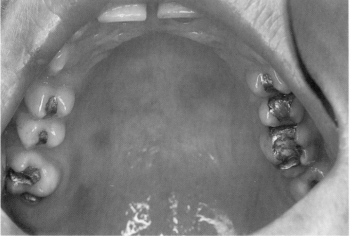

2.142

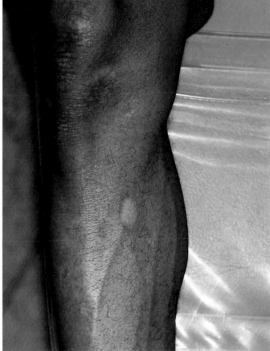

2.143

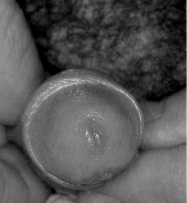

2.144

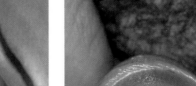

2.145

2.146

YAWS

Non-venereal syphilis, yaws and pinta (the 'endemic' treponematoses) follow a course not dissimilar from syphilis, with primary, secondary and tertiary stages. Yaws, caused by *Treponema pertenue* is seen predominantly in Equatorial regions. The primary lesion (mother yaw) is usually a single, painless papule that appears after 3–6 weeks and ulcerates (**Figure 2.141**).

After a secondary stage with lesions similar to the primary lesions, late lesions present as gummas (**Figure 2.142**), especially on the lower extremities.

The skin may heal with 'tissue paper' scarring and depigmentation (**Figures 2.143 and 2.144**).

REITER'S SYNDROME

Reiter's syndrome is a disease predominantly of young males and may follow gonorrhoea, chlamydial, HIV or enteric infection with *Salmonellae*, *Shigella*, or *Yersinia*. Features include urethritis, uveitis or conjunctivitis, polyarthritis, macular or vesicular lesions on the palms and soles (keratoderma blenorrhagica) and red lesions, sometimes with a whitish border or superficial painful erosions in the mouth (**Figure 2.145**). Rarely, the temporo-mandibular joint is involved in the polyarthritis. Facial palsy may also be seen on rare occasions.

Mucocutaneous lesions are found in up to half the patients but are typically painless initially. Urethritis (**Figure 2.146**) may follow mouth lesions and there may be circinate balanitis.

ACUTE NECROTIZING ULCERATIVE GINGIVITIS (*Vincent's disease*)

Chiefly affecting young adults, acute ulcerative gingivitis (acute necrotizing gingivitis, AUG, ANG, ANUG) is associated with proliferation of *Borrelia vincentii*, fusiform bacilli, and other anaerobes. Ulceration of the interdental papillae is the typical feature of this condition (**Figure 2.147**) which is predisposed by smoking, respiratory infections, poor oral hygiene and immune defects. HIV infection is now a recognized predisposing factor in some patients.

Painful gingival ulceration occasionally spreads from the papillae to the gingival margins (**Figure 2.148**), with sialorrhoea, halitosis and pronounced tendency to gingival bleeding. The gingival bleeding can be profuse and the patient may have malaise, low fever and regional lymph node enlargement. Occasional patients have primary herpetic stomatitis complicated by ANUG (**Figure 2.149**; note ulcer in upper vestibule).

CANCRUM ORIS (*Noma*)

Although usually a trivial illness in healthy persons, ANUG in malnourished, debilitated, or immunocompromised patients may extend onto the oral mucosa and skin with gangrenous necrosis (cancrum oris, noma) (**Figure 2.150**). Anaerobes, particularly *Bacteroides* species, have been implicated, and the condition is especially seen in malnourished patients from the developing world.

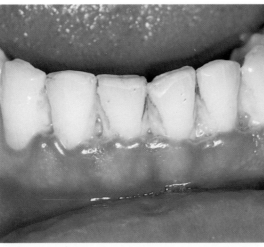

2.147

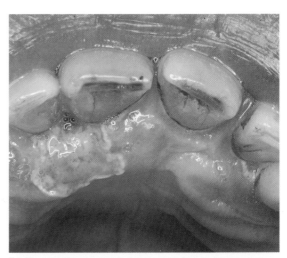

2.148

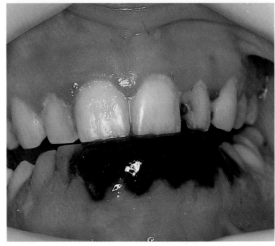

2.149

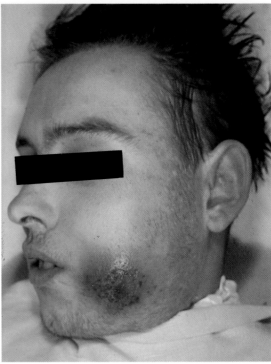

2.150

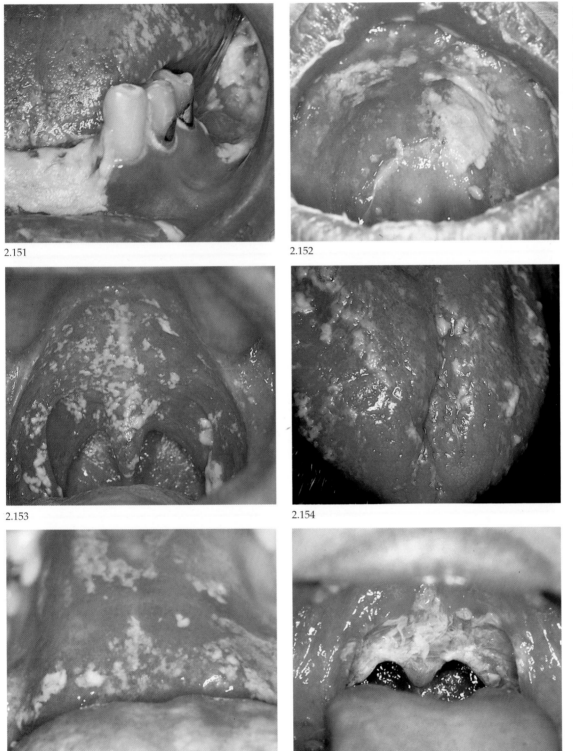

2.151

2.152

2.153

2.154

2.155

2.156

ACUTE CANDIDOSIS
(Thrush, candidiasis, acute pseudo-membranous candidosis, moniliasis)

Candida species are common oral commensals. *Candida albicans* is the most common and virulent species, which can act as an opportunistic pathogen, causing thrush (**Figure 2.151**).

Thrush appears as white flecks or plaques, which are easily removed with gauze to leave an erythematous base (**Figure 2.152**). Apart from neonates, who have no immunity to *Candida* species, thrush indicates an immunocompromised patient, or a local disturbance in oral flora, such as that caused by xerostomia, antibiotic treatment or corticosteroids.

Thrush can affect any oral site, typically the palate or upper buccal vestibule posteriorly (**Figure 2.153**). The yellow colour is caused by amphotericin. It is a feature in many immune defects, especially leukaemia (**Figure 2.154**), and particularly where there has also been radiotherapy affecting the mouth and salivary glands.

In severely immunocompromised patients, there may also be other fungal infections, such as *Aspergillus*, *Mucor* or *Trichosporon* species.

Thrush can be an early feature of HIV (**Figure 2.155**) or related disease. Orogenital and anogenital transmission of *Candida* is also possible.

Local causes of thrush should always be excluded: the use of corticosteroid inhalers may produce faucial and oropharyngeal thrush (**Figure 2.156**; *see also* **Figure 17.22**).

ACUTE ATROPHIC CANDIDOSIS (*Antibiotic sore tongue*)

Broad spectrum antimicrobials such as tetracycline or ampicillin, and corticosteroids, predispose to an acute atrophic candidosis that causes soreness or a burning sensation, especially of the tongue (**Figure 2.157**).

CHRONIC ATROPHIC CANDIDOSIS (*Denture-induced stomatitis*)

Chronic atrophic candidosis is common beneath complete upper dentures, especially in the elderly (**Figure 2.158**). Although termed denture sore mouth, it is usually asymptomatic. Characteristically the erythema is limited to the denture-bearing area (**Figure 2.159**). It is rare below lower dentures. Occasionally the lesion is complicated by the development of papillary hyperplasia (*see* page 216).

Patients with denture-induced stomatitis are usually otherwise healthy. The lesion is caused by *Candida* proliferating on the denture surface, especially when it is worn during sleep. Inadequate dentures predispose to the lesion in some patients.

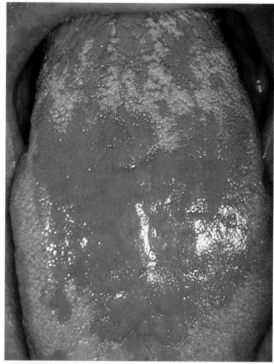

2.157

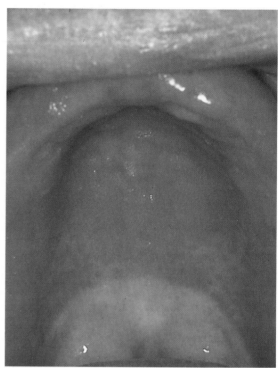

2.158

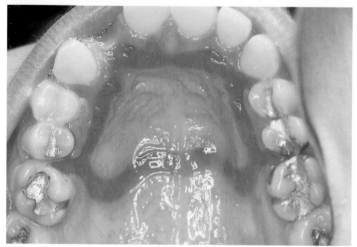

2.159

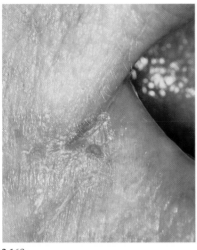

2.160

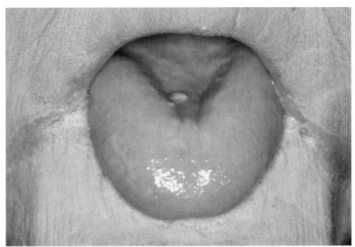

2.161

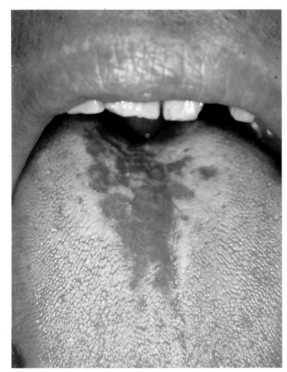

2.162

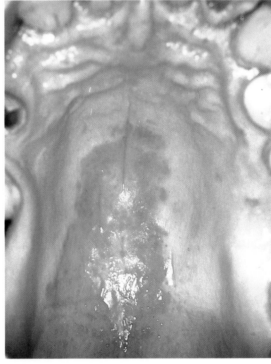

2.163

ANGULAR STOMATITIS (*Angular cheilitis, cheilosis, perleche*)

Denture-induced stomatitis may predispose to angular stomatitis, which is bilateral and produces erythema, fissuring or ulceration which can be painful and disfiguring (**Figure 2.160**; *see also* **Figures 5.1** and **5.2**).

Rarely, angular stomatitis is a manifestation of iron deficiency (**Figure 2.161**), or of vitamin deficiency — when there may also be glossitis and mouth ulcers, or of an immune defect (*see* **Figure 2.59**). Although *Candida albicans* is the prevalent organism, *Staphylococcus aureus* and other microorganisms may sometimes be isolated.

MEDIAN RHOMBOID GLOSSITIS

Median rhomboid glossitis, although originally thought to be a developmental lesion, is rarely seen in children and may be chronic focal candidosis (**Figure 2.162**). It is a fairly common lesion and predisposed by diabetes, cigarette smoking, the wearing of dentures and HIV infection. (*See also* pages 223 and 308.)

MULTIFOCAL CHRONIC CANDIDOSIS

Focal chronic candidosis may occur in apposition to the tongue lesion — the 'kissing lesion' (**Figure 2.163**).

Multifocal chronic candidosis may appear as red, white or mixed lesions and is usually seen in smokers.

CANDIDAL LEUKOPLAKIA

Chronic hyperplastic candidosis, or candidal leukoplakia, is a firm white adherent plaque, usually seen inside the commissures (**Figure 2.164**), or on the tongue. These leukoplakias have a higher premalignant potential than many forms of keratosis.

Candidal leukoplakia may be a speckled red and white lesion (**Figure 2.165**). HIV infection or deficiencies of haematinics may underlie chronic candidosis.

CHRONIC MUCOCUTANEOUS CANDIDOSIS

Chronic mucocutaneous candidosis (CMC) is a heterogeneous group of syndromes characterized by recurrent or persistent cutaneous, oral and other mucosal candidosis, usually from early life. Early lesions are of thrush, as here (**Figure 2.166**) in one variant (candidosis-endocrinopathy syndrome: Wells' type 3 CMC) that also includes hypoparathyroidism (note dental defects) and often hypo-adrenocorticism, hypothyroidism and diabetes mellitus. *Candida albicans* is the usual cause of candidosis but *C. tropicalis*, *C. parapsilosis*, *C. guilliermondii* and *C. krusei* may also be implicated.

Enamel hypoplasia may also be seen in CMC (**Figure 2.167**). This shows the same patient as in **Figure 2.166**, at a later age.

(Contd)

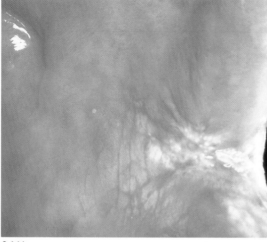

2.164

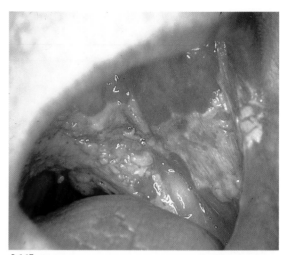

2.165

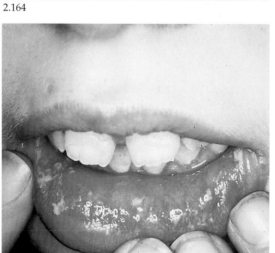

2.166

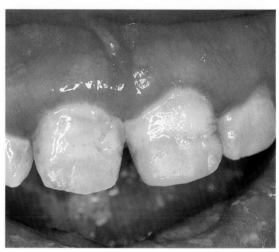

2.167

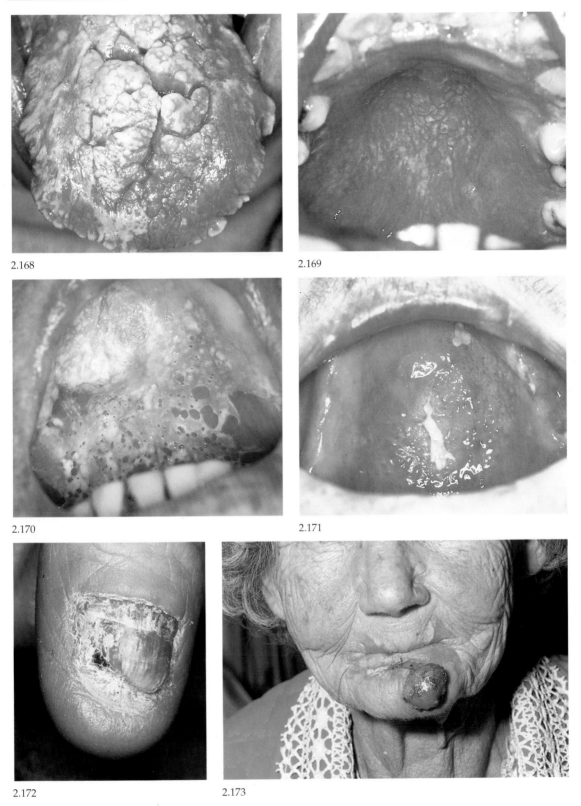

2.168

2.169

2.170

2.171

2.172

2.173

The white plaques eventually become widespread, thick and adherent, and the tongue fissured (**Figure 2.168**). The CMC extends over the palate and into the oropharynx (**Figures 2.169** and **2.170**). Chronic oral candidosis is often associated with malignant thymoma in this type (Good's syndrome). Antifungal treatment is at least transiently effective (**Figure 2.171** is the same patient as that in **Figure 2.170**).

In CMC, the nails are usually involved, but both cutaneous and nail involvement vary in severity (**Figure 2.172**).

Granulomas may be seen in the diffuse variant of CMC (**Figure 2.173**). These patients also have chronic oral candidosis, and candidosis may affect the larynx and eyes. There can be a familial pattern and early onset of disease.

HISTOPLASMOSIS

Rare in Europe, oral histoplasmosis may be seen in immunocompromised patients. Oral lesions appear as mucosal nodules or non-specific indurated ulcers (**Figure 2.174**). There may be associated low-grade fever, lymphadenopathy and hepatosplenomegaly. (*See also* **Figures 2.90** and **2.91**.)

BLASTOMYCOSES

North American blastomycosis (Gilchrist's disease) is a rare fungal disease. Caused by *Blastomyces dermatitidis*, it affects mainly the lungs and skin. Nearly 25 per cent have oral or nasal lesions — usually an ulcer with a warty surface which may simulate a neoplasm (**Figure 2.175**).

The oral lesions of South American blastomycosis (paracoccidioidomycosis, Lutz's disease) are similar to those of the North American form of the fungal disease (**Figure 2.176**). The causal organism, *Paracoccidioides brasiliensis*, may enter the body through the lungs or periodontium and cause granulomatous or ulcerative lesions and lymphadenopathy.

MUCORMYCOSIS (*Phycomycosis: zygomycosis*)

Despite the fact that *Rhizopus*, *Mucor* and *Absidia* are fungi ubiquitous in decaying vegetation and some sugary foods, infection is rare and seen almost exclusively in immunocompromised patients. Nasal and paranasal sinus mucormycosis is seen in poorly-controlled diabetics, and in particular presents resembling sinusitis. However, it may invade orbit, frontal lobe, palate (**Figure 2.177**) and elsewhere.

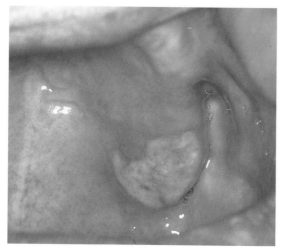

2.174

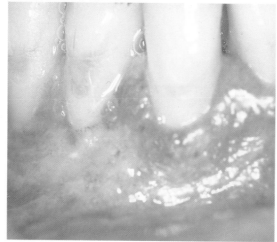

2.175

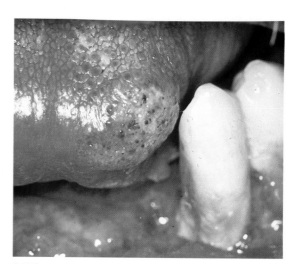

2.176

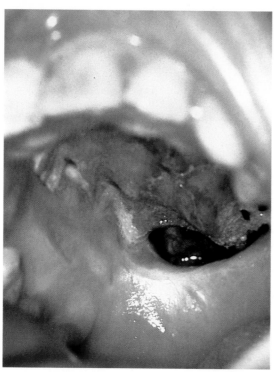

2.177

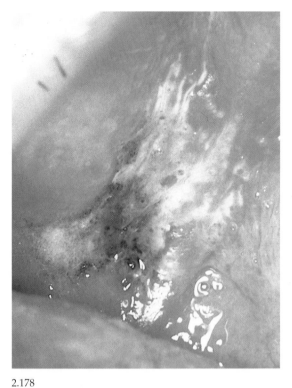

2.178

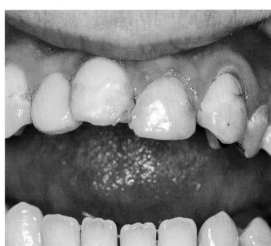

2.179

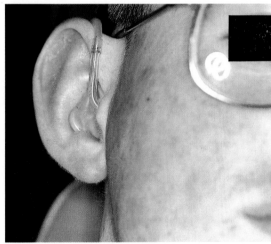

2.180

ASPERGILLOSIS

Infection with *Aspergillus* species, usually *Aspergillus fumigatus*, but also *A. flavus* and *A. niger*, can present in several ways. The most serious is systemic aspergillosis, or respiratory tract *Aspergillus* infection in immunocompromised patients. In *Aspergillus* sinusitis, there are normally non-invasive fungus balls, but infection of the antrum may rarely invade the palate (**Figure 2.178**), orbit or brain.

It has been reported that antral aspergillosis can be precipitated by overfilling maxillary root canals with endodontic material containing zinc oxide and paraformaldehyde.

TOXOPLASMOSIS

Toxoplasmosis is an infection by the protozoan *Toxoplasma gondii*, contracted mainly by the ingestion of the parasite from infected meat (especially pork) or material contaminated with cat faeces. *T. gondii* can also cross the placenta, and can be transmitted in blood, tissues or organs.

Lymphadenopathy is the most common manifestation of toxoplasmosis, typically being seen in the neck. Chorioretinitis is a serious manifestation. Immunocompromised persons are especially liable also to pneumonitis, myocarditis, pericarditis, hepatitis, polymyositis, or encephalitis or meningoencephalitis.

Congenital toxoplasmosis may cause intrauterine death, or severe foetal damage, and may present with enamel hypoplasia (**Figure 2.179**) and deafness (**Figure 2.180**).

MYIASIS

Myiasis (*Myia* means 'fly' in Greek) is the infestation of body tissues of animals by the larvae, commonly known as maggots, of two-winged flies — the Diptera. Oral myiasis has only rarely been reported in the English-language literature. Flies can affect a tooth-extraction site (**Figure 2.181**).

LARVA MIGRANS

Nematodes that are not normally parasitic to man often fail to develop fully if they infect humans, and may wander, causing one of several forms of 'larva migrans' before they die. The syndrome of *visceral* larva migrans is synonymous with toxocariasis — infection by larvae from roundworms of dogs, cats or wild carnivores. The syndrome of *cutaneous* larva migrans (creeping eruption) is caused by the larvae from hookworms of various animals, mainly dogs and cats.

Cutaneous larva migrans is characterized by itchy serpiginous tracks, affecting mainly the feet, hands or buttocks. It is common in tropical countries and in Central and South America. The nematode *Ancyclostoma brasiliense* is the main aetiological agent. Cutaneous larva migrans is now being seen increasingly in persons visiting the developing world.

Although common in the skin, larva migrans is rare in the mouth, with very few reports in the literature. As in the skin, the mouth infection probably mainly occurs by direct contact with contaminated sand, but ingestion of contaminated food may also be responsible.

Larva migrans in this patient involved the tongue, lips, cheeks, floor of the mouth, palate and oropharynx (**Figures 2.182** and **2.183**), but not the skin.

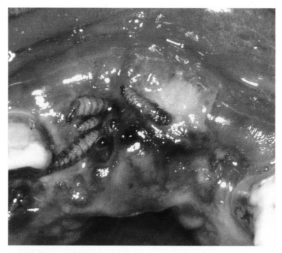

2.181

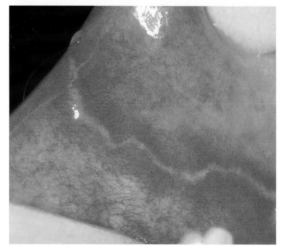

2.182

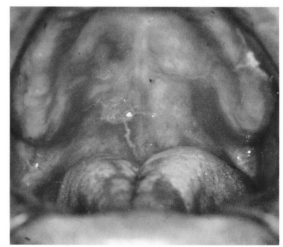

2.183

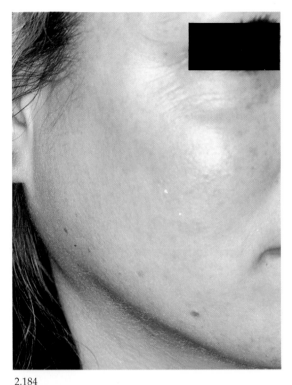

2.184

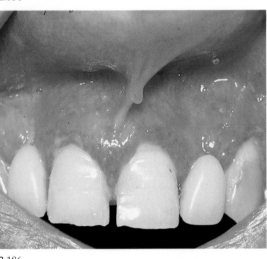

2.186

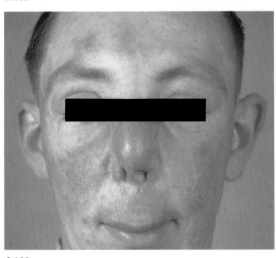

2.188

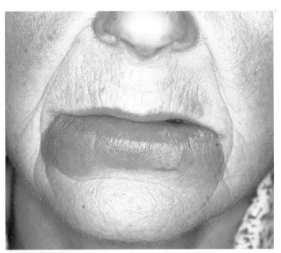

2.185

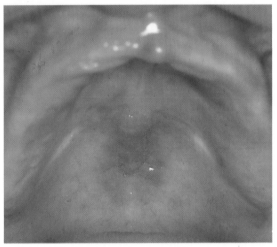

2.187

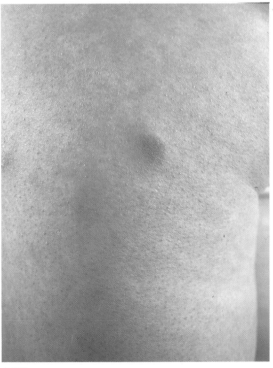

2.189

SARCOIDOSIS
(*Boeck's sarcoid*)

Sarcoidosis is a multi-system non-caseating granulomatous condition of unknown aetiology that affects mainly the lungs, lymph nodes and eyes but seldom produces oral lesions. Acute sarcoidosis usually manifests as hilar adenopathy with erythema nodosum (HAEN). The salivary glands may be affected (**Figure 2.184**) with firm, painless swelling and xerostomia and, rarely, with fever, uveitis, and facial palsy (Heerfordt's syndrome, uveoparotid fever).

Chronic swelling of the lip may be a feature of sarcoidosis (**Figure 2.185**) and difficult to differentiate from oral Crohn's disease and variants thereof, such as Melkersson–Rosenthal syndrome, orofacial granulomatosis and cheilitis granulomatosa.

Obvious oral lesions are uncommon but include red nodules which may affect any oral site, including the gingiva (**Figure 2.186**). The tongue is rarely involved but sarcoid may be seen in the palate (**Figure 2.187**). Palatal biopsy even from an apparently normal palate may show granulomas in sarcoidosis.

Lupus pernio (**Figure 2.188**) — large, persistent, red or violaceous infiltrations of the skin — is a typical feature of chronic sarcoidosis, and may be associated with pulmonary fibrosis.

Multiple small, purple–brown dermal macules, papules or nodules are common in early active sarcoidosis but may be transient (**Figure 2.189**). Arthropathy is a prominent early feature, associated with fever and erythema nodosum. Chronic periarticular swelling affects the fingers and toes especially and there may be bony changes.

Sarcoidosis may be rarely associated with primary biliary cirrhosis, Crohn's disease, coeliac disease or amyloidosis, and some patients develop lymphomas. It is as yet unclear which, if any, of these associations are true overlap syndromes.

ORF (*ecthyma contagiosum*)

Orf is a parapoxvirus infection of sheep which rarely affects those in contact. It starts as a small firm reddish papule that becomes umbilicated. Occasional cases affect the lip (**Figure 2.190**).

KAWASAKI DISEASE (mucocutaneous lymph node syndrome)

Of uncertain but probably infective origin, this condition can cause cardiac involvement together with lymphadenopathy, a 'strawberry' tongue cheilitis and desquamation of the palms and soles.

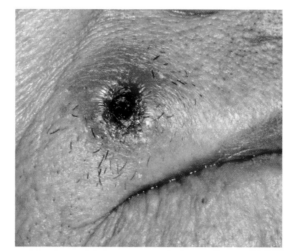

2.190

3 NEOPLASMS AND HAMARTOMAS

104

CARCINOMA OF LIP

Oral carcinoma accounts for less than 3 per cent of cancer deaths in Western countries but in some developing countries, particularly parts of India, oral cancer accounts for more than one third of admissions to cancer hospitals. Most oral malignant neoplasms are squamous cell carcinomas. Patients with carcinoma of the lip tend to present early and the prognosis is usually good. Oral carcinoma in this site is seen especially in male Caucasians living in sunny climes. Predisposing factors include chronic sun exposure, possibly smoking, and immunosuppression. The overall incidence is decreasing.

Early carcinoma presents with an asymptomatic red or white lesion, small indurated lump, or erosion with crusts developing (**Figures 3.1** and **3.2**).

Typically located at the mucocutaneous junction the neoplasm spreads within the vermilion and on to the skin (**Figure 3.3**).

In extreme examples, a deep ulcer with an irregular surface and rolled edges results (**Figure 3.4**). Metastasis is primarily to submental and submandibular lymph nodes.

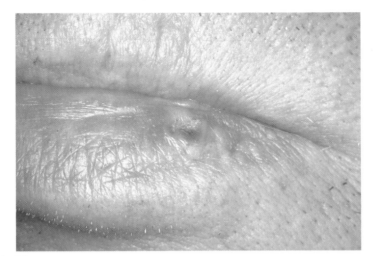

3.1

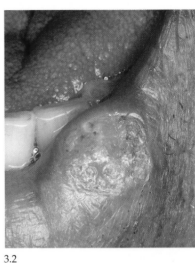

3.2

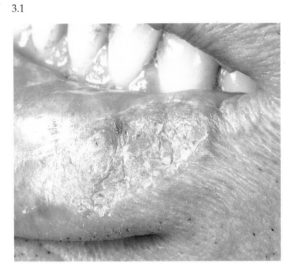

3.3

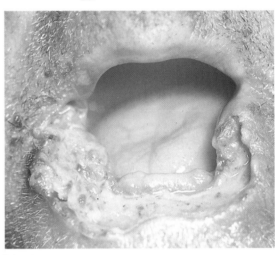

3.4

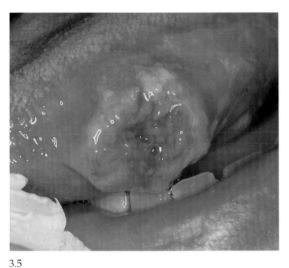

3.5

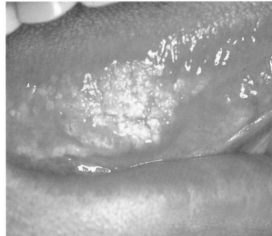

3.6

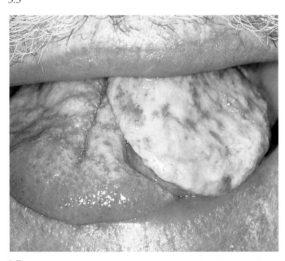

3.7

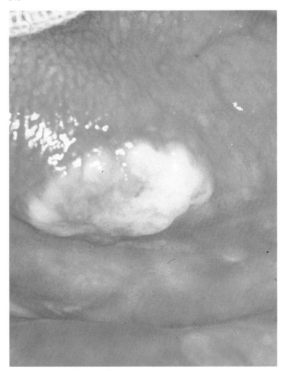

3.8

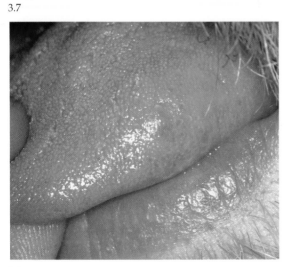

3.9

CARCINOMA OF TONGUE

The tongue is the most common intraoral site of carcinoma. Most tumours are on the lateral margin extending on to the ventrum (**Figure 3.5**). Tobacco or alcohol use and infections such as tertiary syphilis and chronic candidosis are predisposing factors. The incidence of tongue cancer is now increasing.

A lesion predominantly of elderly males, carcinoma presents as a red or white lesion, nodule, erosion or an ulcer (**Figure 3.6**). The lesion is indurated, usually sited on the posterolateral margin, and often associated with enlarged submandibular or jugulodigastric lymph nodes, sometimes bilaterally. The tumour tends to metastasize early and the patients present late.

On rare occasions the carcinoma is exophytic and extends on to the dorsum of the tongue (**Figure 3.7**).

Carcinoma may present as, or in, a white lesion (**Figure 3.8**). Leukoplakia of the floor of the mouth/ventrum of tongue may have a high premalignant potential — the so-called 'sublingual keratosis' (*see* page 212).

SARCOMA OF TONGUE

Apart from carcinoma, malignant oral soft tissue lesions are rare. They include melanoma, Kaposi's sarcoma, fibrosarcoma, malignant fibrous histiocytoma, alveolar soft part sarcoma (**Figure 3.9**), lymphoproliferative disorders, soft tissue metastases and others. In most malignant neoplasms, the clinical features are insufficiently specific to give a reliable diagnosis. Biopsy is invariably indicated.

106

CARCINOMA OF GINGIVA

Carcinoma of the gingiva is rare. It may present as a lump or as a more obvious vegetating mass (**Figure 3.10**).

Suspicious red lesions, white lesions, ulcers or mixed lesions (**Figure 3.11**), should be biopsied to exclude carcinoma. Tobacco-chewing predisposes to carcinoma of the gingiva, buccal mucosa and the floor of the mouth.

CARCINOMA OF ALVEOLAR RIDGE

Carcinoma of lower alveolus: the variation in the clinical appearance of carcinomas is illustrated in **Figures 3.12** to **3.15**. In **Figure 3.12**, there is an obvious malignant ulcer with rolled edges and a red base, within an area of keratosis. There is an association between carcinoma in the floor of the mouth and cirrhosis.

Figure 3.13 shows a vegetating mass extending from the lower alveolus on to the floor of the mouth.

Figure 3.14 is a carcinoma on the alveolus, but more aggressive in appearance and extending on to buccal mucosa.

Figure 3.15 is a carcinoma of the upper alveolus: the speckled appearance of the exophytic mass is a common finding in oral carcinoma. This is an oral squamous cell carcinoma but occasionally an antral carcinoma or lymphoma invades the alveolus or palate to present in a similar manner.

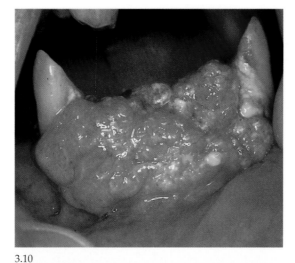

3.10

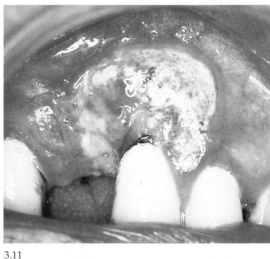

3.11

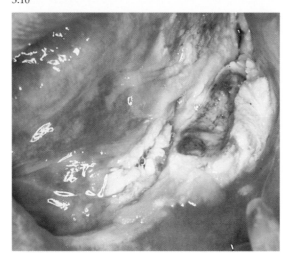

3.12

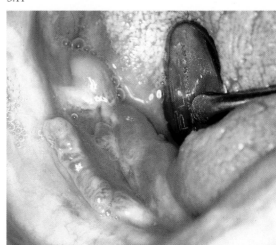

3.13

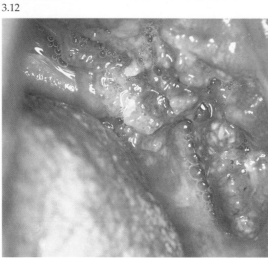

3.14

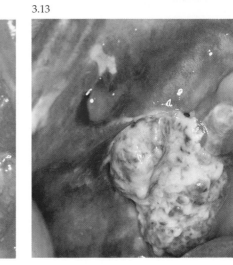

3.15

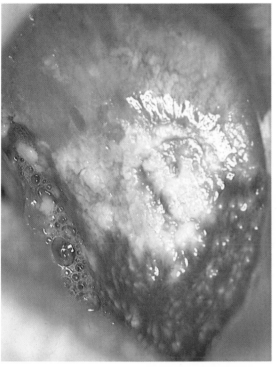

3.16

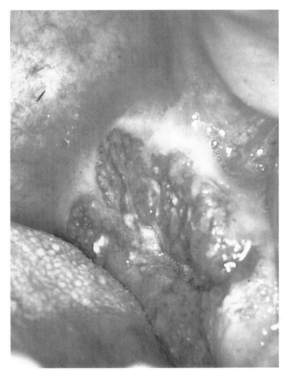

3.17

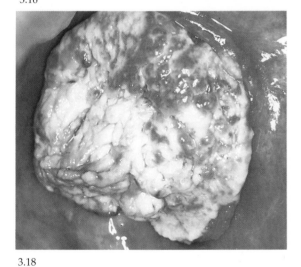

3.18

CARCINOMA OF BUCCAL MUCOSA

Habits such as snuff-taking or tobacco-chewing (including the use of smokeless tobacco) may predispose to buccal carcinoma.

The particular example shown in **Figure 3.16** is diffuse rather than exophytic and has red (erythroplasia) and white (leukoplakia) components. Erythroplasia is often highly dysplastic or malignant (*see* page 214).

An ulcerated exophytic malignant ulcer is shown in **Figure 3.17**. This is verrucous carcinoma, a variant of squamous cell carcinoma, which is predominantly exophytic, slow-growing, and of relatively good prognosis. Most common in elderly males, typically it affects the buccal mucosa and has a pebbly surface (**Figure 3.18**). A clinically similar condition, verrucous hyperplasia, is probably a variant.

CARCINOMA OF PALATE

Palatal carcinoma (**Figure 3.19**) is very rare in the West, but is fairly common in parts of the world where reverse cigarette smoking is practised.

CARCINOMA OF ANTRUM

Carcinoma of the maxillary antrum is a rare neoplasm, found especially in those who work with wood, for example, in the furniture industry, and in those who work in the shoe and boot industry. Snuff use also appears to predispose to antral carcinoma. Initially asymptomatic, antral carcinoma eventually invades the palate, nose or orbit. Antral carcinoma often presents clinically as a swelling in the palate or alveolus, usually in the premolar molar region. The swelling may ulcerate (**Figure 3.20**). Occipitomental radiography shows opacity and invasion with loss of the bony walls of the antrum (**Figure 3.21**).

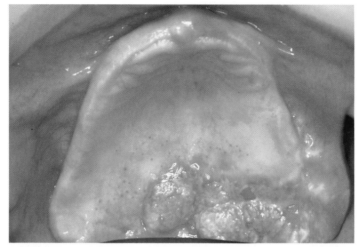

3.19

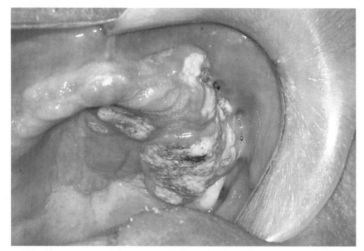

3.20

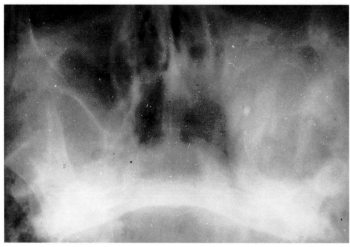

3.21

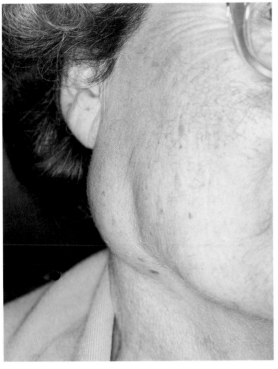

3.22

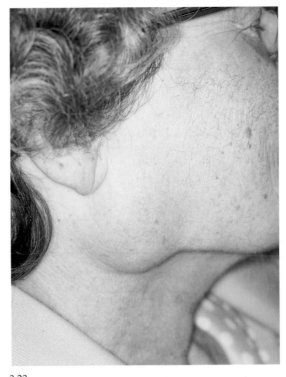

3.23

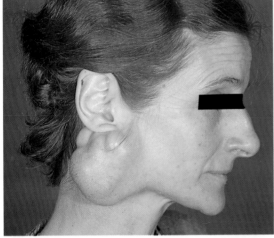

3.24

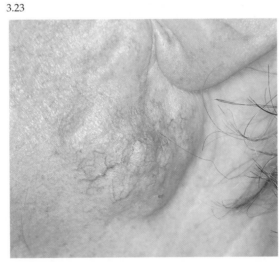

3.25

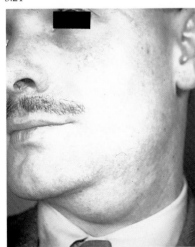

3.26

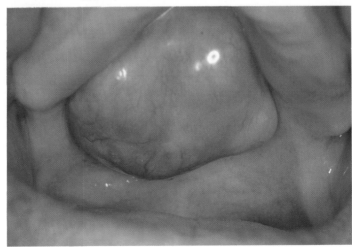

3.27

PLEOMORPHIC SALIVARY ADENOMA (*Mixed salivary tumour*)

Salivary gland neoplasms are uncommon and of unknown aetiology, although there is increased incidence in those exposed to atomic or therapeutic irradiation and possibly an association with breast carcinoma. The most common is pleomorphic salivary adenoma (PSA), a benign neoplasm which typically affects middle-aged or elderly persons. There is a slight female predominance and the neoplasm is found mainly in the parotid (**Figure 3.22**).

The majority of salivary neoplasms are benign, most are PSA and most affect the parotid. Swellings of the parotid gland typically appear behind and over the angle of mandible and evert the lobe of the ear (**Figure 3.23**).

PSA is usually painless and has no effect on the facial nerve, despite an often intimate relationship. PSA frequently has a lobulated surface and is slow-growing (**Figur 3.24**).

Malignant change, although uncommon, is suggested by pain, rapid growth, facial palsy, increased vasculature (**Figure 3.25**) or ulceration. Metastases are rare.

In some cases, the submandibular gland may be the site of PSA (**Figure 3.26**).

Intraoral salivary gland neoplasms are most common in the palate, usually in the region of the junction of the hard and soft palate (**Figure 3.27**).

(Contd)

PLEOMORPHIC SALIVARY ADENOMA

(Contd)

PSA is not only the most common neoplasm of major salivary glands but also of the minor salivary glands of the lip (**Figure 3.28**), palate and elsewhere. A nodule or sometimes a cystic mass, especially in the upper lip, should be considered as a salivary neoplasm until histologically proved otherwise (**Figure 3.29**, showing same patient as **Figure 3.28**).

Ulceration is uncommon in PSA, even where the lesion has impinged on a denture (**Figures 3.27** and **3.30**).

ADENOID CYSTIC CARCINOMA

Adenoid cystic carcinoma is the most common malignant neoplasm of minor salivary glands and is usually seen in the palate as a fairly slow-growing lump which eventually ulcerates (**Figure 3.31**). Nevertheless, it is invasive, especially perineurally, and has a poor prognosis.

MUCOEPIDERMOID TUMOUR

Neoplasms are rare in the sublingual gland (**Figure 3.32**), but are typically malignant, such as acinic cell tumour, mucoepidermoid tumour, adenoid cystic tumour, malignant PSA, or adenocarcinoma.

Mucoepidermoid tumour appears to be the most common malignant tumour of salivary glands induced by previous irradiation.

MONOMORPHIC SALIVARY ADENOMA

Monomorphic adenomas may occur intraorally (**Figure 3.33**).

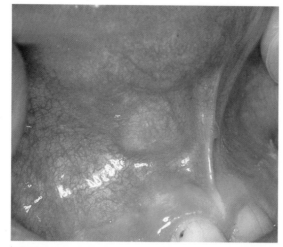

3.28

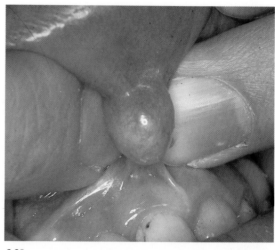

3.29

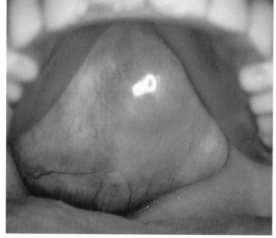

3.30

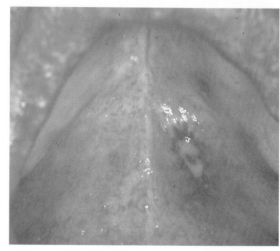

3.31

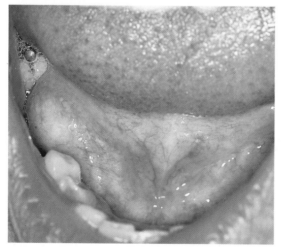

3.32

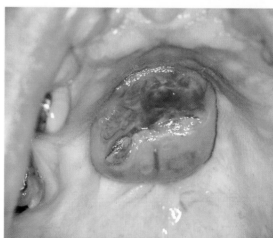

3.33

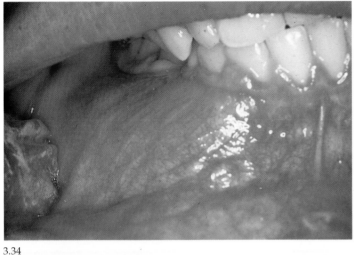

3.34

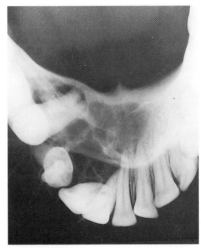

3.35

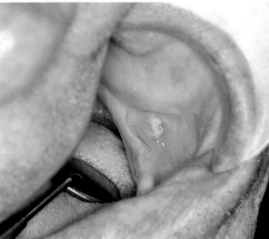

3.36

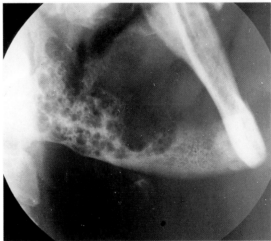

3.37

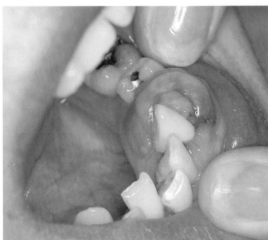

3.38

MYXOMA

Myxomas may have an odontogenic origin (odontogenic myxoma), usually affect the mandible, and are most commonly seen in young people (**Figure 3.34**). They are slow growing, but pain may be a feature.

Bony expansion with cortical destruction, displacement of teeth without root resorption, and a multilocular, or honeycomb appearance, are typical radiographic features (**Figure 3.35**).

AMELOBLASTOMA (*Adamantinoma*)

This locally invasive odontogenic tumour affects the mandible four times more frequently than the maxilla, and 75 per cent of mandibular lesions are at the angle. Although the lesion may appear at any age, it usually presents in middle age. It grows insidiously, and rarely causes neuropathy or mucosal breakdown. Ulceration (**Figure 3.36**) may be caused by trauma from a denture.

The plain radiographic appearance of ameloblastoma is generally of a cystic multilocular radiolucency (**Figure 3.37**). Bony expansion may be seen. A unilocular appearance is not uncommon, however.

ADENOMATOID ODONTOGENIC TUMOUR (*Adeno-ameloblastoma*)

This benign odontogenic tumour is more common in the maxillary canine region, although **Figure 3.38** shows a lesion in the mandible.

MALIGNANT MELANOMA

Primary oral melanoma is rare. It affects both sexes equally, is more common in coloured patients, and usually appears in or after middle age. Most arise in the palate and many are preceded by melanosis. Some vegetate profusely (**Figure 3.39**, a rather extreme example), others remain flattish and spread more deeply. Not all are pigmented. The prognosis is very poor.

It has recently been suggested that patients with melanoma may present with facial erythema.

METASTATIC NEOPLASMS

Blood-borne metastases are rare in the oral soft tissues and most are seen in the mandible, especially the angle and body. They virtually all present with pain or anaesthesia, expansion of the jaw, or loosening of the teeth. Metastases to the jaws are usually from carcinomas of the breast or bronchus, thyroid, kidney, colo-rectum, stomach, prostate or uterus. **Figure 3.40** was a metastatic carcinoma of the bronchus.

Metastatic lymphatic spread is a particular feature of carcinomas of the oral and perioral regions, and is a poor prognostic finding. The patient in **Figure 3.41** had a carcinoma of the tongue, and the cervical lymph node swelling was the presenting feature.

Rarely, metastases in cervical lymph nodes ulcerate the skin (**Figure 3.42**).

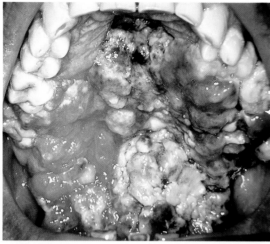

3.39

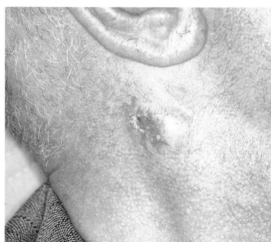

3.40

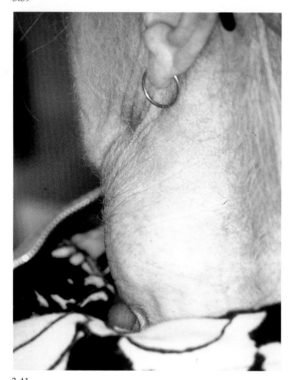

3.41

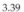

3.42

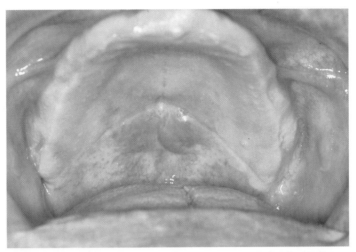

3.43

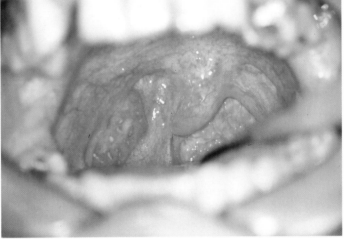

3.44

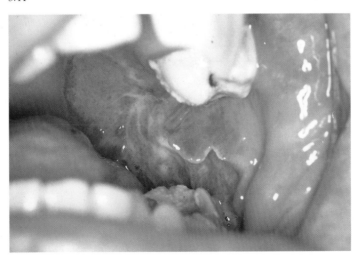

3.45

LYMPHOMAS

Lymphomas are rare in the mouth, although cervical lymph node involvement is common. Usually lymphomas present as ulcers or swellings (**Figure 3.43**).

Non-Hodgkin's lymphoma (**Figure 3.44**) often appears in the fauces. It also commonly affects the tonsillar region, and usually presents as a diffuse painless swelling that eventually ulcerates (**Figure 3.45**). There is an increased prevalence in HIV infection (*see* **Figure 2.92**). (*See also* Sjögren's syndrome, page 262.)

(*Contd*)

114

LYMPHOMAS
(*Contd*)

African Burkitt's lymphoma is associated with Epstein–Barr virus and typically affects children before the age of 12–13 years. The jaws, particularly the mandible, are common sites of presentation (**Figure 3.46**). Massive swelling, which ulcerates in the mouth, may be seen. Radiographically, the teeth may appear to be 'floating in air'.

The jaws are less frequently involved in non-African Burkitt's lymphoma. Discrete radiolucencies in the lower third molar region, destruction of lamina dura and widening of the periodontal space may be seen on radiography. In **Figure 3.47** it presents as an ulcerated lump arising from the mandible, but the disease may also cause oral pain, paraesthesia or increasing tooth mobility.

The association of non-African Burkitt's lymphoma with Epstein–Barr virus is tenuous and the disease is less common.

The initial sign of a non-Hodgkin's lymphoma is often diffuse progressive local swelling, seen in **Figure 3.48** over the mandibular angle. Growth can be very rapid and blood-borne metastasis widespread.

Patients with lymphocytic lymphomas are also predisposed to develop squamous carcinomas of the head and neck, possibly owing at least partly to the chemotherapy.

MIDLINE GRANULOMAS

These are discussed in Chapter 8, page 154.

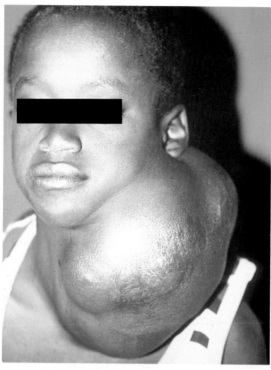

3.46

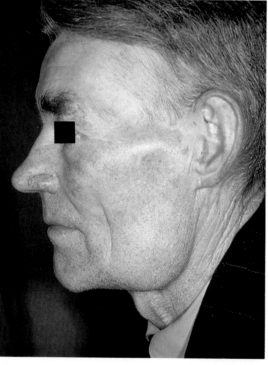

3.47

3.48

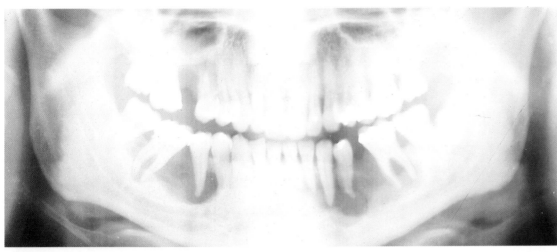

3.49

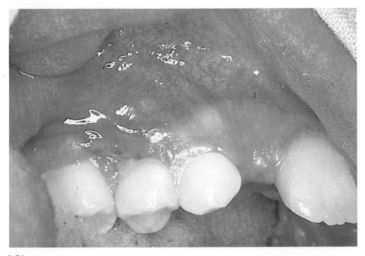

3.50

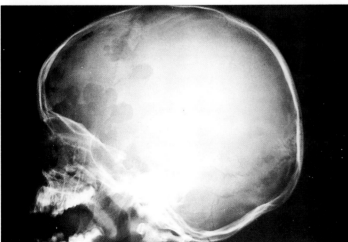

3.51

LANGERHAN'S CELL HISTIOCYTOSES

Langerhan's cell histiocytoses are a group of disorders, formerly termed histiocytosis X, arising from Langerhan's cells.

Hand–Schüller–Christian disease (**Figure 3.49**) appears at 3–6 years of age with disseminated bone lesions including osteolytic jaw lesions and loosening of teeth (floating teeth), diabetes insipidus and exophthalmos.

Eosinophilic granuloma is a localized benign form of histiocytosis where there are painless osteolytic bone lesions and, sometimes, mouth ulcers (**Figure 3.50**). The affected teeth may loosen.

Letterer–Siwe disease is an acute disseminated and usually lethal form of histiocytosis in children under the age of 3 years. There are destructive bone lesions (**Figure 3.51**), skin lesions, fever, lymphadenopathy and hepatosplenomegaly.

MYCOSIS FUNGOIDES

Mycosis fungoides is a predominantly cutaneous T-cell neoplasm that may produce oral plaques (**Figure 3.52**), infiltrates or ulcers, especially on the tongue, vermilion of the lips or buccal mucosa. Incidentally, this patient also has erythema migrans.

MULTIPLE MYELOMA (*Myelomatosis*)

Myelomatosis is a malignant disorder of plasma cells, affecting predominantly the bone marrow. Most commonly found in males over 50 years of age, it particularly affects the skull and axial skeleton. The jaws may be involved but soft tissue lesions (**Figure 3.53**) are rare.

The symptomatic stage is preceded by the presence in plasma of an M-type (monoclonal) plasma protein, raised ESR, and proteinuria. Renal dysfunction may eventually arise.

Clinically there may be anaemia, bone pain, swelling, paraesthesia or, occasionally, pathological fractures. Radiography shows multiple punched-out radiolucencies (**Figure 3.54**).

Ultimately, there may be circulatory impairment, Raynaud-type phenomena or bleeding tendency caused by the paraproteins. Amyloidosis may be seen. There is a predisposition to recurrence of varicella zoster virus infection.

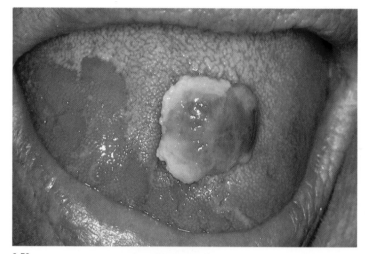

3.52

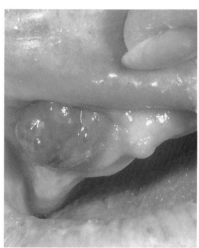

3.53

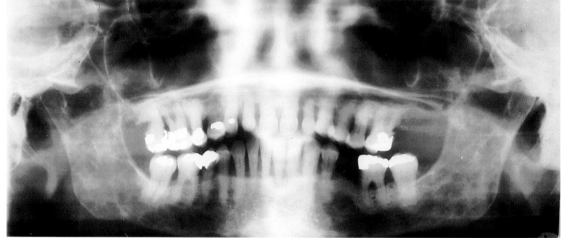

3.54

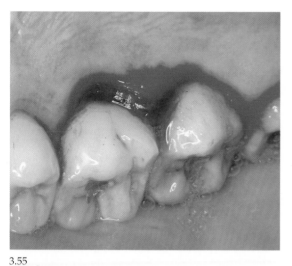

3.55

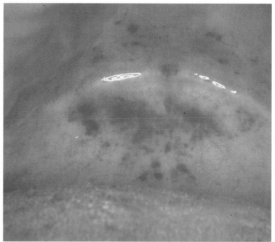

3.56

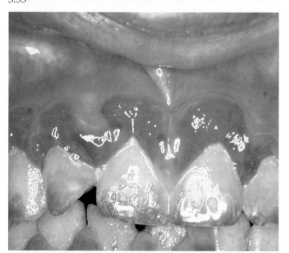

3.57

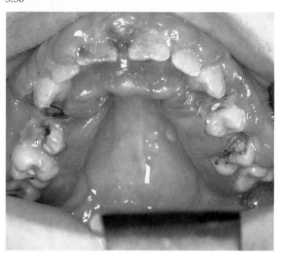

3.58

LEUKAEMIAS

Replacement of bone marrow by leukaemic tissue leads to crowding out of other cellular elements and consequent anaemia and thrombocytopenia. Spontaneous gingival haemorrhage is common (**Figure 3.55**).

Oral purpura is also common, particularly where there is trauma, such as the suction exerted by an upper denture (**Figure 3.56**). Chemotherapy may aggravate the bleeding tendency.

Gingival haemorrhage can be so profuse as to dissuade the patient from oral hygiene, but this simply aggravates the problem as the gingivae then become inflamed, more hyperaemic (**Figure 3.57**) and bleed more profusely.

Leukaemic deposits in the gingivae occasionally cause gingival swelling (**Figure 3.58**). This is a feature especially of myelomonocytic leukaemia (a variant of acute myeloid leukaemia, **Figure 3.59**).

(Contd)

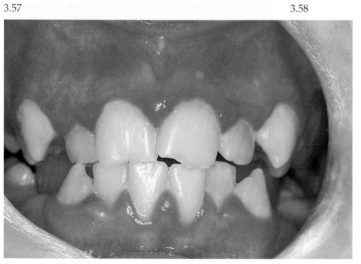

3.59

118

LEUKAEMIAS
(Contd)

Simple odontogenic infections can spread widely and be difficult to control (**Figure 3.60**).

Non-odontogenic oral infections are common in leukaemic patients and involve a range of organisms including *Staphylococcus aureus*, *Pseudomonas aeruginosa*, *Klebsiella pneumoniae*, *Staphylococcus epidermidis*, *Escherichia coli*, enterococci, herpes simplex or varicella-zoster viruses, *Candida* species, *Aspergillus*, *Mucor* and, occasionally, other opportunists.

Mouth ulcers are common in leukaemia and often lack an inflammatory halo (**Figure 3.61**). Some are associated with cytotoxic therapy, some with viral or bacterial infection, and some are non-specific.

Erythroleukaemia or Di Guglielmo's disease is a rare disorder, now recognized as a variant of myeloid leukaemia, characterized by proliferation of erythropoietic cells, with anaemia and hepatosplenomegaly but no lymphadenopathy. Oral ulceration and pallor (**Figure 3.62**) and purpura are the main features.

Microbial infections are common in the mouth and can be a significant problem to the leukaemic patient. Candidosis is extremely common (**Figure 3.63**). Of the viral infections, recurrent intraoral herpes simplex is also common. The patient in **Figure 3.63** has a dendritic ulcer, caused by herpes simplex virus.

Recurrent herpes labialis is common in leukaemic patients. The lesions can be extensive and, because of the thrombocytopenia, there is often bleeding into the lesion (**Figure 3.64**).

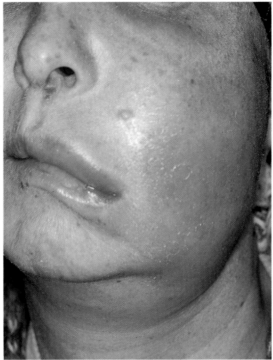

3.60

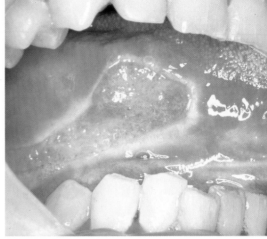

3.61

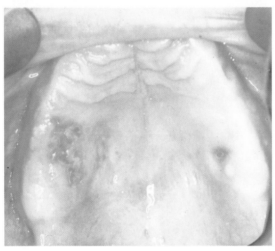

3.62

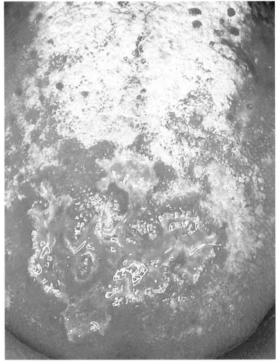

3.63

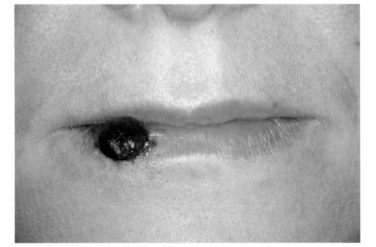

3.64

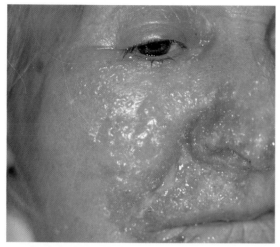

3.65

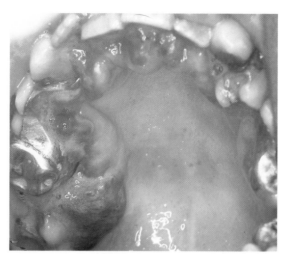

3.66

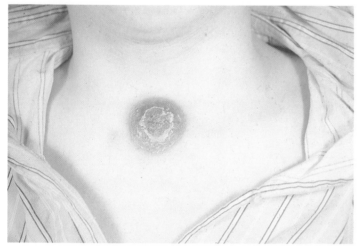

3.67

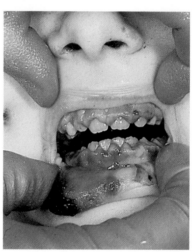

3.68

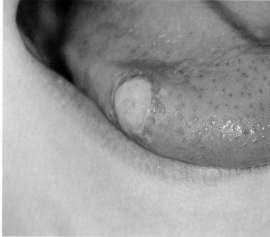

3.69

Zoster is also common in leukaemic patients (**Figure 3.65**) and hairy leukoplakia may rarely be seen.

Bacterial infections, however, are uncommon (**Figure 3.66**) but a wide range of organisms may be involved, including various enteric organisms such as *Klebsiella* and *Escherichia coli* and septicaemia may originate from oral lesions.

Leukaemic deposits may appear in the mouth, or on the face and neck (**Figure 3.67**), but are uncommon. The most common manifestation in the neck of leukaemic patients is cervical lymph node enlargement.

Figure 3.68 shows pallor, gingival haemorrhage and herpetic infection in a child with terminal leukaemia. However, the prognosis in childhood leukaemias is now greatly improved.

Finally, infiltration of the oral mucosa (**Figure 3.69**) is most typical of acute myeloid leukaemia although it has been rarely reported in chronic lymphocytic leukaemia. The precise reason for the variable infiltration of the oral mucosa with different leukaemias is unknown.

CONGENITAL EPULIS

Congenital epulis of the newborn is a rare lesion seen mostly in females and in the maxilla. **Figure 3.70** shows an infant with a lump over the anterior mandible. Histologically similar to the granular cell tumour, the congenital epulis is a distinct benign entity, possibly of neural origin. The lesion does not grow after birth and may resolve spontaneously. It may need to be removed if it interferes with feeding.

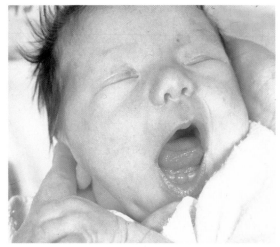

3.70

LIPOMA

Lipoma is a relatively rare benign intraoral tumour, generally found in adults. The appearance is typical with thin epithelium over the yellowish tumour and prominent superficial blood vessels (**Figure 3.71**). Lipomas may be very soft on palpation (semi-fluctuant) and mistaken for cysts.

LEIOMYOMA

This benign tumour of smooth muscle is rare in the oral cavity (**Figure 3.72**), and usually found on the tongue.

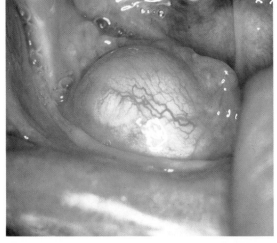

3.71

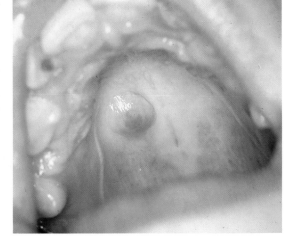

3.72

GRANULAR CELL TUMOUR
(*Abrikssoff's tumour; granular cell myoblastoma*)

This rare benign lesion of controversial origin may arise in many sites in the body but is most common in the tongue, presenting as a firm, submucosal, painless nodule (**Figure 3.73**). Some have a whitish surface and occasionally this appearance, with pseudoepitheliomatous hyperplasia on histology, leads to a misdiagnosis of carcinoma.

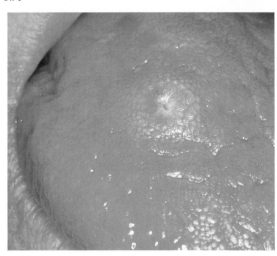

3.73

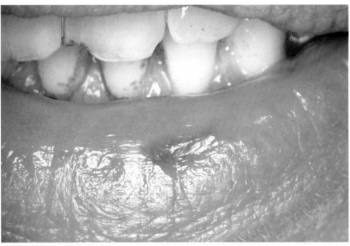

3.74

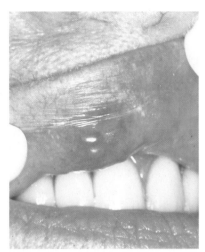

3.75

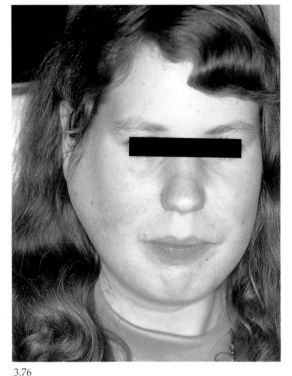

3.76

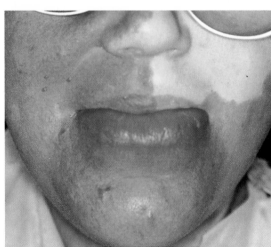

3.77

EPHELIS (*Freckle*)

These circumscribed melanotic macules, typically smaller than 0.5 cm, appear on sun-exposed areas in childhood, owing to a local increase in melanin production, in a normal number of melanocytes. Although usually affecting the skin, ephelides may occasionally involve mucous membranes (**Figure 3.74**).

HAEMANGIOMA

Haemangiomas are fairly common hamartomas in the mouth, especially on the lip (**Figure 3.75**).

Facial disfiguration in **Figure 3.76** was caused by an haemangioma, although the appearance simulates a parotid swelling.

Extensive haemangiomas may sometimes be seen (**Figure 3.77**). Some of these may result in partial enlargement of the soft tissues and underlying bone (Klippel–Trenaunay or angio-osteohypertrophy syndrome) and others may be part of the von Hippel–Lindau syndrome (involving retina, cerebellum, spinal cord, kidneys, pancreas, liver but not the mouth), or the Sturge–Weber syndrome (*see* page 294). Facial haemangiomas may rarely be associated with posterior fossa brain abnormalities often of the Dandy–Walker type.

MAFFUCCI'S SYNDROME

Haemangiomas are typically in the tongue in Maffucci's syndrome, when they are associated with multiple enchondromas elsewhere, particularly in cartilage bones such as in the hands and feet. Haemangiomas also can involve skin, other mucosae and viscera. **Figure 3.78** shows cavernous haemangiomas in the buccal mucosa, adjacent to the parotid papilla.

LYMPHANGIOMA

Lymphangioma is an hamartoma most common in the anterior tongue (**Figure 3.79**) or lip.

The typical 'frogspawn' appearance of the surface is seen in **Figure 3.80**, a lymphangioma of the buccal mucosa.

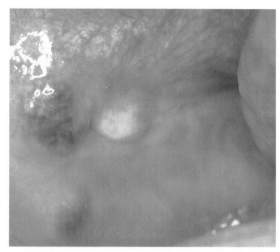

3.78

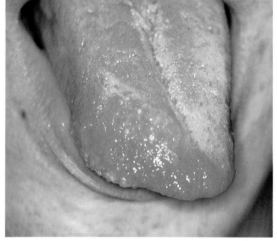

3.79

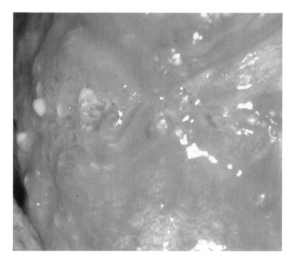

3.80

4 ENDOCRINE, NUTRITIONAL AND METABOLIC DISEASES AND IMMUNITY DISORDERS

CONGENITAL HYPOTHYROIDISM (*Cretinism*)

Short stature, mental handicap, and coarse facies (**Figure 4.1**) are the most obvious features of cretinism. Oral changes include macroglossia, delayed eruption and hypoplasia of the teeth.

DIABETES MELLITUS

The oral changes in diabetes are non-specific and seen mainly in severe insulin-dependent diabetics. Parodontal abscesses, infections, and rapid periodontal breakdown are the most obvious features. **Figure 4.2** shows gingivitis in the lower anterior region and an abscess above the right lateral incisor which proved to be a periapical abscess related to the non-vital and discoloured central incisor.

Figure 4.3 shows severe periodontal breakdown in a diabetic (there is a healing lesion of herpes labialis on the upper lip).

Other oral lesions in diabetes may include sialosis, median rhomboid glossitis, glossodynia, and lichenoid lesions induced by hypoglycaemic drugs. Dry mouth may be caused by dehydration in diabetes. Mucormycosis is a rare complication (*see* **Figure 2.177**). Diabetic angiopathy rarely presents with palatal petechiae and diabetes has rare associations with acanthosis nigricans (*see* page 256). Autonomic neuropathy may cause xerostomia or gustatory sweating. Hyperglycaemia may cause pronounced halitosis.

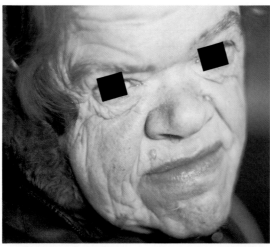

4.1

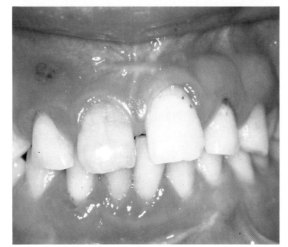

4.2

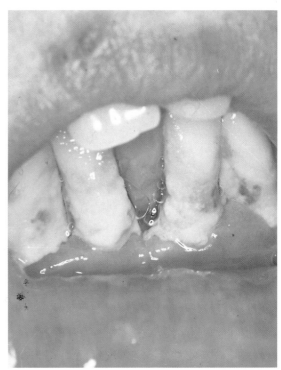

4.3

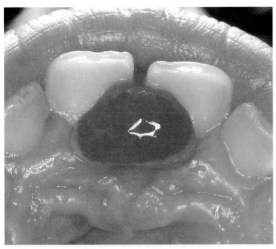

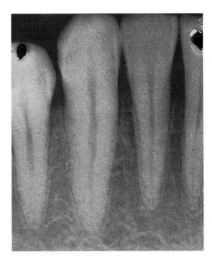

4.4

4.5

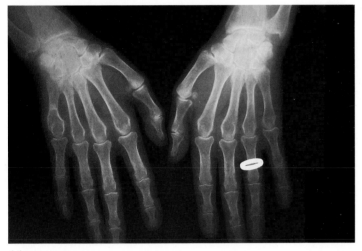

4.6

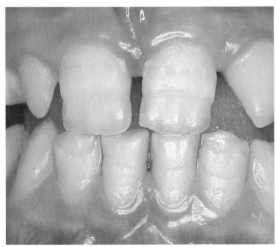

4.7

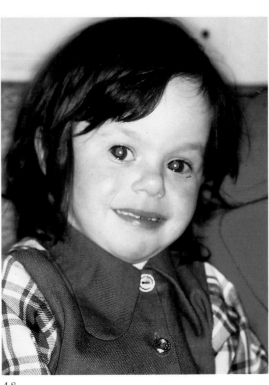

4.8

HYPER-PARATHYROIDISM

Giant-cell granulomas are occasionally associated with hyperparathyroidism (**Figure 4.4**).

Skeletal changes in primary hyperparathyroidism typically include generalized rarefaction, and sometimes lytic lesions (osteitis fibrosa cystica), but an almost pathognomonic oral change is the loss of the lamina dura (**Figure 4.5**). Almost all patients with primary hyperparathyroidism have skeletal lesions microscopically indistinguishable from the central giant cell granuloma of bone (brown tumours). Skull and jaw involvement is a late complication.

The characteristic radiographic sign of the condition is subperiosteal bone resorption, and 'tufting' of terminal phalanges (**Figure 4.6**).

CONGENITAL HYPO-PARATHYROIDISM

In congenital hypo-parathyroidism, there may be severe hypoplasia of the teeth (**Figure 4.7**), shortened roots and retarded eruption.

Rare patients with candidosis-endocrinopathy syndrome and with Di George syndrome also have chronic mucocutaneous candidosis (*see* page 96), as well as hypoparathyroidism.

Acquired hypo-parathyroidism in adult life produces facial tetany but no oral manifestations.

PSEUDOHYPO-PARATHYROIDISM

Elfin facies (**Figure 4.8**), short stature, short metatarsals and metacarpals, calcified basal ganglia and enamel hypoplasia are features of this rare, complex, dominant disorder, possibly sex-linked (*see also* **Figure 10.32**). Parathyroid hormone is secreted, but the end organs are unresponsive. There is also an association with other endocrine disorders, particularly hypothyroidism.

126

ACROMEGALY

Acromegaly results from increased growth hormone secretion by a pituitary adenoma.

Mandibular prognathism, generalized thickening of soft tissues (**Figure 4.9**) and spacing of the teeth (**Figure 4.10**) are typical of acromegaly. Another feature is large hands (**Figure 4.11**).

Enlarged pituitary fossa, as a result of the causal pituitary adenoma, and enlarged supraorbital ridges and mandible may be obvious on radiography (**Figure 4.12**). Headache and tunnel vision (bitemporal hemianopia) may result eventually as the pituitary neoplasm enlarges. An enlarged tongue may be seen (**Figure 4.13**).

CARCINOID SYNDROME

Flushing of the face and neck with telangiectasia and sometimes periorbital oedema may be seen in carcinoid syndrome.

GLUCAGONOMA

Oral ulceration, glossitis and angular stomatitis can be seen in glucagonoma.

ADDISON'S DISEASE (*Hypo-adrenocorticism*)

Addison's disease is hypo-adrenocorticism, often of autoimmune aetiology, but may be caused by tumour, tuberculosis or, rarely, cytomegalovirus or histoplasmosis. Lower plasma cortisol levels result in increased pituitary secretion of adrenocorticotrophic hormone (ACTH) and precursor hormones with MSH-like activity.

Oral hyperpigmentation of a brown, grey or black colour, especially at sites of trauma such as the buccal mucosae or tongue, is typical of Addison's disease (**Figure 4.14**), although most patients with oral hyperpigmentation prove to have other causes.

(Contd)

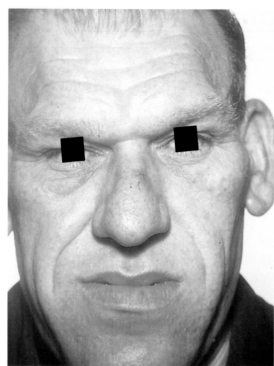

4.9

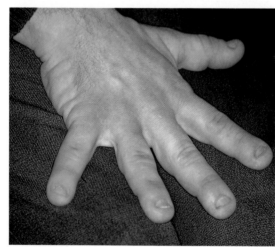

4.11

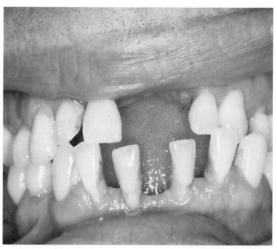

4.10

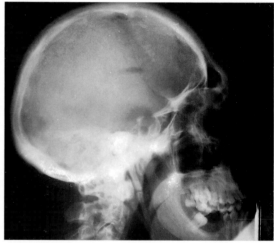

4.12

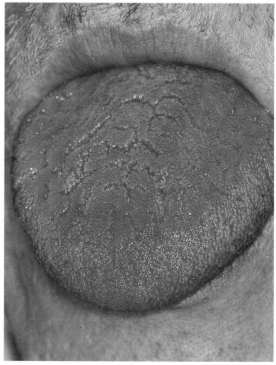

4.13

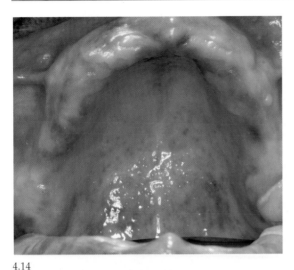

4.14

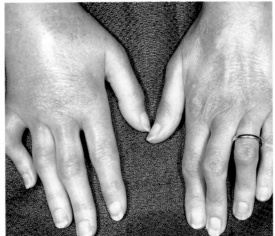

4.15

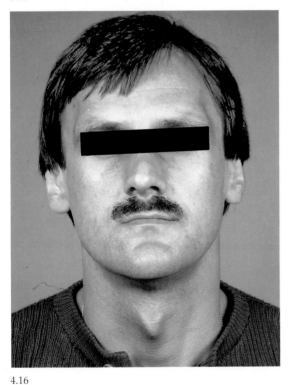

4.16

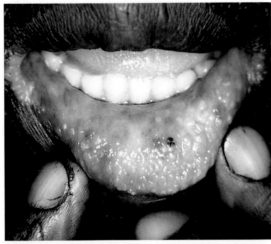

4.17

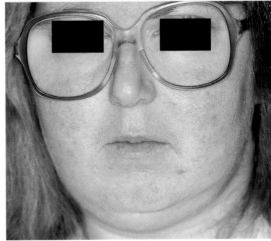

4.18

Generalized skin hyperpigmentation is also seen (**Figure 4.15**). The skin pigmentation is mainly in sun-exposed or traumatized sites, the areolae and genitalia (**Figure 4.16**). Similar hyperpigmentation is also seen in Nelson's syndrome (increased ACTH production after bilateral adrenalectomy).

There are occasional associations of Addison's disease with other diseases, particularly autoimmune diseases, such as the probable TASS syndrome of thyroiditis, Addison's disease, Sjögren's syndrome and sarcoidosis. The patient in **Figure 4.15** also has incidental Dupuytren's contractures.

MULTIPLE ENDOCRINE ADENOMA SYNDROME TYPE III

Oral mucosal neuromas (**Figure 4.17**) are associated with medullary cell carcinoma of the thyroid, phaeo-chromocytoma and, occasionally, hyperpara-thyroidism in the type 2b multiple endocrine adenoma syndrome. Patients may have a Marfanoid habitus and may have macroglossia.

Mucosal neuromas may be seen on the lips, tongue, nasal and pharyngeal mucosae, conjunctivae and cornea.

CUSHING'S SYNDROME

Cushing's syndrome arises when glucocorticoid levels are increased from any source, including iatrogenically. Cushing's disease is the consequence of a pituitary adenoma oversecreting ACTH, thus stimulating excess adrenocortical activity.

Truncal and facial obesity, hypertension, weakness, hirsutism, purplish abdominal striae, osteoporosis, amenorrhoea and glycosuria are the typical features. The 'moon-face' appearance is typical (**Figure 4.18**).

VITAMIN B DEFICIENCY

Figure 4.19 shows atrophic glossitis in a child with malabsorption syndrome. The tongue is completely depapillated and smooth (*see also* **Figure 10.310**). Oral ulcers and angular stomatitis are also common features. This particular child had coeliac disease, associated with selective IgA deficiency (*see* page 132).

Angular stomatitis is seen particularly in vitamin B$_{12}$ deficiency (**Figure 4.20**) and in riboflavin deficiency, and is also seen in iron or folate deficiency. The most common cause of angular stomatitis, however, is candidosis (*see* page 95).

VITAMIN B$_{12}$ DEFICIENCY

In Western countries, vitamin B$_{12}$ deficiency is rarely dietary in origin. Usually it is due to pernicious anaemia, gastric or small intestinal disease. Gastric bypass surgery for morbid obesity is a cause recently described.

Atrophic glossitis (**Figure 4.21**) or red lines or red patches on the tongue (Moeller's glossitis), **Figure 4.22**, are fairly typical of early vitamin B$_{12}$ deficiency.

Pernicious anaemia is characterized often by premature greying of the hair and blue eyes (**Figure 4.23**) and may progress to neurological damage, especially subacute combined degeneration of the spinal cord.

DEFICIENCY OF HAEMATINICS

Deficiency of haematinics (iron, vitamin B$_{12}$, or folic acid) can manifest with glossitis, angular stomatitis and mouth ulcers (**Figure 4.24**). A significant proportion of patients with classical clinical aphthae prove to be deficient in an haematinic.

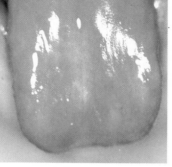
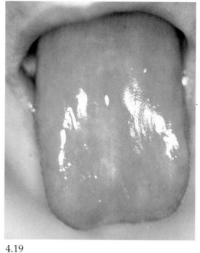

4.19

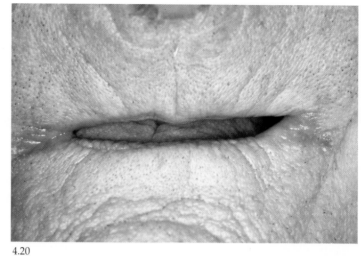

4.20

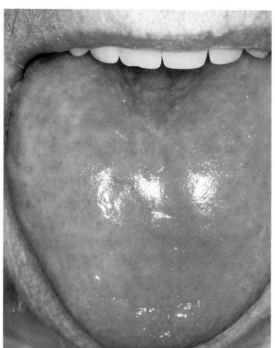

4.21

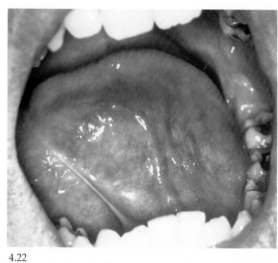

4.22

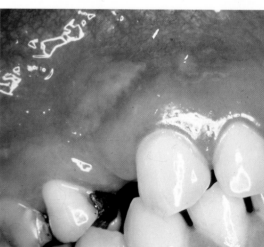

4.24

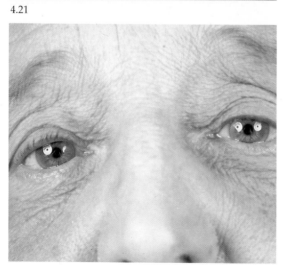

4.23

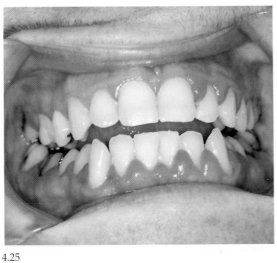

4.25

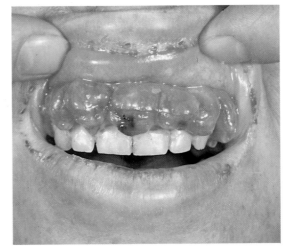

4.26

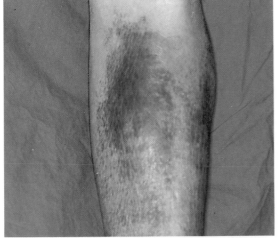

4.27

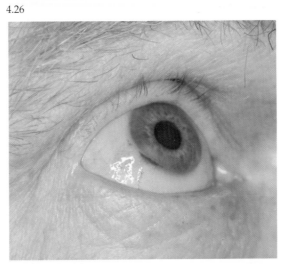

4.28

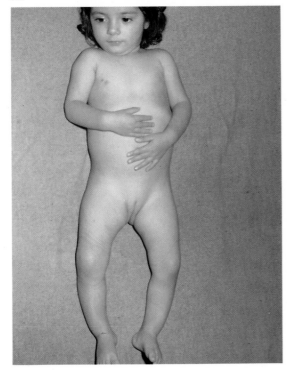

4.29

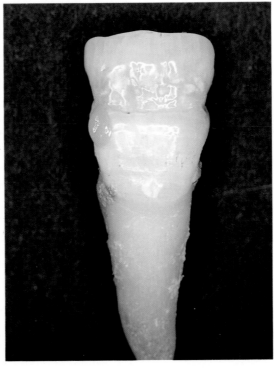

4.30

SCURVY (*Vitamin C deficiency*)

Although rare in Western countries, scurvy is an occasional cause of gingival hyperplasia (**Figure 4.25**). Most patients develop scurvy because they have an abnormal diet, lacking in fresh vegetables.

Gingival hyperplasia with purpura in severe scurvy (**Figure 4.26**) is reminiscent of leukaemia.

Perifollicular haemorrhages are typical of scurvy but occasionally there may be more severe purpura (**Figure 4.27**). Cutaneous bleeding is most obvious on the legs and buttocks. Small subconjunctival haemorrhages may also be seen (**Figure 4.28**).

RICKETS (*Vitamin D deficiency*)

Rickets (**Figure 4.29**) is uncommon in Western countries, but has been recorded in Asian patients living in environments where they are exposed to relatively little sunlight and with a diet rich in phytate (found in chuppatti flour), which chelates dietary calcium.

Enamel hypoplasia has been seen only in extremely severe rickets (**Figure 4.30**) where tooth eruption may also be retarded (*see also* renal rickets, page 235).

AMYLOIDOSIS

Amyloidosis is a group of diseases in which one of a range of materials is deposited in tissues. Deposits are sufficiently large in size to give a characteristically fibrillar structure on electron microscopy, and green birefringence on polarization microscopy after Congo Red staining. Amyloid L arises from immunoglobulin light chains, amyloid A, from amyloid A protein, and others are from prealbumin, gamma-trace protein, or beta-2-microglobulin.

Primary amyloidosis (that associated with plasma cell dyscrasias) particularly affects males over the age of 50 years and is the type of amyloid most commonly associated with deposits in the oral mucosa and sub-endocardium. Macroglossia is typical. The tongue is large, firm and indurated and may show red nodules and/or petechiae, especially at the lateral margins (**Figure 4.31**). Petechiae, ecchymoses or blood-filled blisters may be seen (**Figure 4.32**), as there is an acquired deficiency of blood coagulation factor X in patients with the light chain type of amyloid found in plasma cell dyscrasias.

Figure 4.33 shows subconjunctival haemorrhage in the patient shown in **Figure 4.32**, who subsequently died from amyloid nephropathy, detected through his heavy proteinuria and glycosuria.

Secondary types of amyloidosis — most of those associated with deposits other than of light chains — rarely affect the mouth.

The tongue may be involved in beta-2-microglobulin amyloidosis in patients on long-term haemodialysis.

HEAVY CHAIN DISEASE

The palate may be red and swollen in Franklin's gamma heavy-chain disease.

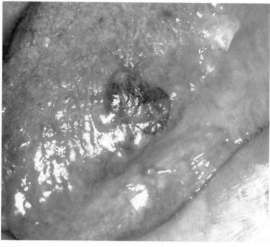

4.31

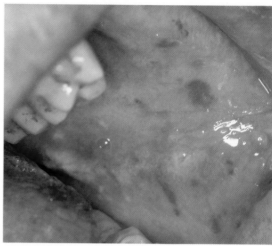

4.32

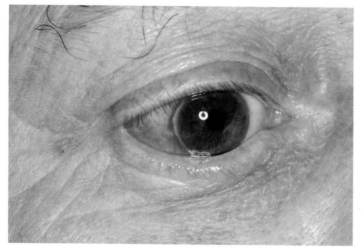

4.33

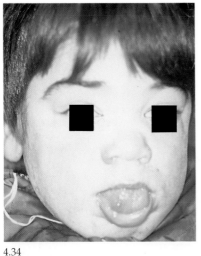

4.34

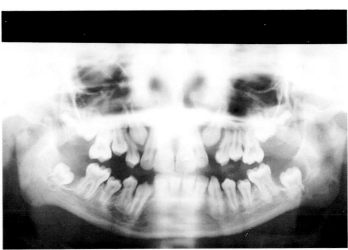

4.35

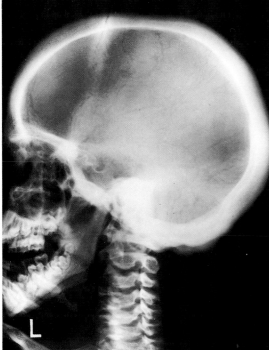

4.36

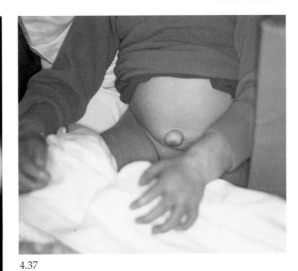

4.37

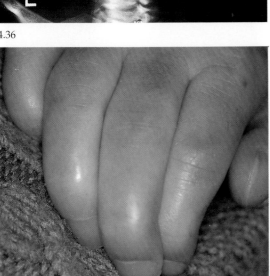

4.38

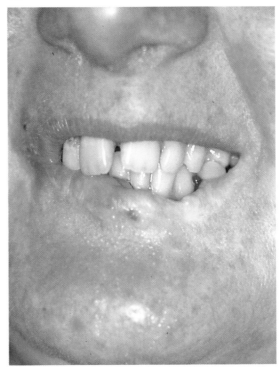

4.39

MUCOPOLY-SACCHARIDOSES

Deficiency of mucopolysaccharidases leads to the accumulation of mucopolysaccharides (glycosaminoglycans) and to one of a number of syndromes, characterized by dwarfism, hirsutism, coarse features, and macroglossia, often with mental handicap, deafness, cardiac failure and corneal clouding. Hurler's syndrome or gargoylism (**Figure 4.34**) is the most common of these disorders.

Hurler's syndrome manifests in early childhood with deteriorating mental and physical development. There are frequent upper respiratory infections, cardiomegaly and murmurs. Delayed or incomplete eruption of teeth (**Figure 4.35**) and radiolucent lesions around the crowns of the lower second molars may be seen, as well as temporo-mandibular joint anomalies.

The head is large with premature closure of sagittal and metopic sutures. The pituitary fossa is boot- or slipper-shaped (**Figure 4.36**). Hepatosplenomegaly causes abdominal swelling, and umbilical hernia is common (**Figure 4.37**).

Characteristic 'claw hand' occurs because the joints cannot be fully extended (**Figure 4.38**). There are also flexion contractures in many other joints. Talipes is common.

LESCH–NYHAN SYNDROME

Sex-linked hyperuricaemia, owing to deficiency of the enzyme hypoxanthine guanine phosphoribosyl transferase, is associated with mental handicap, choreoathetosis, and self-mutilation especially of the tongue and lip (**Figure 4.39**).

SELECTIVE IgA DEFICIENCY

Selective IgA deficiency is the most common primary (genetically determined) immune defect. Some patients are healthy but those who also lack IgG$_2$ suffer recurrent respiratory infection, autoimmune disorders and atopy. Many have mouth ulcers (**Figure 4.40**), and there may be a reduced protection against dental caries.

AGAMMA-GLOBULINAEMIA (*Bruton's syndrome*)

Panhypoimmunoglobulin-aemia affects males almost exclusively, and presents mainly with recurrent pyogenic respiratory infections. Several patients with mouth ulcers have been recorded (**Figure 4.41**).

Severe infections in the neonate can disturb odontogenesis, causing enamel hypoplasia. In the past, tetracycline treatment caused tooth discoloration (**Figure 4.42**).

CELL-MEDIATED IMMUNODEFICIENCY

Chronic oral candidosis, which may present with angular stomatitis, is an early and prominent feature in any cell-mediated immune defect (**Figure 4.43**), and there is a predisposition to recurrent lesions of herpes simplex and varicella-zoster virus.

Oral thrush (**Figure 4.44**) is an early feature of many T-lymphocyte defects.

Herpes labialis is often reactivated during immunosuppression of the cellular response, as in this patient (**Figure 4.45**) on systemic corticosteroids.

(*See* Chapter 2, pages 74–81 for discussion of HIV disease.)

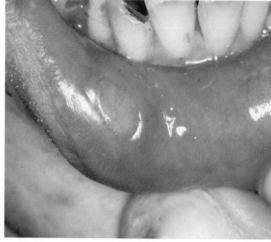

4.40

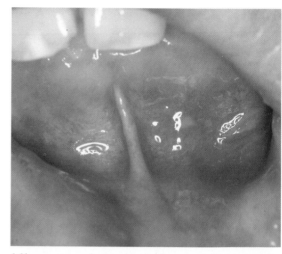

4.41

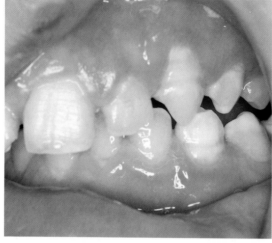

4.42

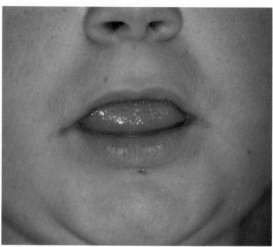

4.43

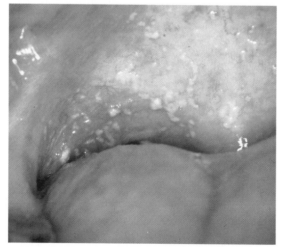

4.44

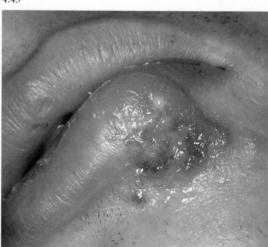

4.45

5 DISEASES OF THE BLOOD AND BLOOD-FORMING ORGANS

IRON DEFICIENCY

The most common cause of iron deficiency in Western countries is chronic haemorrhage. When bone marrow iron stores are depleted, there is a stage of iron deficiency without anaemia (sideropenia) before red cell changes are evident. Angular stomatitis (**Figure 5.1**) is one oral manifestation which may be seen in the pre-anaemic stage as well as in anaemia.

Angular stomatitis is soreness and sometimes fissuring at the commissure (**Figure 5.2**). Usually of local aetiology, related to candidosis beneath an upper denture, it is occasionally precipitated by a deficiency of iron, folate or vitamin B (*see also* page 128).

Although deficiency of iron or other haematinics can cause sore tongue with atrophic glossitis (**Figure 5.3**), many haematinic deficient patients with a sore tongue have no obvious organic lesion. Oral ulceration is sometimes a manifestation of iron deficiency.

Spoon-shaped nails (koilonychia) which tend to split are typical of iron deficiency anaemia (**Figure 5.4**).

Other deficiency anaemias are discussed in Chapter 4.

HAEMO-GLOBINOPATHIES

Haemoglobinopathies such as sickle-cell anaemia and thalassaemias may present with maxillary hyperplasia owing to marrow overgrowth.

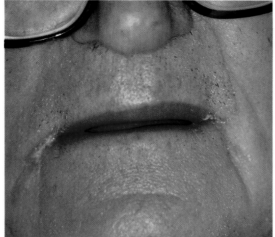

5.1

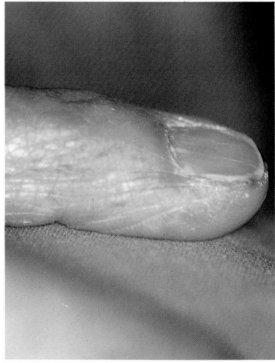

5.2

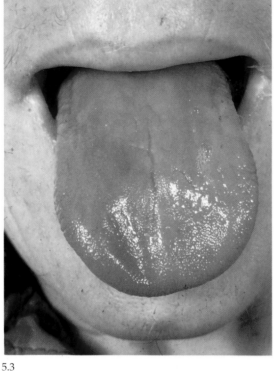

5.3

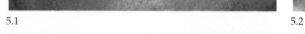

5.4

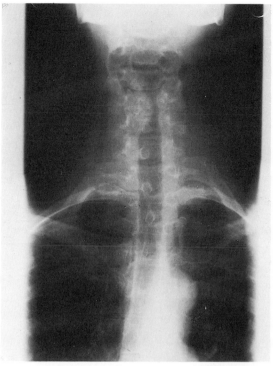

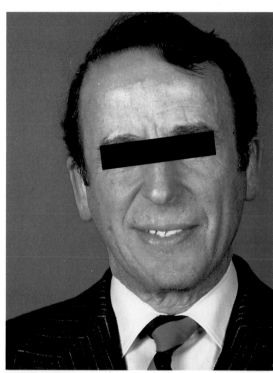

5.5

5.6

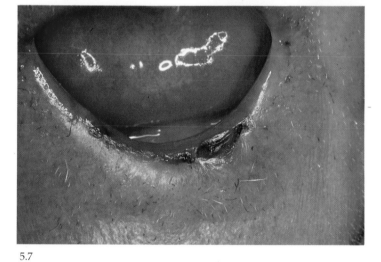

5.7

PLUMMER–VINSON SYNDROME (*Patterson–Kelly syndrome*)

In this syndrome (sideropenic dysphagia), patients typically are middle-aged with dysphagia caused by an oesophageal web, often with candidosis, hypochromic microcytic anaemia, koilonychia and a depapillated tongue. There is a predisposition to post-cricoid carcinoma (**Figure 5.5**) and to oral carcinoma.

POLYCYTHAEMIA RUBRA VERA

Polycythaemia rubra vera is a primary myeloproliferative disorder characterized by increased numbers of red cells (giving a plethoric appearance, **Figure 5.6**), increased granulocytes, and increased but dysfunctional platelets. Oral purpura or haemorrhage may be seen.

Cytotoxic therapy of the disease may lead to neutropenic oral ulceration and an increased bleeding tendency (**Figure 5.7**). Secondary polycythaemia is associated with compensatory or inappropriate erythropoietin release in cardiorespiratory disease, heavy smoking, or in association with a variety of tumours, such as renal carcinoma, cerebellar haemangioblastoma and malignant·fibrous histiocytoma of the parotid gland.

MYELODYSPLASTIC SYNDROME

In this group of disorders there is a functional neutropenia as a result of disordered granulopoiesis. The ulcers notably lack an inflammatory halo (**Figure 5.8**).

APLASTIC ANAEMIA

Clinical features of aplastic anaemia depend on the predominant cell type affected and aplastic anaemia may therefore present with signs and symptoms of thrombocytopenia, leukopenia, anaemia or a combination of all three (pancytopenia). Profound and spontaneous purpuric or ecchymotic haemorrhages of the skin and mucous membrane can be the presenting features (**Figure 5.9**).

Leukopenia (particularly neutropenia) leads to decreased resistance to infection, manifest as severe ulceration, often associated with opportunistic organisms. Typically there is, as in agranulocytosis, only a minimal red inflammatory halo around the ulcers (**Figure 5.10**).

Bone marrow transplantation (*see* page 141) is often the treatment for aplastic anaemia. Oral complications include mucositis, candidosis, parotitis, graft-versus-host disease with lichenoid or sclerodermatous reactions, and infections with herpes viruses or fungi, such as *Aspergillus* (*see* page 99). Xerostomia predisposes to caries.

LEUKAEMIAS AND LYMPHOMAS

See Chapter 3, pages 113–120.

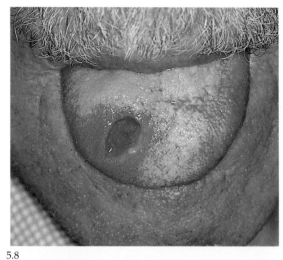

5.8

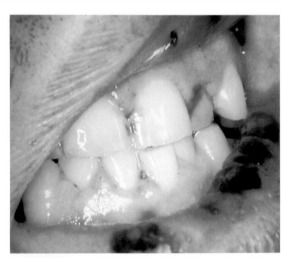

5.9

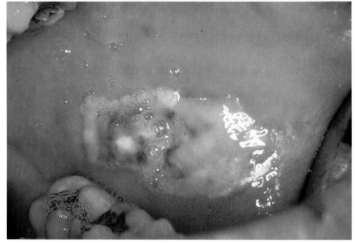

5.10

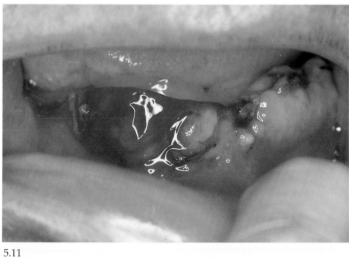

5.11

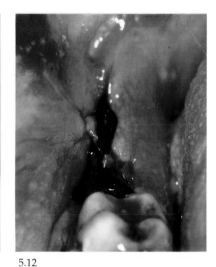

5.12

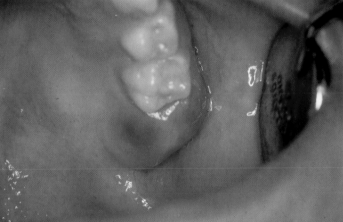

5.13

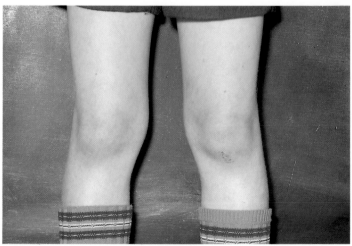

5.14

HAEMOPHILIAS

Defects of blood coagulation factors, unlike thrombocytopenia, do not predispose to spontaneous gingival haemorrhage, oral petechiae or ecchymoses. Any breach of the mucosa, however, especially tooth extraction, can lead to persistent bleeding (**Figure 5.11**) that is occasionally fatal. Haemorrhage after extraction here, a case of haemophilia A, was controlled with factor VIII replacement. Surgery must only be carried out with adequate factor VIII levels.

One danger is that haemorrhage into the fascial spaces, especially from surgery in the lower molar region, can track into the neck and embarrass the airway.

The combined factor VIII defect and platelet abnormality in von Willebrand's disease (**Figure 5.12**) can sometimes be more serious than classic haemophilia A (deficiency of factor VIII).

Tooth eruption and exfoliation are usually uneventful but, occasionally, there can be a small bleed into the follicle (**Figure 5.13**).

Haemophilia A (classic haemophilia) is ten times as common as haemophilia B (Christmas disease) where factor IX is deficient. Deep haemorrhage is a serious complication of both. Trauma predisposes to bleeding, though it can be spontaneous. Haemarthrosis (**Figure 5.14**) can be crippling.

HIV or hepatitis viruses infection may be seen in patients given blood transfusions, or factor replacement before screening or heat-treated factors were available.

THROMBO-CYTOPENIA

Oral petechiae and ecchymoses appear (**Figures 5.15 and 5.16**) mainly at sites of trauma but can be spontaneous. Petechiae appear mainly in the buccal mucosa, on the lateral margin of the tongue, and at the junction of hard and soft palates — sites readily traumatized.

Spontaneous gingival bleeding (**Figure 5.17**) is often an early feature in platelet deficiencies or defects. Post-extraction bleeding may be a problem.

Petechiae and ecchymoses also appear readily on the skin (**Figure 5.18**), especially if there is trauma. Even the pressure from a sphygmomanometer can cause petechiae during the measurement of blood pressure.

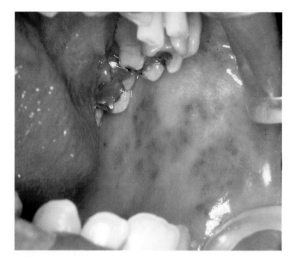

5.15

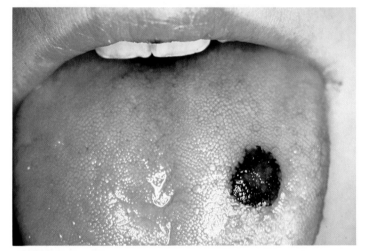

5.16

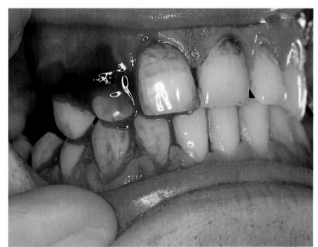

5.17

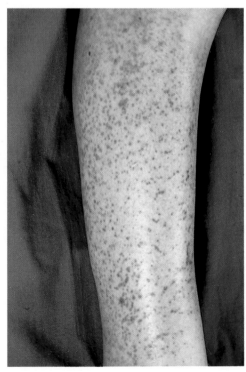

5.18

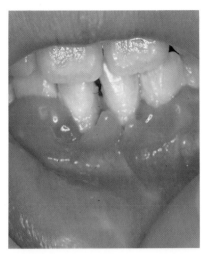

5.19

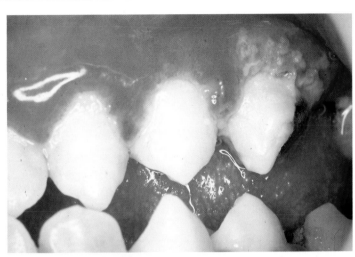

5.20

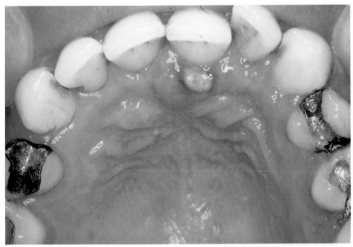

5.21

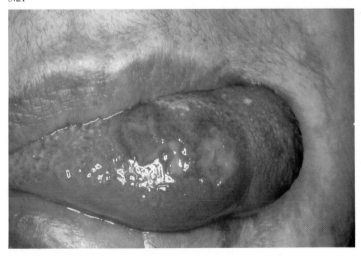

5.22

CHRONIC NEUTROPENIA

Neutropenias predispose to gingivitis, rapidly destructive periodontal disease (**Figure 5.19**) and to oral ulceration.

CYCLIC NEUTROPENIA

Neutropenia may be cyclical with a drop in polymorphonuclear neutrophil count, and sometimes other leukocytes, every 21 days. Destructive periodontal disease, recurrent ulcerative gingivitis and recurrent mouth ulcers are frequent manifestations (**Figure 5.20**), together with recurrent pyogenic infections. Palatal ulceration (**Figure 5.21**) is rare in aphthae and in this case suggested an immune defect which proved to be neutropenia.

Recurrent mouth ulcers in neutropenias, leukaemias, and some cell-mediated immune defects are sometimes due to intraoral herpes simplex recurrences (**Figure 5.22**) or other viral infections such as CMV (*see* **Figure 2.89**).

Gangrene may be seen in patients with neutropenia or rare neutrophil defects such as acatalasia (seen mainly in Japan, Korea, Israel and Switzerland).

CHRONIC GRANULOMATOUS DISEASE (*CGD*)

This predominantly sex-linked leukocyte defect in which neutrophils and monocytes are defective at killing catalase-positive micro-organisms, presents typically with cervical lymph node enlargement and suppuration (a submandibular node abscess has been drained in **Figure 5.23**).

Recurrent infections in early childhood may result in enamel hypoplasia (**Figure 5.24**). The tooth loss here, however, was from a road traffic accident. CGD also predisposes to oral ulceration and periodontal destruction.

Other types of neutrophil defect also predispose to ulcers and accelerated periodontitis.

IDIOPATHIC PLASMACYTOSIS

Idiopathic plasmacytosis is an uncommon disorder clinically characterized by the development of painful, diffuse, red granular lesions on the free and attached gingivae (**Figure 5.25**). Gingival lesions can be localized or generalized and there can also be involvement of other oral mucosal surfaces, particularly the lips and tongue. Rarely, there is involvement of the pharynx and supraglottic larynx as in this patient who had widespread oral, pharyngeal and laryngeal plasmacytosis (**Figure 5.26**).

Plasmacytosis probably represents an atypical hypersensitivity reaction to a variety of agents including chewing gum, other confectionery and toothpastes.

In the past, plasma-cell gingivitis was seen and probably again represented a hypersensitivity reaction.

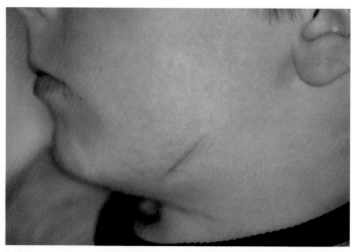

5.23

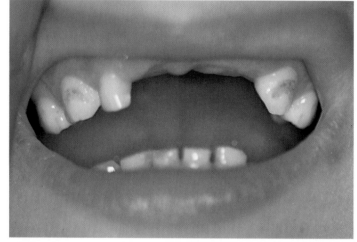

5.24

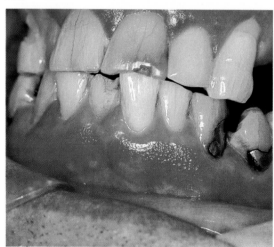

5.25

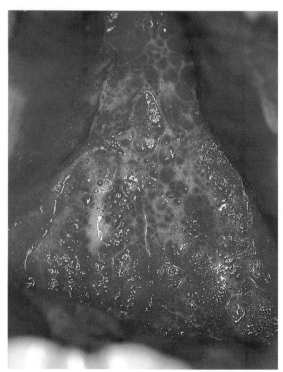

5.26

BONE-MARROW TRANSPLANTATION

Oral complications are common and can be a major cause of morbidity following bone-marrow transplantation (BMT). Mucositis (**Figure 5.27**), infections (**Figure 5.27** also shows candidosis), bleeding, xerostomia and loss of taste result from the effects of the underlying disease, chemo- and/or radiotherapy, and graft-versus-host disease (GVHD). The ventrum of the tongue, buccal and labial mucosae (**Figure 5.28**) and gingiva may be affected by ulceration.

Acute GVHD manifests with painful mucosal desquamation and ulceration, and/or cheilitis, and lichenoid plaques or striae. Small white lesions affect the buccal and lingual mucosa early on, but clear by day 14. Erythema and ulceration are most pronounced at 7–11 days after BMT. Oral candidosis and herpes simplex stomatitis are common (occasionally zoster), and there may be oral purpura.

The oral lesions in chronic GVHD are coincident with skin lesions, and include generalized mucosal erythema, lichenoid lesions, mainly in the buccal mucosa (**Figure 5.29**), and xerostomia with depressed salivary IgA levels in minor gland saliva. Xerostomia is most significant in the first 14 days after transplantation and is a consequence of drug treatment, irradiation and/or GVHD.

The chronic immunosuppression needed following organ transplantation predisposes to candidosis other mycoses (*see* **Figure 2.178**) and viral infections. Some patients develop white lesions (keratoses) or hairy leukoplakia. Cyclosporin may induce gingival hyperplasia (*see* page 234). Rarely, oral malignant neoplasms have been recorded.

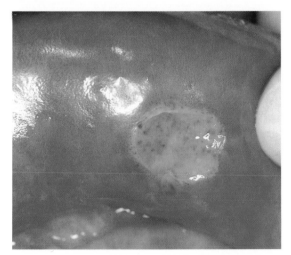

5.27

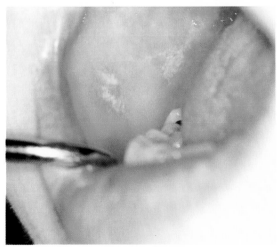

5.28

5.29

6 MENTAL DISORDERS

ORAL DYSAESTHESIA (*Burning mouth syndrome, glossopyrosis, glossodynia*)

A burning sensation in the mouth, especially the tongue, may be caused by infection such as candidosis, vitamin or iron deficiency, diabetes, drugs such as captopril or lesions such as erythema migrans. In some patients, no organic cause can be established, the tongue appears normal (**Figure 6.1**), and there may be a psychogenic basis. Affected patients are often females of middle age or older and the burning sensation *may* be relieved by eating. Anxiety about cancer is found in many.

ATYPICAL FACIAL PAIN

Persistent, dull, boring pain, especially in the maxilla, in the absence of identifiable organic disease, is seen in some psychiatric disorders, such as depression. Most patients affected with this atypical facial pain are females of middle age or older. **Figure 6.2** is an extreme example of a patient who is wearing a large bandage to help 'relieve' the pain, perhaps an attention-seeking device.

Patients with psychogenically-related orofacial symptoms not infrequently bring in diaries, graphs or notes outlining their complaints, which are often of pain, bad taste in the mouth, non-existent slime, lumps, dry or wet mouth, and are often multiple. A 'syndrome of oral complaints' has even been described.

PSYCHOGENIC ORAL DISEASE

A feature sometimes seen in these patients is a remarkable degree of tongue protrusion to the extent that the epiglottis can be seen (**Figure 6.3**).

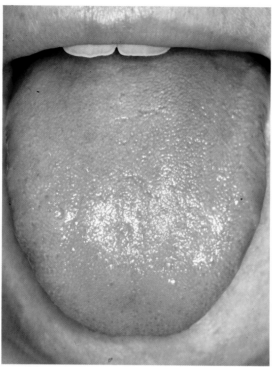

6.1

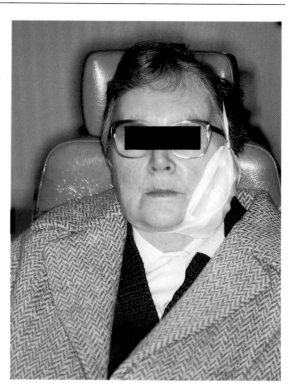

6.2

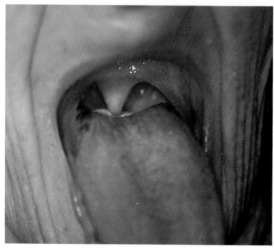

6.3

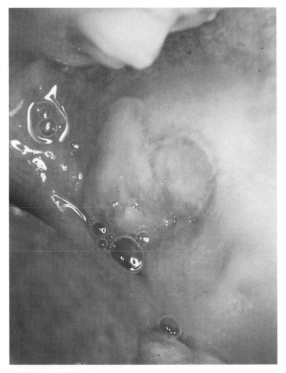

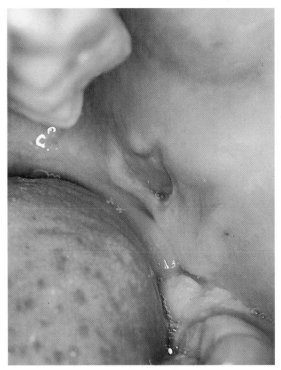

SELF-MUTILATION

Factitious or artefactual lesions are seen in some disturbed or mentally handicapped patients; in patients with Lesch–Nyhan syndrome (*see* page 131); in Gilles de la Tourette syndrome (tic, coprolalia and copropraxia); where there is sensory loss in the area (*see* page 148) and where there is congenital indifference to pain as in familial dysautonomia (Riley–Day syndrome).

Figure 6.4 shows an oral ulcer in a child whose father had just left home to be away for some weeks. The ulcer began to heal just after the father returned home (**Figure 6.5**).

(*See also* pages 183 and 221.)

6.4

6.5

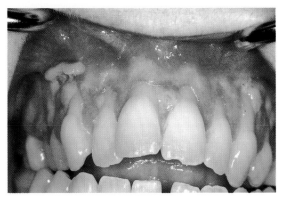

6.6

ANOREXIA NERVOSA

Anorexia nervosa is a syndrome characterized by severe weight loss due to self-starvation and is mainly a disease of previously healthy adolescent girls.

The disorder, which is regarded as an hysterical neurosis, is associated with a preoccupation to be thin. The body image appears to be so distorted that, even when emaciated, the patient still regards herself as too fat.

These patients usually refuse to eat or, if forced to do so, often induce vomiting. Menstrual upset is an early feature. Peripheral cyanosis and coldness with bradycardia and amenorrhoea are common, as are depression which lacks the classic features of depression in adults, and obsessional features.

Anorexia nervosa may be complicated by anaemia, endocrine disturbances, peripheral oedema and electrolyte depletion (especially hypokalaemia). Parotid enlargement (sialosis) and angular cheilitis may develop, as in other forms of starvation. The parotid swellings tend to subside if and when the patient returns to a normal diet. Erosion of teeth (perimylolysis) may result from repeated vomiting. The erosion is usually most pronounced on lingual, palatal and occlusal surfaces. Oral ulcers or abrasions may be caused by fingers or other objects used to induce vomiting.

Some patients cannot control their voluntary food restriction and have episodes in which they gorge food (bulimia) and then force vomiting. Bulimics, in contrast to anoretics, may have normal or near-normal weight. Uncontrolled and unpredictable ingestion of huge amounts of foods (usually soft sweet or starchy foods) is followed by vomiting. Bulimia may occur in isolation, or in anorexia nervosa, and appears to be a stress-related disorder. Erosion of the teeth, sore throat, angular cheilitis and painless swelling of the parotid glands may be seen and there may be xerostomia and an increase in caries.

Self mutilation (**Figure 6.6**), ulcers in the palate caused by using the fingers to induce retching, tooth erosion (*see* **Figures 10.79** and **10.80**) and sialosis may thus be seen in anorexia nervosa/bulimia.

146

MUNCHAUSEN'S SYNDROME

Munchausen's syndrome is the term used for persons who fabricate symptoms such as to result in unwarranted operative intervention. Patients with Munchausen's syndrome typically present with apparently acute illnesses supported by plausible histories, later often found to be full of falsifications. They have usually been seen by multiple clinicians and/or in several hospitals. Patients also frequently discharge themselves from care, sometimes after arguments with their clinical attendants.

The symptomatology of Munchausen's syndrome is highly varied but may be centred on particular areas, though few patients have been described with Munchausen's syndrome presenting with oral complaints. **Figure 6.7** shows one patient who complained of multiple odontalgia eventually persuading several clinicians to perform unnecessary interventions (**Figure 6.8**).

ORAL ARTEFACTUAL DISEASE

Oral self-inflicted lesions are often bizarre, typically destructive, may involve hard or soft tissues (*see* **Figures 6.4** and **6.6**) and may be a feature of mental handicap or psychiatric disorder.

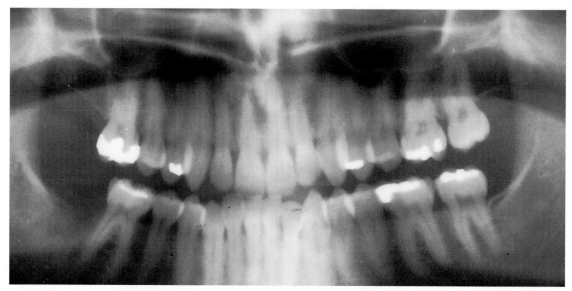

6.7

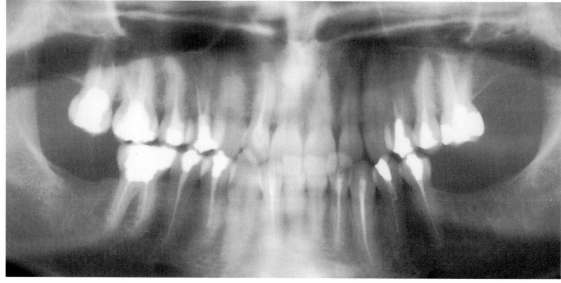

6.8

7 DISEASES OF THE NERVOUS SYSTEM

TRIGEMINAL NEURALGIA (*Paroxysmal trigeminal neuralgia*)

Neuralgia in the trigeminal region can have many causes. Multiple sclerosis, intracranial neoplasms and vascular anomalies, and connective-tissue disorders are the main recognizable causal diseases. If such organic causes cannot be demonstrated it is termed benign paroxysmal trigeminal neuralgia. This affects mainly the middle-aged or elderly and causes intermittent lancinating pain, usually in one division or branch in the sensory distribution of the trigeminal nerve. There are no organic manifestations but, if there is a trigger zone on the face, patients are understandably reluctant to touch the area — as in **Figure 7.1**, a patient who was reluctant to shave his right upper lip.

Treatment is usually medical (typically carbamazepine) but surgery such as cryoanalgesia may be required. Neurosurgery is rarely required and then may leave a sensory deficit. The patient in **Figure 7.2** was left with a numb left cheek and nose after neurosurgery and constantly traumatizes the area.

SENSORY LOSS IN THE TRIGEMINAL AREA

The trigeminal nerve emerges from the pons and runs through the posterior and middle cranial fossa. The most common causes of sensory loss are iatrogenic — for example, local anaesthesia, after which the patient accidentally traumatizes the lip (**Figure 7.3**). Removal of lower third molars, and mandibular osteotomies are other common iatrogenic causes.

(Contd)

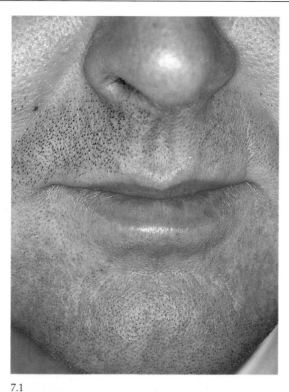

7.1

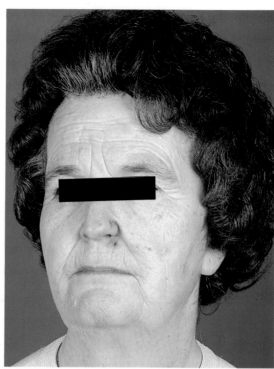

7.2

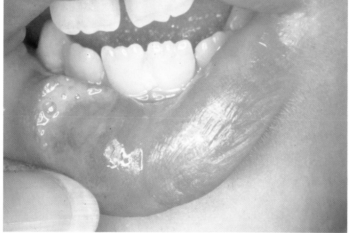

7.3

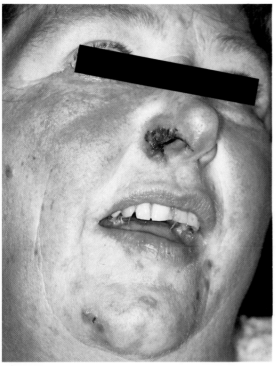

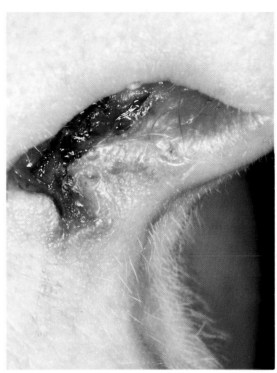

7.4

7.5

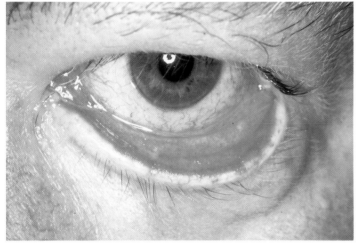

7.6

Sensory loss may be central in origin (cerebrovascular disease and anomalies, syringobulbia, cerebral neoplasm, or trauma) or peripheral (trauma, neoplasm or infection). **Figures 7.4** and **7.5** show a patient who had a cerebral neoplasm resulting in lesions of cranial nerves V and VI. Subsequently she repeatedly traumatized her nose and mouth on the right side. Trophic ulceration has also been reported.

Other causes include bone disease; drugs; neuropathy; a premonitory feature in the occasional patient with trigeminal neuralgia; an acute spontaneously resolving idiopathic neuropathy; and neuropathy associated with HIV infection, systemic sclerosis, mixed connective tissue disease or other autoimmune states.

PARKINSONISM

There are no specific oral lesions in parkinsonism but there can be oral neglect and salivary dysfunction, or facial dyskinesias can result from drug therapy (*see* Section 1.5, page 56).

CEREBRO-VASCULAR ACCIDENT

One of the most common causes of facial palsy is stroke, when there is often unilateral facial palsy with ipsilateral hemiplegia. An upper motor neurone lesion as in a stroke, causes paralysis mainly of the contralateral lower face, but involuntary movement is preserved: for instance, laughing can still produce facial movement. Perhaps the greatest danger from facial palsy is to the eye on the affected side, since poor eyelid closure and defective corneal reflex exposes the cornea to damage (**Figure 7.6**).

BELL'S PALSY

Bell's palsy is an acute lower motor neurone facial palsy of unknown aetiology, possibly viral. **Figures 7.7** and **7.8** show a patient during, and **Figure 7.9** after, an attack of right-sided palsy.

Typically, Bell's palsy affects young or middle-aged patients and is acute and unilateral, often preceded by mild pain around the ear region and sometimes a degree of hypo-aesthesia. The mouth droops on the side affected — the patient's right in **Figure 7.7**.

Although usually a mononeuropathy, Bell's palsy may be part of a more widespread cranial or even peripheral polyneuropathy. There are occasional associations with diabetes and with lymphoma.

One complete side of the face is paralysed. Attempts to smile or to whistle reveal the motionless affected side (**Figure 7.8**). The eyelids cannot be closed tightly on that side. Absence of the efferent arc of the corneal reflex presents a hazard to the eye.

Most cases resolve spontaneously in a few weeks (**Figure 7.9**) but it may be prudent to give a short course of systemic corticosteroids to try and avoid permanent nerve damage.

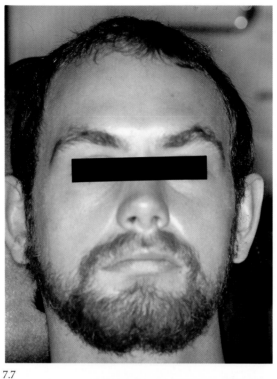

7.7

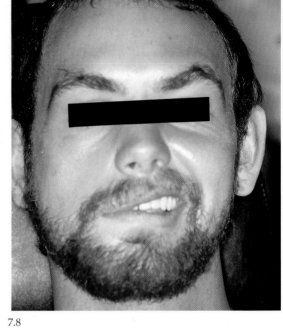

7.8

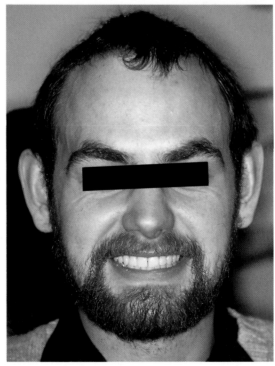

7.9

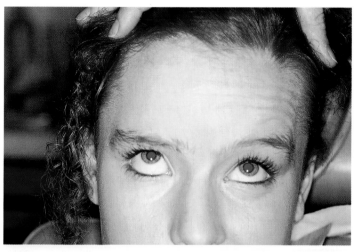

7.10

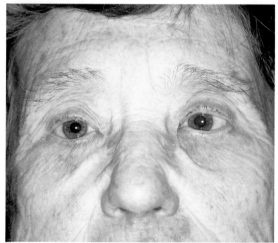

7.11

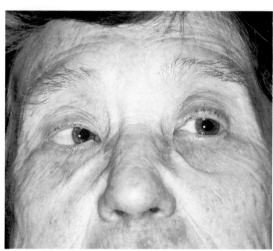

7.12

OTHER LOWER MOTOR NEURONE FACIAL LESIONS

Lower motor neurone (LMN) facial palsy is a rare disorder which may be congenital (Moebius' syndrome); or caused by varicella-zoster virus (Ramsay-Hunt syndrome, *see* page 68) or by HIV; or seen in association with sarcoidosis (Heerfordt's syndrome, *see* page 101), Melkersson–Rosenthal syndrome (*see* page 227), Guillain–Barré syndrome, leprosy (*see* page 63), Kawasaki disease (mucocutaneous lymph node syndrome) or Lyme disease (tick-borne infection with *Borrelia burgdorferi*).

LMN facial palsy is characterized by unilateral paralysis of all muscles of facial expression for voluntary and emotional responses. The forehead is unfurrowed and the patient unable to close the eye on that side. Upon attempted closure the eye rolls upwards (Bell's sign) (**Figure 7.10**).

ABDUCENT NERVE LESION

The abducent (cranial nerve VI) arises from the pons, has the longest intracranial course of any cranial nerve, and can be damaged by lesions in the posterior or middle cranial fossae, or the orbit. Abducent nerve palsy can be an early feature of an aneurysm on the circle of Willis. The nerve supplies the lateral rectus muscle which abducts the eye. **Figure 7.11** shows a patient with a left abducent nerve palsy looking forwards. **Figure 7.12** demonstrates that when the patient tries to look to her left, the left eye cannot abduct.

GLOSSO-PHARYNGEAL AND VAGUS NERVE PALSY

In glossopharyngeal and vagus nerve palsy the palatal sensation and, therefore, the gag reflex are impaired. The uvula deviates away from the affected side (**Figure 7.13**). This patient had deficits of cranial nerves IX to XII inclusive (bulbar palsy) from a posterior cranial fossa neoplasm.

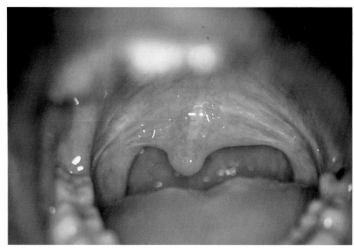

7.13

LATERAL MEDULLARY SYNDROME

Occlusion of the inferior artery of the lateral medulla oblongata, or occasionally of the posterior inferior cerebellar artery or vertebral artery, produces a syndrome of contralateral impairment of pain and thermal sense (damage to the spinothalamic tract); ipsilateral Horner's syndrome (damage to the sympathetic tract); hoarseness, dysphagia, and ipsilateral palatal palsy, as shown in **Figure 7.14** (IX and X cranial nerve palsies); sensory loss over the ipsilateral face (damage to V nerve nuclei); vestibular signs; and loss of taste (damage to tractus solitarius).

Asymmetry of the soft palate is demonstrated in **Figure 7.14** by the naso-gastric tube which marks the midline.

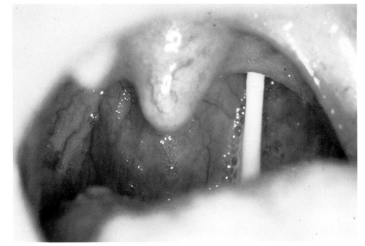

7.14

HYPOGLOSSAL NERVE LESION

The hypoglossal nerve arises from the medulla and supplies motor fibres to most tongue muscles. Lower motor neurone lesions are rare but cause paralysis and wasting of the ipsilateral half of the tongue (**Figure 7.15**). On protrusion, the tongue often deviates to the affected side. Rarely, lingual carcinoma may involve the hypoglossal nerve.

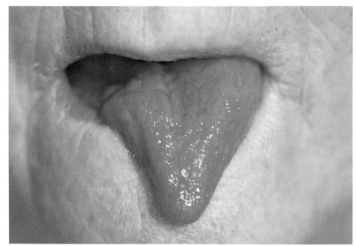

7.15

8 DISEASES OF THE CIRCULATORY SYSTEM

154

PERIARTERITIS NODOSA (*Polyarteritis nodosa*, PAN)

Periarteritis nodosa is a necrotizing vasculitis of small- and medium-sized arteries, affecting mainly males and often related to previous infection with hepatitis B virus. Arthralgia, angina, hypertension and renal disease are the main features. Oral nodules, bleeding or ulcers (**Figure 8.1**) may be seen.

WEGENER'S GRANULOMATOSIS

This is a rare disorder with granulomatous lesions in the respiratory tract, generalized necrotizing vasculitis and, later, focal necrotizing glomerulo-nephritis. Gingival swelling, mucosal ulcers or delayed wound healing are the main oral features. Up to 5% have oral lesions: the most pathognomonic is gingival swelling with a resemblance to a ripe strawberry (gingival hyperplasia with petechiae) (**Figure 8.2**).

Occasionally, a limited form of the disease, involving only one or two organ systems, is seen.

MIDLINE GRANULOMA (*Idiopathic midfacial granuloma syndrome*)

This is a group of rare disorders, now recognized as being lymphomas, starting in the nasal or paranasal tissues, causing destruction of the facial bones (**Figure 8.3**). This clinical syndrome can result from Stewart's granuloma, lymphomatoid granulomatosis or polymorphic reticulosis.

SUBLINGUAL VARICES

Dilated lingual veins give rise to varices, common in the elderly (**Figure 8.4**), and are of no special significance. There are occasional associations with varices elsewhere in the body, including the jejunum and scrotum.

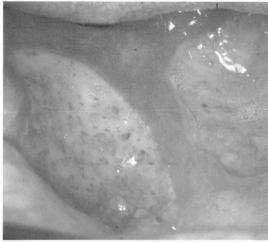

8.1

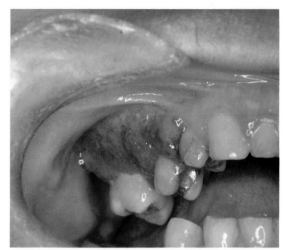

8.2

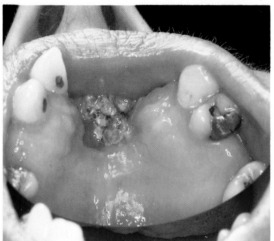

8.3

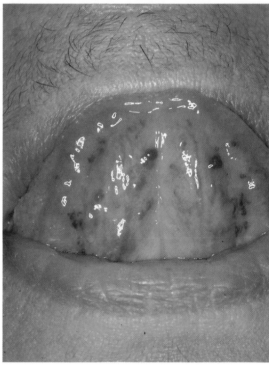

8.4

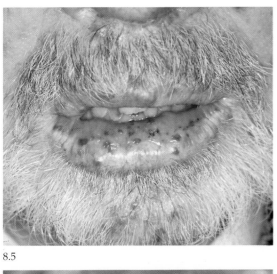

8.5

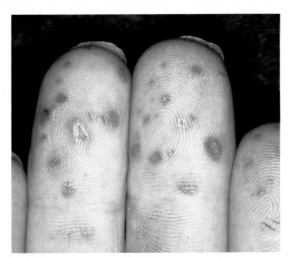

8.6

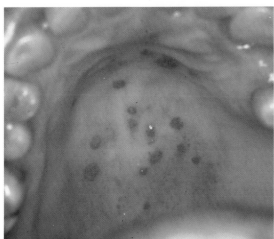

8.7

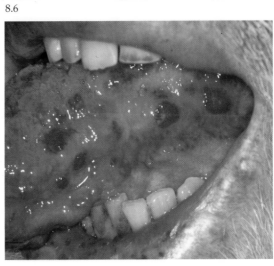

8.8

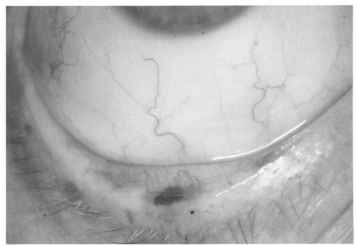

8.9

HEREDITARY HAEMORRHAGIC TELANGIECTASIA (*Osler–Rendu–Weber syndrome*)

Hereditary haemorrhagic telangiectasia (HHT) is an autosomal dominant condition characterized by mucosal and cutaneous telangiectases which appear on the lips and periorally, often well after birth (**Figure 8.5**). Occasional telangiectases appear on the extremities; particularly on the palmar surfaces of the digits (**Figure 8.6**). The mucosal telangiectases are found in the mouth (**Figure 8.7**), nasal, and alimentary mucosa.

The telangiectases may result in repeated haemorrhage (**Figure 8.8**), leading eventually to severe anaemia and even cardiac failure.

Occasional telangiectases affect other mucosae, such as the conjunctiva (**Figure 8.9**). Retinal telangiectases predispose to intraocular bleeding. Pulmonary arteriovenous fistulae, central nervous system and hepatic vascular anomalies predispose to complications.

HHT has occasional associations with von Willebrand's disease, and with IgA deficiency.

156

GIANT-CELL ARTERITIS

Giant-cell, or temporal, arteritis is a granulomatous arteritis, sometimes termed Horton's disease, which involves medium and larger arteries, particularly branches of the aortic arch, and is found mainly in older women. It is closely related to polymyalgia rheumatica.

Apart from low-grade fever, anorexia, weight loss and generalized aches and pains, there are often manifestations in the head and neck including temporal pain and tenderness and headache, and neuro-ophthalmic features, particularly sudden blindness. Patients may also have jaw or masseteric pain, or may have pain in the tongue, particularly during chewing. Lingual arteritis is common, presenting as pain or ulceration (**Figure 8.10**).

Although the tongue has an excellent blood supply and usually survives, lingual necrosis has now been described in several patients with giant cell arteritis. The lingual necrosis is almost invariably unilateral, and only very rare cases of bilateral necrosis (**Figure 8.11**) have been reported. Labial gangrene (**Figure 8.12**) is another rare complication of giant-cell arteritis.

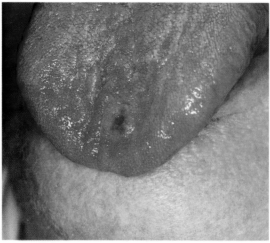
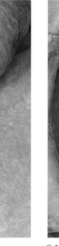
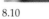

8.10

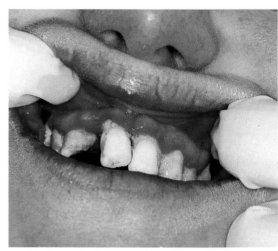

8.11

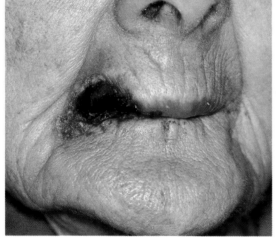

8.12

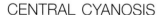

8.13

CENTRAL CYANOSIS

Central cyanosis is readily demonstrable in the oral soft tissues (**Figure 8.13**; *see also* **Figures** 16.3 and **16.4**).

ISCHAEMIC HEART DISEASE

Angina occasionally produces pain which radiates to the jaw or palate. Use of calcium-channel blockers such as nifedipine may lead to gingival hyperplasia (**Figure 8.14**). Beta-blockers may cause lichenoid lesions.

HEART TRANSPLANTATION

Drugs used after cardiac transplantation may produce oral adverse side-effects. The most common are gingival hyperplasia (cyclosporin or nifedepine, *see* **Figure 17.10**) and candidosis (corticosteroids). Other oral complications may include hairy leukoplakia — as in persons with other organ transplants (*see* page 76).

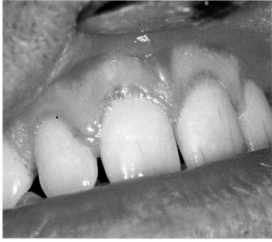

8.14

9 DISEASES OF THE RESPIRATORY SYSTEM

STREPTOCOCCAL TONSILLITIS

Caused by *Streptococcus pyogenes* (Lancefield Group A beta haemolytic streptococcus), the incubation period of 2–4 days is followed by sore throat, dysphagia and fever. Usually children are affected. The uvula, tonsils and pharynx are diffusely red, with punctate white or yellow tonsillar exudates (**Figure 9.1**). Complications are rare but can include otitis media, quinsy, sinusitis, rheumatic fever or glomerulonephritis.

Any form of tonsillitis can cause halitosis.

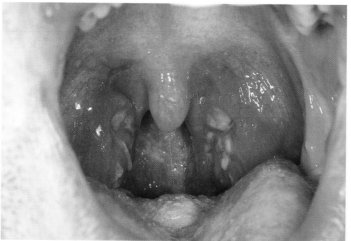
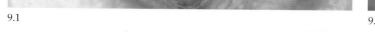

9.1

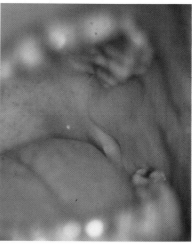

9.2

QUINSY (*Peritonsillar abscess*)

Peritonsillar abscess, although usually following *Streptococcus pyogenes* infection, typically contains a variety of oropharyngeal micro-organisms. The abscess causes severe pain, dysphagia and trismus before pointing (**Figure 9.2**) and discharging.

INFLUENZA

Oral lesions have not often been reported in influenza but ulcers (**Figure 9.3**), pericoronitis, gingivitis and soft palate hyperaemia have been described.

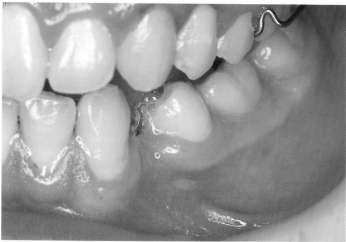

9.3

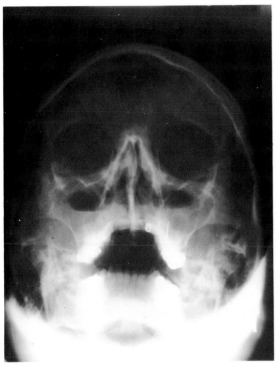

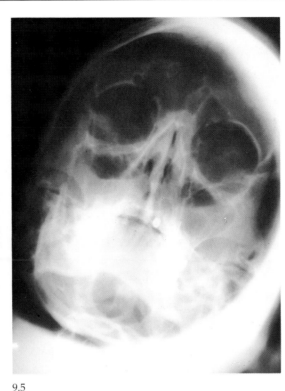

9.4

9.5

MAXILLARY SINUSITIS

Acute sinusitis is usually preceded by an upper respiratory tract viral infection but occasionally follows an oroantral fistula or displacement of a tooth or root into the sinus. Pain is felt over the antrum, especially on moving the head, and the ipsilateral premolars and molars may be tender to percussion. There may be halitosis. Transillumination or occipitomental radiography show opacities in the affected antra (**Figure 9.4**).

Tilting the head (**Figure 9.5**) shows that the bilateral antral opacities in this case are fluid.

Sinusitis is also a complication of cystic fibrosis, Kartagener's syndrome (immobile cilia and dextrocardia), HIV disease and various other immunodeficiencies. Such patients may also have enamel hypoplasia.

ANTRAL CARCINOMA

See page 108 and **Figures 3.20** and **3.21**.

CYSTIC FIBROSIS

Cystic fibrosis, which produces serious pulmonary and pancreatic disease, may result also in sinusitis and xerostomia.

LUNG CANCER

Oral changes are rare in lung cancer but may include metastases (*see* **Figure 3.40**), orofacial pain, or hyperpigmentation — particularly of the soft palate.

10 DISEASES OF THE DIGESTIVE SYSTEM

HYPODONTIA

Isolated hypodontia is fairly common, may have a genetic basis, and affects mainly the permanent dentition, particularly third molars, second premolars or upper lateral incisors (**Figure 10.1**). The right upper deciduous lateral incisor is retained (**Figure 10.1**), a common occurrence when the permanent successor is missing.

Teeth may be apparently missing in many cases because they are impacted and thus fail to erupt. Rarely, eruption is delayed because of systemic disease, such as cretinism or Down's syndrome or because of radio- or chemotherapy.

Figures 10.2 and **10.3** show congenital absence of several teeth. In **Figure 10.2** the retained lower deciduous central incisors are discoloured because they are non-vital, having been worn down by attrition which has caused pulpal exposure, as shown, and pulp necrosis. The permanent central incisors in **Figure 10.3** are congenitally absent.

Figure 10.4 shows a radiograph showing several missing teeth in an otherwise healthy person (same patient as in **Figure 10.1**).

Hypodontia is a feature of local disorders such as cleft palate, and of many systemic disorders. In some, the teeth are present but fail to erupt; in others, such as ectodermal dysplasia (**Figure 10.5**), or incontinentia pigmenti, they are truly missing (*see* page 288). Rarely, all teeth are absent (anodontia).

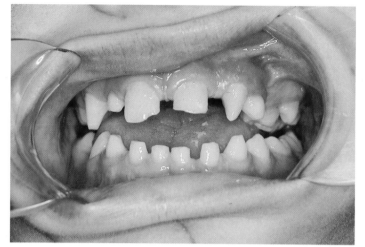

10.1

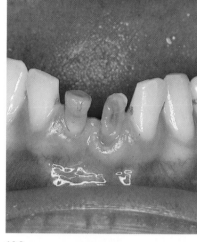

10.2

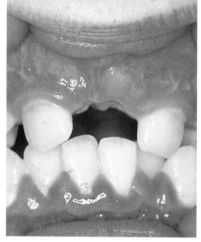

10.3

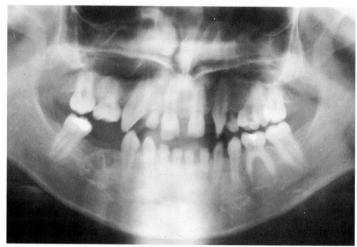

10.4

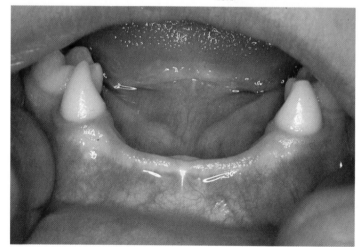

10.5

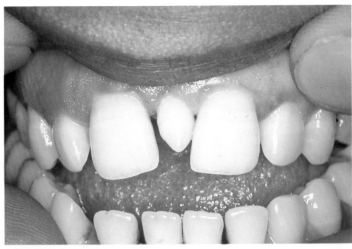

10.6

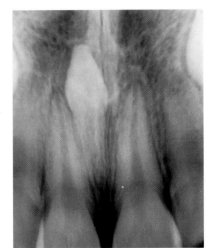

10.7

HYPERDONTIA

Additional teeth are usually of simple conical shape (supernumerary) and are most common in the upper incisor region. If midline (**Figure 10.6**) the tooth is termed a mesiodens. Supernumerary teeth may cause malocclusion, occasionally impede tooth eruption, or, rarely, are the site of cyst formation.

Although a mesiodens may erupt, sometimes it is inverted (**Figure 10.7**).

Additional teeth often erupt in an abnormal position (**Figure 10.8**). This malocclusion may predispose to caries or periodontal disease.

Extra maxillary molars resemble normal teeth and are thus termed supplemental (or sometimes distodens) (**Figure 10.9**).

Supernumerary teeth are usually seen in otherwise healthy patients but occasionally are a manifestation of a systemic disorder such as cleidocranial dysplasia (*see* page 278) or Gardner's syndrome (*see* page 200).

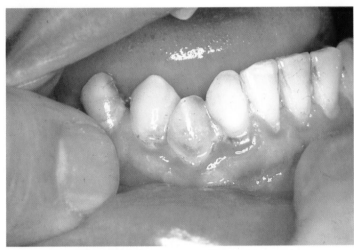

10.8

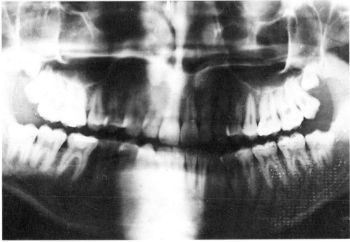

10.9

FUSION

Fusion (union of two normally separate, adjacent tooth germs) gives rise to a large tooth with one tooth obviously missing from the series (**Figure 10.10**), unless the fusion is with a supernumerary tooth.

Fusion may be complete along the length of the teeth (**Figure 10.11**) or may involve roots alone.

Fused or geminated teeth may give rise to poor aesthetics (**Figure 10.12**) and sometimes malocclusions.

GEMINATION (*Geminated odontome*)

An odontome is a developmental malformation of dental tissues. Gemination is a result of incomplete attempted division of a tooth germ. Usually seen in the incisor region, the crowns may be separate or divided by a shallow groove (**Figure 10.13**). However, the root is shared.

It is often difficult to differentiate gemination from fusion (**Figure 10.14**): the terms 'double tooth' or 'twinning' are therefore sometimes used.

Double teeth are seen most commonly, but not invariably, in the incisor and canine regions and may be seen elsewhere (**Figure 10.15**) and in the deciduous and permanent dentitions.

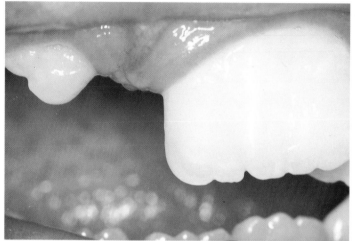

10.10

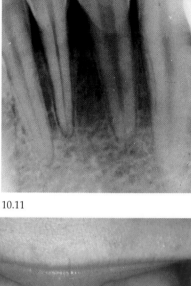

10.11

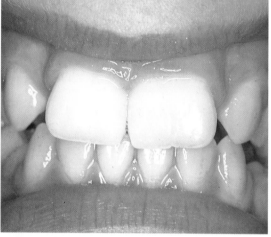

10.12

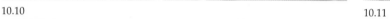

10.13

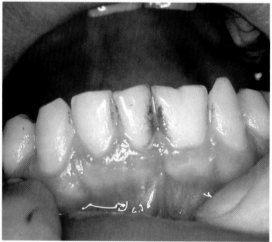

10.14

10.15

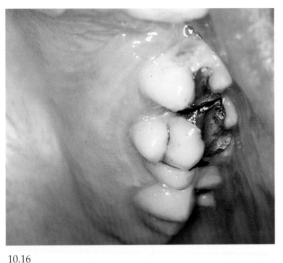

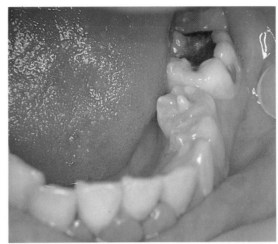

CUSP OF CARABELLI

This is an anatomical variant — a palatal cusp on the upper first molar (**Figure 10.16**).

EVAGINATED ODONTOME (*Dens evaginatus*)

A small occlusal nodule is seen, especially in mongoloid races (**Figure 10.17**). Since the nodule contains a pulp horn, pulpitis is not uncommon when there is attrition.

10.16

10.17

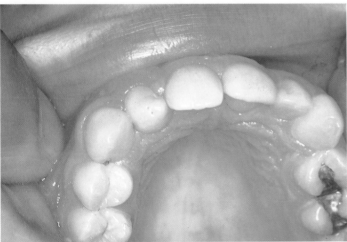

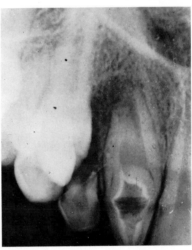

INVAGINATED ODONTOME (*Dilated odontome, dens in dente*)

Invagination of enamel and dentine in the *dens in dente* may also dilate the affected tooth (**Figure 10.18**).

Ameloblasts invaginate during development to form a pouch of enamel such that a radiograph shows what resembles a tooth within a tooth (**Figure 10.19**). This odontome is prone to caries development in the abnormal pouch.

10.18

10.19

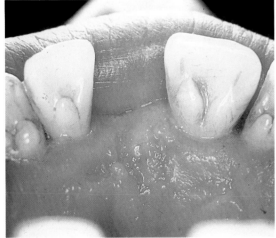

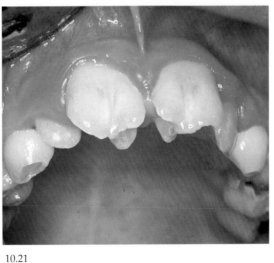

PROMINENT TUBERCULES OR CUSPS

Prominent tubercles are shown in **Figure 10.20**.

Teeth are occasionally malformed with a large palatal cusp, to the extent that they have a talon cusp configuration (**Figure 10.21**).

10.20

10.21

PEG-SHAPED LATERAL INCISOR

This is the most common anomaly of tooth shape and produces a cosmetic problem (**Figure 10.22**)

ENAMEL NODULE (*Enameloma, enamel pearl*)

A small circular mass of enamel is seen on the tooth surface near the cemento–enamel junction (**Figure 10.23**)

Sometimes the enamel nodule contains dentine and pulp. Nodules are most common on maxillary teeth (**Figure 10.24**).

TAURODONTISM

Taurodontism is the term applied to teeth that clinically look normal but on radiograph resemble those of ungulates (hence the Latin origin, *taurus*, a bull). The crown is long, the roots short (**Figure 10.25**). Taurodontism is usually a simple racial trait but may rarely be associated with some chromosome anomalies such as Klinefelter's syndrome; tricho–dento–osseous syndrome; orofacial–digital syndrome; ectodermal dysplasia; or amelogenesis imperfecta. In the tricho–dento–osseous syndrome there is also enamel hypoplasia, curly hair and thickening of cortical bone.

Taurodont teeth lack a pronounced constriction at the neck of the tooth and are parallel-sided. The floor of the pulp chamber is lower than normal and the pulp appears extremely large (**Figure 10.26**). Taurodontism usually affects permanent molars, especially the lower second molar, sometimes only one in the arch, but may affect teeth in the deciduous dentition.

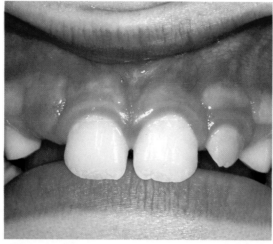

10.22

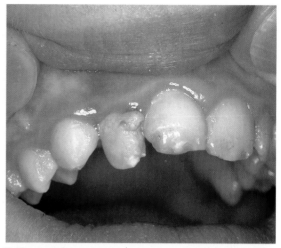

10.23

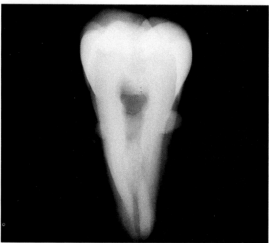

10.24

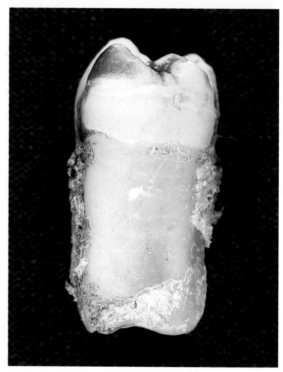

10.25

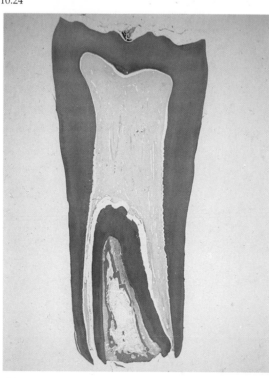

10.26

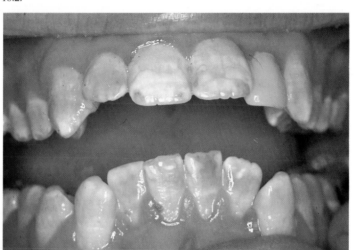

10.27

FLUOROSIS

Mottling of the enamel may be seen where the fluoride in drinking water exceeds about 2 ppm or excess fluoride is taken via other sources, although in the mildest form it may not produce a cosmetic defect. Mottling in mild fluorosis is usually seen as white flecks or patches (**Figure 10.27**). The mottling here is enough to require the cosmetic crowning of the upper anterior teeth. An example of mottling more severe than in **Figure 10.27** is shown in **Figure 10.28**.

Severe fluorosis causes opacity and brown and white staining and pitting of the entire enamel (**Figure 10.29**). This can be difficult clinically to differentiate from amelogenesis imperfecta (*see* page 169).

NON-FLUORIDE ENAMEL OPACITIES

Whitish flecks are not uncommon (**Figure 10.30**) and are often idiopathic.

10.28

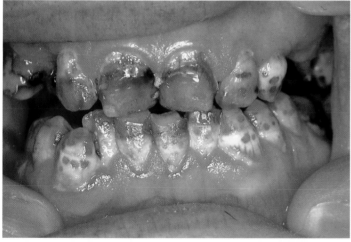

10.29

10.30

ENAMEL HYPOPLASIA

Tooth development can be disturbed by constitutional disturbances in childhood, such as fevers, coeliac disease, cystic fibrosis, gastroenteritis and radiotherapy or chemotherapy, producing a linear pattern of defects corresponding to the site of amelogenesis at the time ('chronological' hypoplasia). Horizontal pits or grooves are usually seen in the incisal third of the crowns of permanent teeth (**Figure 10.31**). Intrauterine infections such as rubella, or metabolic disturbances, may cause hypoplasia of the deciduous dentition.

In **Figure 10.32**, mottling and hypoplasia of the deciduous dentition was caused by intrauterine disease — here by pseudohypoparathyroidism (*see* page 125). Enamel hypoplasia may also appear in the absence of any identifiable cause.

DILACERATION

Trauma to a developing tooth may produce distortion and dilaceration — a bend (**Figure 10.33**).

ISOLATED HYPOPLASIA (*Turner tooth*)

Infection of, or trauma to, a deciduous tooth, may cause hypoplasia of the underlying permanent successor (**Figure 10.34**).

In **Figure 10.35**, the lower second premolar was deformed after an abscess on the predecessor deciduous molar. The malformed Turner tooth has subsequently become carious.

In **Figure 10.36**, comparison of a normal premolar (on the reader's left) with a Turner tooth shows the degree of deformity that can result.

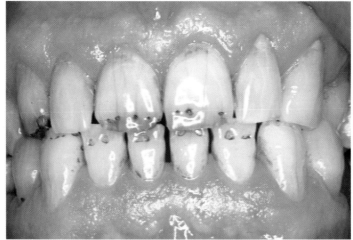

10.31

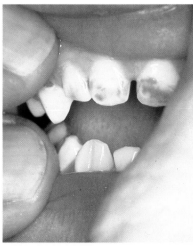

10.32

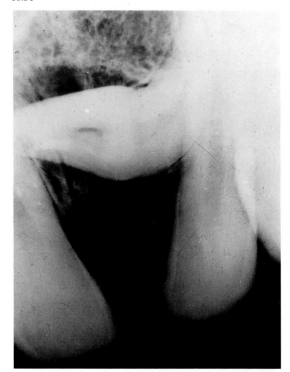

10.33

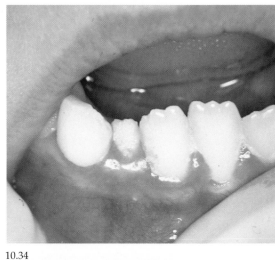

10.34

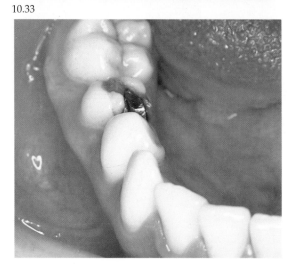

10.35

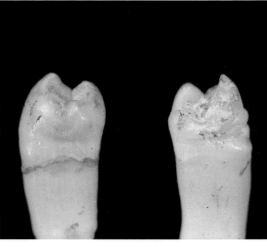

10.36

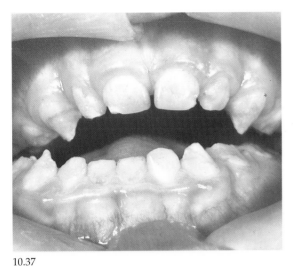

10.37

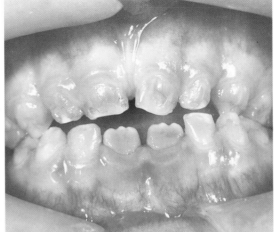

10.38

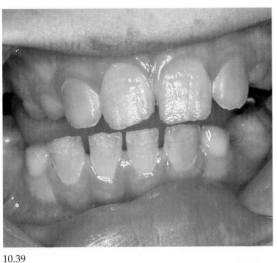

10.39

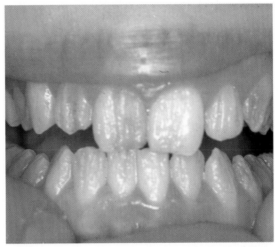

10.40

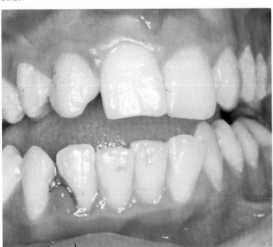

10.41

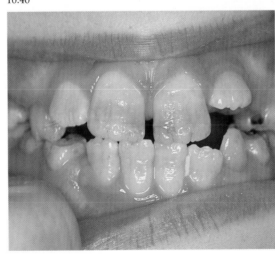

10.42

AMELOGENESIS IMPERFECTA

Amelogenesis imperfecta is the term applied to a number of rare genetically-determined disorders of enamel formation. **Figure 10.37** shows an affected primary dentition.

There are three main types of amelogenesis imperfecta: in hypoplastic types the enamel is thin; in hypocalcified types it is of normal thickness but weak and soft; and in hypomaturation types it can be pierced with a probe.

Figure 10.38 is of a sibling of the patient in **Figure 10.37**, and shows the genetic basis and the fact that the primary and secondary dentitions (the permanent central incisors are erupting) are both affected.

Figure 10.39 shows an example of hereditary enamel hypoplasia of an autosomal dominant type. The enamel matrix is defective, although calcification is normal (note the vertical ridging). **Figure 10.40** shows a more extreme example: a sex-linked dominant type.

Pitting and grooving is seen in some types of hereditary enamel hypoplasia (**Figure 10.41**). **Figure 10.42** shows a more extreme example of the type of hereditary enamel hypoplasia shown in **Figure 10.41**.

(Contd)

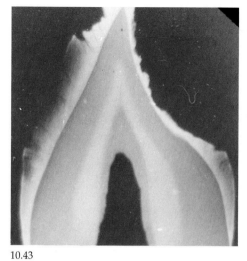

10.43

AMELOGENESIS IMPERFECTA
(Contd)

Radiographs show enamel deficiencies in hereditary enamel hypoplasia (**Figures 10.43** and **10.44**).

Hereditary enamel hypocalcification is the second main type of amelogenesis imperfecta — the matrix is normal but calcification defective. The soft enamel may wear away rapidly to leave only the dentine core (**Figure 10.45**). In **Figure 10.46**, there is almost complete breakdown of the dentition, and incidental calculus deposition.

The third main type of amelogenesis imperfecta is hereditary enamel hypomaturation. **Figure 10.47** shows opaque white flecks or patches in an autosomal dominant variety ('snow capped' teeth), whilst **Figure 10.48** shows a variant affecting permanent first molars only.

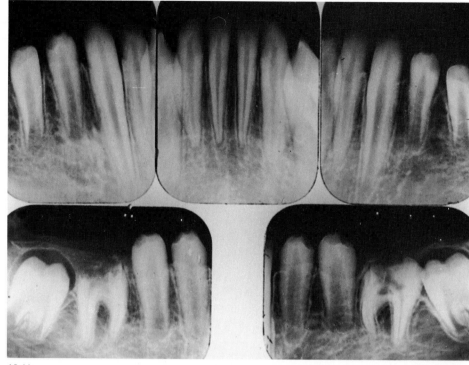

10.44

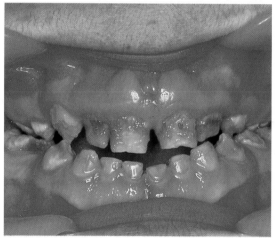

10.45

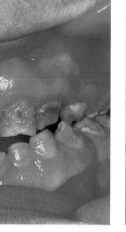

10.46

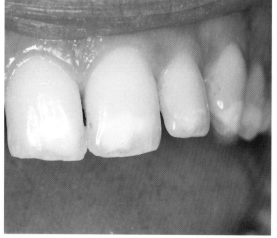

10.47

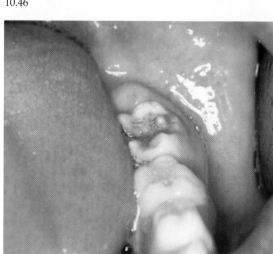

10.48

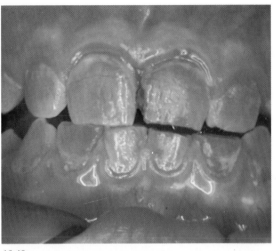

10.49

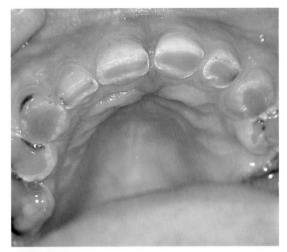

10.50

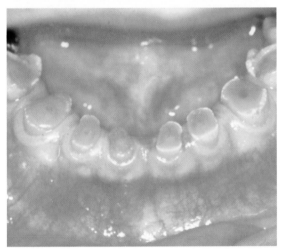

10.51

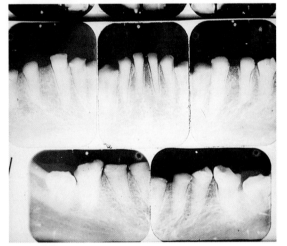

10.52

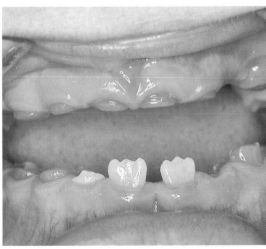

10.53

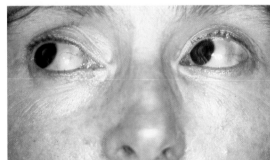

10.54

DENTINOGENESIS IMPERFECTA

Dentinogenesis imperfecta is an autosomal dominant condition in which the dentine is abnormal in structure and is translucent. **Figure 10.49** shows Type I dentinogenesis imperfecta, with translucent brown teeth, but teeth may vary in colour from grey to blue or brown.

The tooth crowns are bulbous and the roots short. The enamel, though normal, is poorly adherent to the abnormal dentine and chips and wears (**Figure 10.50**).

Ultimately the teeth are worn flat by attrition (**Figure 10.51**) but, fortunately, the pulp chambers are obliterated by secondary dentine and, therefore, are not exposed. The roots, however, fracture easily. Pulp obliteration can be seen on radiography (**Figure 10.52**).

The deciduous dentition is often more severely affected than the permanent, especially in coronal dentine dysplasia or Type II dentine dysplasia (**Figure 10.53**). Radiographs show flame-shaped pulp chambers and narrow pulp canals. There may be several pulp stones in most teeth. Hereditary opalescent dentine is an alternative term for Type II dentinogenesis imperfecta.

Type III dentinogenesis imperfecta is associated with osteogenesis imperfecta. The deciduous dentition is more severely affected than the permanent teeth. Dentinogenesis imperfecta appears frequently in those patients with osteogenesis imperfecta who have normal, rather than blue sclerae (**Figure 10.54**).

(Contd)

DENTINOGENESIS IMPERFECTA
(Contd)

In Type IV dentinogenesis imperfecta, dentine formation ceases after the initial mantle layer, leaving teeth that are shell-like (**Figure 10.55**).

NATAL TEETH

Rarely, teeth are present at, or soon after, birth and have been described even at 26 weeks' gestation. They may cause no trouble but may ulcerate the tongue (**Figure 10.56**), or the breast if suckling. Usually the teeth involved are lower incisors of the normal primary dentition: occasionally they are supernumeraries. Rarely, there are associations with Ellis–van Creveld syndrome; pachyonychia congenita; Hallermann–Streiff syndrome, or steatocystoma multiplex.

If there are problems from natal teeth, radiographs should be taken before extractions are contemplated (**Figure 10.57**). Extractions are best restricted to those teeth that are supernumeraries or are very loose and in danger of being inhaled.

TERATOMA

Cystic ovarian teratomas (dermoid) may contain well-formed teeth (**Figure 10.58**).

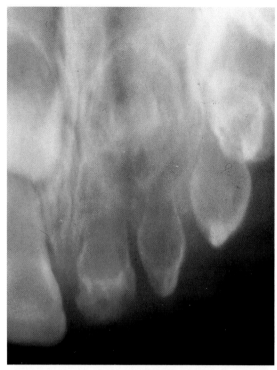

10.55

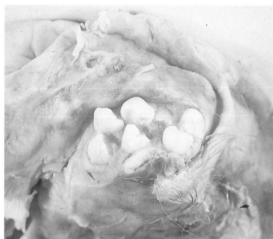

10.56

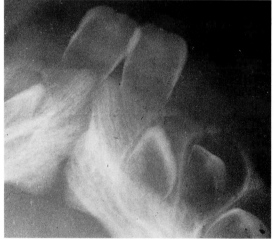

10.57

10.58

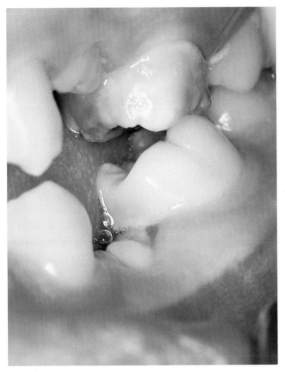

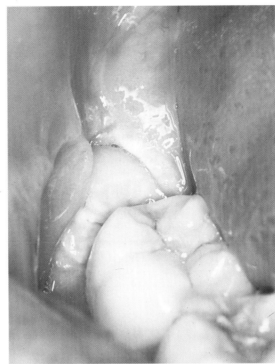

10.59

10.60

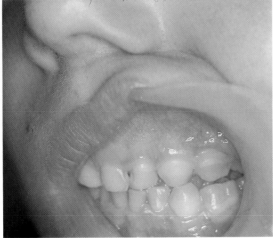

10.61

RETAINED PRIMARY TOOTH

Primary teeth are commonly retained if the successor is missing. Usually this is of little consequence but occasionally, particularly in the case of lower deciduous molars, the tooth fails to maintain its occlusal relationship (infraocclusion or submergence) (**Figure 10.59**).

IMPACTED TEETH

Lower third molars (as here) are the most common teeth to impact, that is, fail to erupt fully because of insufficient space (**Figure 10.60**). Canines and second premolars as well as other teeth also impact commonly. Impacted teeth may well be asymptomatic but occasionally cause pain, usually from caries or pericoronitis, or are the site of dentigerous cyst formation.

BILE PIGMENT STAINING

Haemolytic disease of the newborn (icterus gravis neonatorum) is now rare but more infants survive with hyperbilirubinaemia of other cause. Jaundice in either case may cause enamel hypoplasia in the deciduous dentition, which may have a greenish colour (**Figure 10.61**; *see also* **Figure 11.1**).

Congenital erythropoietic porphyria may cause yellow to brown–red tooth discoloration.

174

TETRACYCLINE STAINING

Tetracyclines are taken up by developing teeth and by bone. If given to pregnant or nursing mothers or to children under the age of 8 years, the tooth crowns become discoloured, initially being yellow but darkening with time. This shows very clearly in **Figure 10.62**, since the permanent teeth that formed after the drug was given in pregnancy have a normal appearance.

Staining of the permanent dentition — yellow and brown bands of staining — is most obvious at the necks of the teeth where the thinner enamel allows the colour of the stained dentine to show through (**Figure 10.63**). Staining is greater the larger the dose of tetracycline, and is worse with tetracycline than with oxytetracycline.

More severe staining of the permanent dentition is seen in **Figure 10.64**. Staining is most obvious in light-exposed anterior teeth. The tooth of normal colour is a supernumerary tooth that clearly developed at a time after tetracyclines had been given.

Even in older children, tetracyclines cause staining but by then most tooth crowns have been formed. The staining then affects the roots — as in the lower third molar (**Figure 10.65**).

Affected teeth may fluoresce bright yellow under ultraviolet light and this helps to distinguish tetracycline staining from dentinogenesis imperfecta. Fluorescence is also seen in undecalcified sections viewed under ultraviolet light (**Figure 10.66**).

Nitrofurantoin has also been reported to cause tooth discoloration.

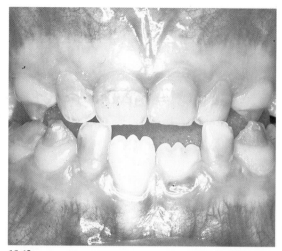

10.62

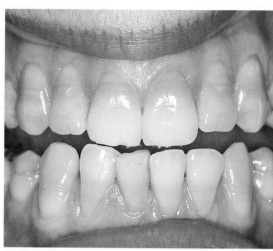

10.63

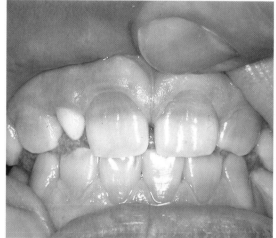

10.64

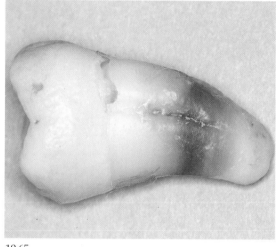

10.65

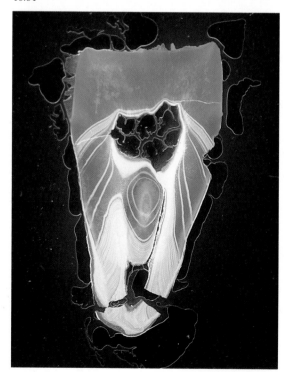

10.66

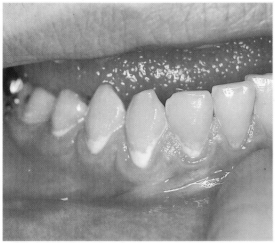

10.67

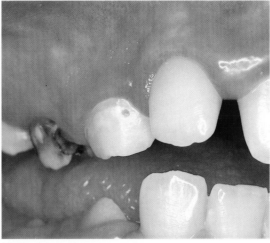

10.68

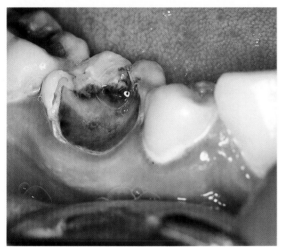

10.69

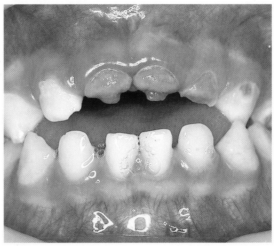

10.70

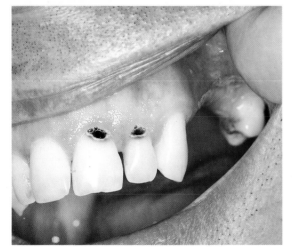

10.71

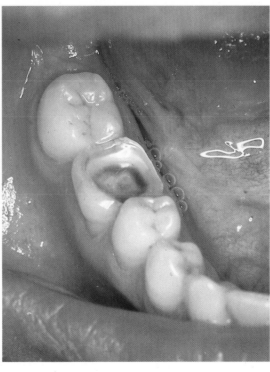

10.72

DENTAL CARIES

Decalcification beneath the bacterial plaque that accumulates in stagnation areas, such as close to the gingival margin, produces an opaque whitish band (**Figure 10.67**). At this early stage, where there is no cavitation, the lesion is reversible if diet is changed and fermentable carbohydrates reduced or excluded. Fluoride aids remineralization.

Figure 10.68 is an upper deciduous canine tooth with early caries. The carious enamel breaks down to form a cavity, as shown.

In **Figure 10.69**, the enamel has been undermined and fractured away. The carious dentine is discolored and this shows through the enamel. Pulpal involvement is inevitable in such carious teeth.

Rampant caries, affecting mainly the upper incisors is typically seen in children using a sugar/fruit juice mix in a bottle to aid sleep at night (**Figure 10.70**).

Change in dietary habits (particularly a reduction in frequency of fermentable carbohydrate intake), fluoride treatment, and improved oral hygiene can arrest the progress of caries. Lesions then darken and become static, as seen in this example at the cervical margins (**Figure 10.71**).

Any change in local environment that makes the various lesions self-cleansing, for example, loss of a tooth adjacent to an interproximal lesion, or fracture of cusps overlying a lesion (**Figure 10.72**), may cause arrest of the caries.

In contrast, xerostomia for any reason significantly predisposes to caries.

ATTRITION

Attrition is wearing away of tooth substance by mastication. It is most obvious where the diet is coarse, the teeth abnormal or where there is a parafunctional habit such as bruxism (**Figure 10.73**). The incisal edges and cusps wear with more loss of dentine than enamel or rarely, in profound vegetative states, Retts syndrome or Fragile X syndrome, leading to a flat or hollowed surface (**Figure 10.74**).

Unless attrition is rapid, the pulp is protected by obliteration with secondary dentine.

ABRASION

Abrasion is wearing away of tooth substance by a habit such as toothbrushing. Brushing with a hard brush and coarse dentifrice may abrade the neck of the tooth. The gingiva recedes but is otherwise healthy. The cementum and dentine wear but the harder enamel survives, resulting in a notch. Eventually, the tooth may fracture (**Figure 10.75**).

LOCALIZED DAMAGE

Seamstress' notch: holding pins, nails, etc, between the teeth can produce a variety of lesions. The patient seen in **Figure 10.76** held pins in her teeth during her work as a seamstress.

Self-mutilation may also occur for aesthetic reasons, according to tribal custom (**Figure 10.77**) (there is also a degree of fluorosis in this case).

EROSION

Erosion is the loss of tooth substance caused by acids. Citrus fruits or carbonated beverages may produce such lesions. Habitual sucking of oranges may cause erosion (**Figure 10.78**). Erosion is also seen where there is gastric regurgitation, such as in alcoholism or anorexia nervosa. Rarely, occupational exposure to acids may produce erosion, and even the low pH of indoor swimming pools may be a cause.

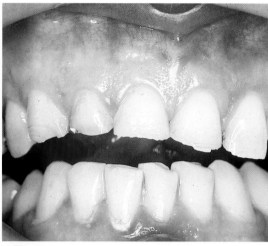

10.73

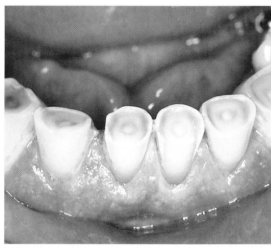

10.74

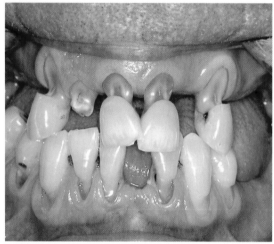

10.75

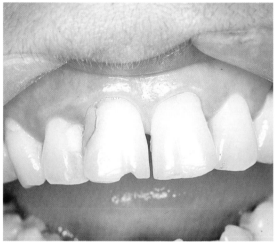

10.76

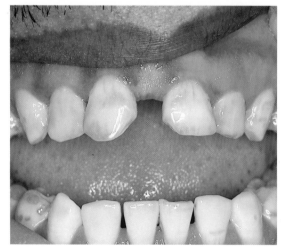

10.77

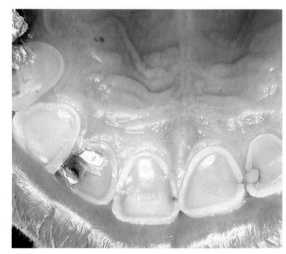

10.78

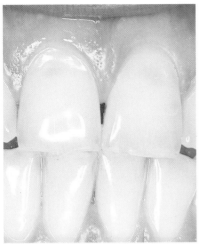

10.79

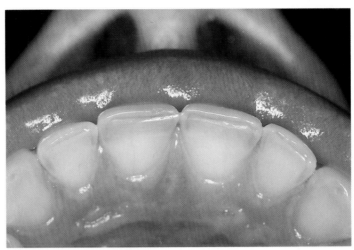

10.80

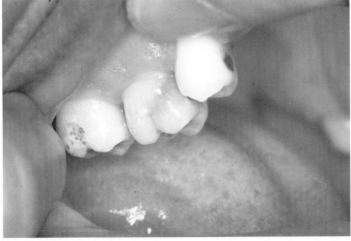

10.81

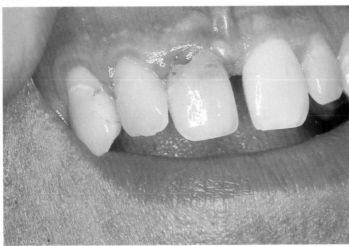

10.82

BULIMIA NERVOSA

Repeated gastric regurgitation over a prolonged period may cause erosion, mainly of the palatal surfaces of the upper teeth. This is seen especially in bulimia nervosa and alcoholism. **Figures 10.79** and **10.80** show a patient with bulimia nervosa.

Other features may include enlargement of salivary glands (mainly parotids) which appears to be sialosis; possible conjunctival suffusion and oesophageal tears (caused by retching); and Russell's sign — abrasions on the back of the hand or fingers caused by using the hand to touch the throat to induce vomiting (*see* page 145).

INTERNAL RESORPTION (*Pink spot*)

In pink spot, dentine is spontaneously resorbed from within and the pulp is eventually exposed (**Figure 10.81**).

Here, the dark brown lesion on the premolar is a result of interproximal caries that has arrested. The lesion on the second molar is a cavity from which the restoration has been lost.

EXTERNAL RESORPTION

Resorption may progress from the external surface, eventually to involve the pulp.

In **Figure 10.82** the maxillary incisor is involved. The canine has a composite restoration. The white semilunar line is decalcification that occurred some years earlier, when the oral hygiene was not so good and the gingiva not so far receded.

178

HYPERCEMENTOSIS

Hypercementosis is usually a consequence of periapical periodontitis, or may affect isolated functionless teeth. Paget's disease of bone may be complicated by hypercementosis (**Figure 10.83**) (*see* page 267).

ANKYLOSIS

Deciduous molars may be retained and in infraocclusion because the permanent successor is absent. (**Figure 10.84** shows bony ankylosis and no evidence of a periodontal ligament.)

POST-ERUPTIVE COLOUR CHANGE OF TEETH

Metal-staining: this is a rare cause of colour change affecting many teeth; it is occupational, affecting workers with chromium (**Figure 10.85**) or lead (*see* pages 59 and 310). Isolated teeth that discolour are usually non-vital or carious.

Non-vital tooth: pulp necrosis from caries or trauma is the usual cause of a non-vital (dead) tooth. The tooth progressively darkens, sometimes to a brownish colour (**Figure 10.86**), and also becomes more brittle.

HYPERPLASTIC PULPITIS
(*Pulp polyp*)

Only when the coronal pulp is widely exposed and there is a very good blood supply does the pulp survive trauma or infection. This situation can occur in young persons, and the pulp becomes hyperplastic and epithelialized (**Figure 10.87**).

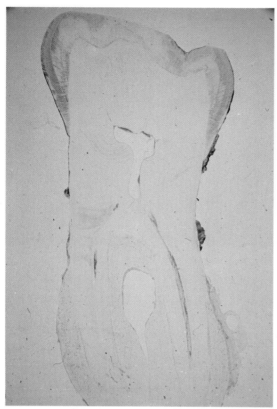

10.83

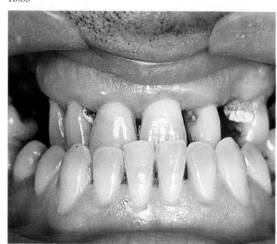

10.85

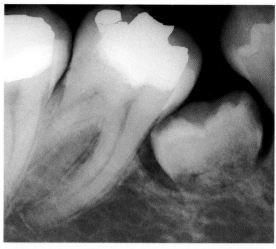

10.84

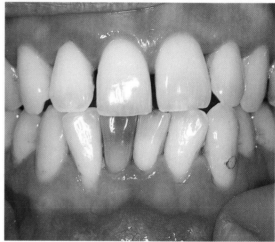

10.86

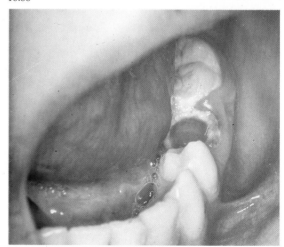

10.87

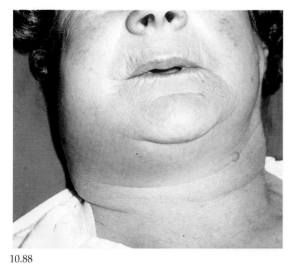

10.88

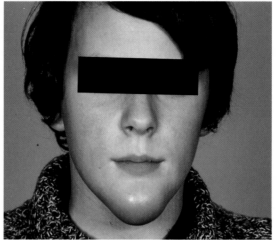

10.89

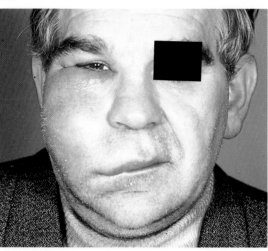

10.90

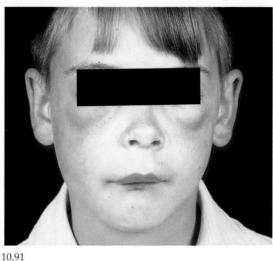

10.91

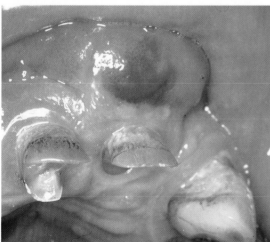

10.92

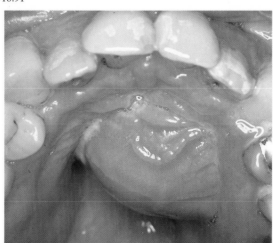

10.93

PERIAPICAL ABSCESS
(*Dental abscess, odontogenic abscess*)

An abscess is often a sequel of pulpitis caused by dental caries, but may arise in relation to any non-vital tooth. A mixed bacterial flora is implicated, although the role of anaerobes such as *Fusobacterium* and *Bacteroides* species is increasingly recognized. Pain and facial swelling, in **Figure 10.88**, from an abscess on a lower molar, are characteristic.

Figure 10.89 shows inflammatory swelling resulting from a dental abscess on a lower incisor. Not all dental abscesses cause facial swelling, however.

Figure 10.90 shows a periapical abscess on an upper premolar causing infraorbital swelling.

Figure 10.91 shows swelling of the infraorbital region and upper lip from a periapical abscess on an upper incisor.

Most dental abscesses also produce an intraoral swelling, typically on the labial or buccal gingiva. In **Figure 10.92**, the large, tender, inflammatory swelling which is about to discharge, is related to pulp exposure from attrition.

Although most periapical abscesses cause swelling buccally, abscesses on maxillary lateral incisors (**Figure 10.93**) and those arising from the palatal roots of the first molar tend to present palatally. The lateral incisor involved here has a deep, carious palatal pit which caused pulp necrosis.

(Contd)

180

PERIAPICAL ABSCESS
(Contd)

Bone destruction caused by a periapical abscess (**Figure 10.94**) on the carious lower permanent molar shows well on this radiograph.

In **Figure 10.95**, the periapical abscess resulted from trauma, rendering the upper deciduous incisor non-vital.

Once the abscess discharges, the acute inflammation, pain and swelling resolve and a chronic abscess develops discharging from a sinus — usually buccally (**Figure 10.96**).

Extraction or endodontic therapy of a tooth affected with a periapical abscess removes the source of infection. **Figure 10.97** shows the pus discharging through the extraction socket.

Occasionally, abscesses — especially those of lower incisors or molars — discharge extraorally (**Figure 10.98**). This sinus arose from a dental abscess on the lower canine. In **Figure 10.99**, the sinus was related to an abscess on the lower first premolar.

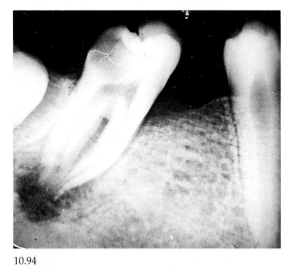

10.94

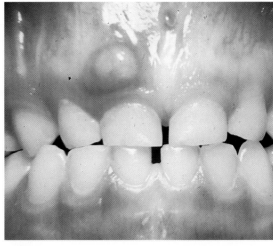

10.95

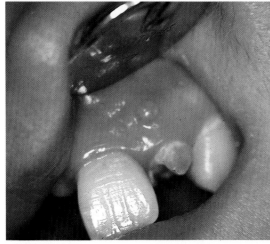

10.96

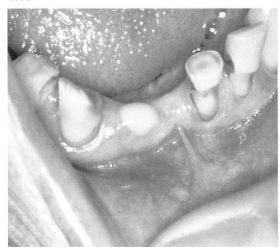

10.97

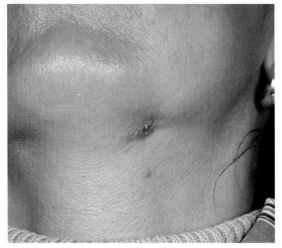

10.98

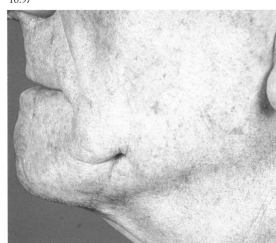

10.99

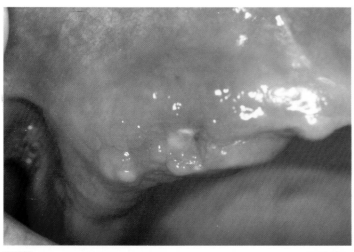

10.100

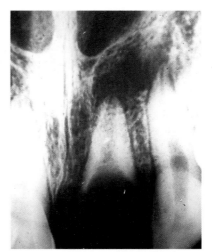

10.101

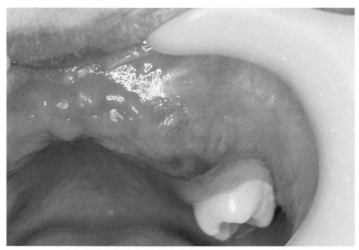

10.102

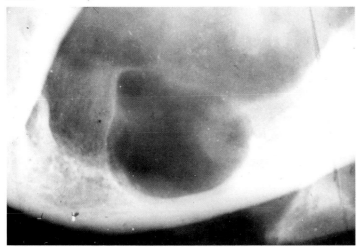

10.103

PERIAPICAL CYST (*Radicular or dental cyst*)

A granuloma may arise at the apex of a non-vital tooth and may occasionally develop into a cyst from proliferation of epithelial rests in the area (cell rests of Malassez). In **Figure 10.100**, there is a retained root in the maxilla with swelling from a cyst. Many periapical cysts involve upper lateral incisors since these not infrequently become carious and the pulp can be involved relatively rapidly.

Most odontogenic cysts are periapical cysts. A periapical cyst may well be asymptomatic and often is a chance radiographic finding. It may present as a swelling (usually in the labial sulcus) or may become infected and present as an abscess. In **Figure 10.101** there is a cyst on the incisor root.

A small periapical cyst may remain attached to, and be extracted with, the causal root or tooth, or resolve with endodontic therapy.

RESIDUAL CYST

A periapical cyst left *in situ* after the causal root or tooth is removed, may continue to expand and is termed a residual cyst. This may produce a bluish swelling (**Figure 10.102**).

A residual cyst is almost invariably unilocular but may expand to an appreciable size. It may be asymptomatic, may be detected as a swelling, a chance radiographic finding (**Figure 10.103**), pathological fracture, or may rarely become infected and present as an abscess.

CHRONIC MARGINAL GINGIVITIS

Most of the population have a degree of gingivitis. Chronic marginal gingivitis (**Figure 10.104**) is caused by the accumulation of dental bacteria plaque on the tooth close to the gingiva. If plaque is not removed it calcifies to become calculus which aggravates the condition by facilitating plaque accumulation.

Inflammation of the margins of the gingiva is painless and often the only features are gingival bleeding on eating or brushing, some halitosis, erythema, swelling (**Figure 10.105**), and bleeding on probing. If left uncorrected this may slowly and painlessly progress to periodontitis and tooth loss.

CHRONIC HYPERPLASTIC GINGIVITIS

Gingivitis may be hyperplastic, especially where there is mechanical irritation, or mouth-breathing, or sometimes with the use of the oral contraceptive or other drugs. Mouth-breathing and poor oral and appliance hygiene are responsible in **Figure 10.106**.

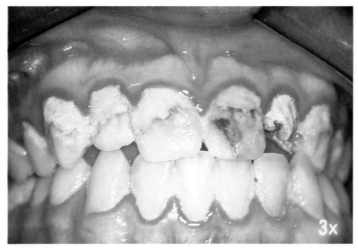

10.104

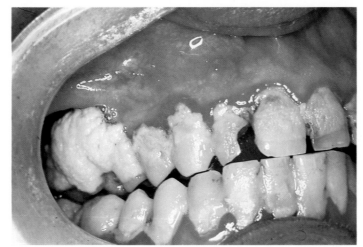

10.105

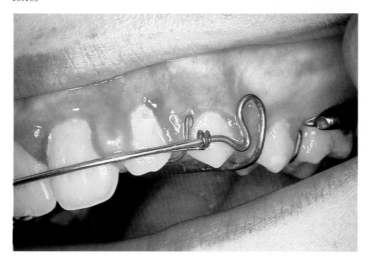

10.106

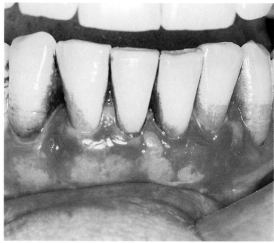

10.107

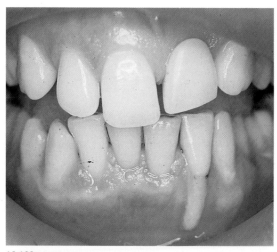

10.108

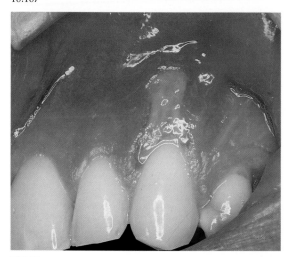

10.109

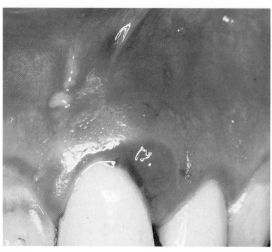

10.110

DESQUAMATIVE GINGIVITIS

Desquamative gingivitis differs from marginal gingivitis in that there is erythema over the attached gingiva, extending into the vestibule: indeed, the gingival margins may be spared (**Figure 10.107**). Mainly seen in middle-aged or elderly females, desquamative gingivitis is typically caused by lichen planus. pemphigoid, or, occasionally, by pemphigus or other vesiculobullous disorders (*see* Chapter 14 and page 15).

LOCALIZED GINGIVAL RECESSION

Isolated recession has exposed the root of the lower lateral incisor in **Figure 10.108**. Incidentally the central incisor has an artificial crown.

ARTEFACTUAL GINGIVAL RECESSION

Self-induced ulcers of the gingival margin are not rare (**Figure 10.109**). The upper canine region seems a common site, and this may be a form of Munchausen's syndrome (*see* page 146).

GINGIVAL ABSCESS

Gingival infection, or a foreign body, may initiate a gingival abscess. **Figure 10.110** is the result of cement pushed into the tissues during cementing the crown on the central incisor.

LATERAL PERIODONTAL ABSCESS (*Parodontal abscess*)

Lateral periodontal abscesses are seen almost exclusively in patients with severe periodontitis, but may follow impaction of a foreign body, or are related to a lateral root canal on a non-vital tooth. Debris and pus cannot escape easily from the pocket and therefore an abscess (**Figure 10.111**), with pain and swelling, results.

Lateral periodontal abscesses usually discharge either through the pocket or buccally, but more coronal than a periapical abscess (**Figure 10.112**).

In **Figure 10.113**, the probe has been gently inserted into a pocket to show continuity with the labial sinus.

ACUTE PERICORONITIS

Inflammation of the operculum over an erupting or impacted tooth is common (**Figure 10.114**). The lower third molar is the site most commonly affected and patients complain of pain, trismus, swelling and halitosis. There may be fever and regional lymphadenitis, and the operculum is swollen, red and often ulcerated.

Acute pericoronitis appears in relation to the accumulation of plaque and trauma from the opposing tooth. Immune defects may predispose.

A mixed flora is implicated and *Fusobacterium* and *Bacteroides* are recognized to be important. Pus usually drains from beneath the operculum but may, in a migratory abscess of the buccal sulcus, track anteriorly (**Figure 10.115**).

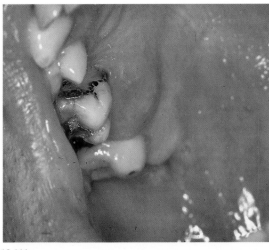

10.111

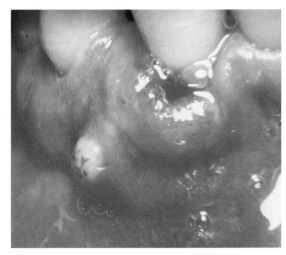

10.112

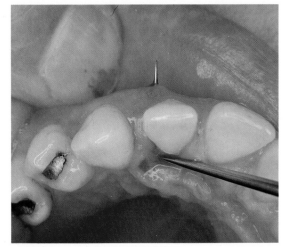

10.113

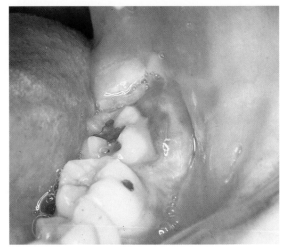

10.114

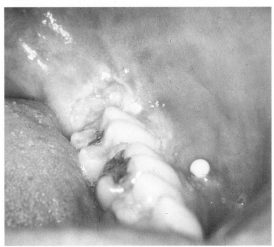

10.115

PERIODONTITIS

Chronic periodontitis is common, related to plaque accumulation, and progresses from marginal gingivitis. The features are often those of marginal gingivitis but, with destruction of alveolar bone support, there is increasing tooth mobility, teeth may drift, and there is deep pocket formation (**Figure 10.116**).

In accelerated periodontitis, patients still develop periodontitis despite good control of plaque (**Figure 10.117**). A range of systemic causes may underlie this accelerated periodontitis, notably diabetes mellitus, white cell dyscrasias including neutrophil defects and neutropenias, and other immune defects including HIV disease.

Rapidly progressive periodontitis (**Figure 10.118**) is the term applied to adults — typically females in their early 30s — who, despite good oral hygiene and general health, develop periodontitis. Minor neutrophil defects may be responsible.

In localized juvenile periodontitis, localized destruction, classically in the permanent incisor (**Figure 10.119**) and first molar regions is seen in some adolescents or young adults in the absence of poor oral hygiene or gross systemic disease. Juvenile periodontitis (periodontosis) is seen especially in females, and in Afro-Asians and may be associated with minor defects of neutrophil function and microorganisms such as *Actinobacillus, actinomycetemcomitans* and capnocytophaga. Similar periodontal destruction can be seen in Down's syndrome, type VIII Ehlers–Danlos syndrome, HIV infection and hypophosphatasia.

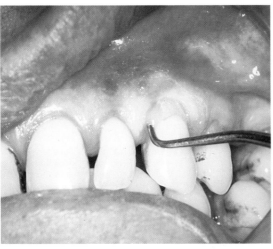

10.116

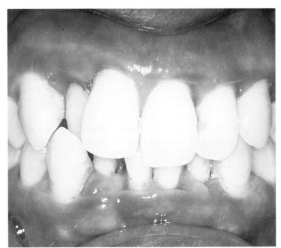

10.117

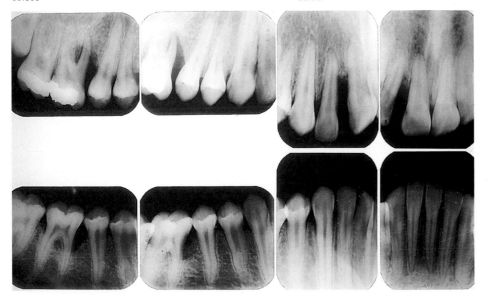

10.118

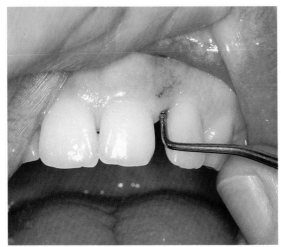

10.119

PAPILLON–LEFÈVRE SYNDROME

The Papillon–Lefèvre syndrome is a rare, genetically-linked disorder of pre-pubertal periodontitis, in association with palmar–plantar hyperkeratosis. Virtually all deciduous teeth are involved and the permanent dentition is usually also affected (**Figure 10.120**).

Most of the deciduous teeth are lost by the age of 4 years, and the permanent teeth by age 16 (**Figure 10.121**).

Skin lesions tend to appear between the ages of 2 and 4 years. The soles are usually affected more severely than the palms (**Figures 10.122** and **10.123**). The dura mater may be calcified as may the tentorium or choroid.

A rare variant of the Papillon–Lefèvre syndrome, not illustrated here, includes arachnodactyly and tapered phalanges as well as the above features.

Other types of palmoplantar hyperkeratosis are discussed on page 284.

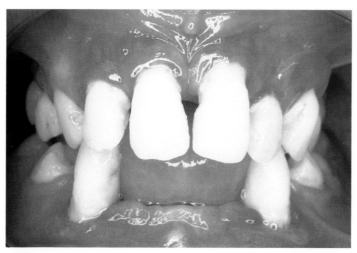

10.120

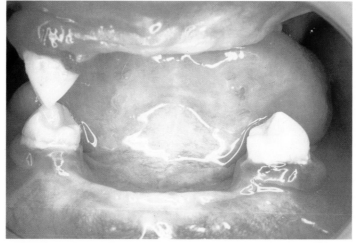

10.121

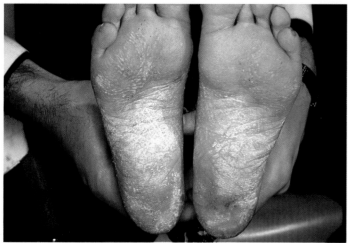

10.122

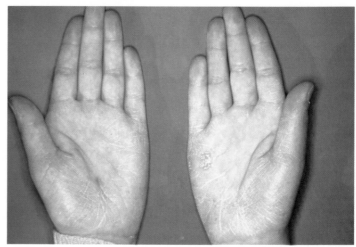

10.123

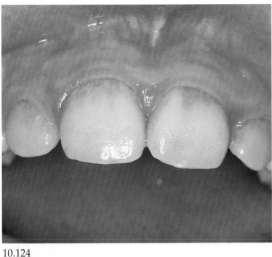

10.124

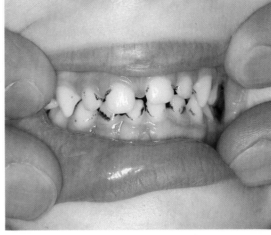

10.125

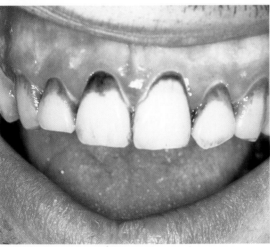

10.126

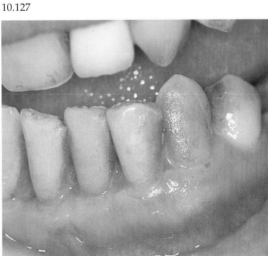

10.127

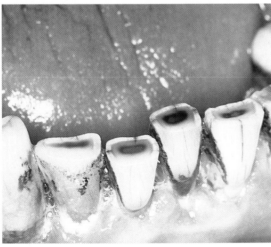

10.128

10.129

EXTRINSIC TOOTH STAINING

Extrinsic staining of the teeth can be of various colours and is more likely to appear where oral hygiene is poor or where coloured foods/drinks are taken.

Orange stain (**Figure 10.124**) is believed to be caused by chromogenic bacteria.

Brown stain is shown in **Figure 10.125**. Extrinsic staining is concentrated mainly where plaque accumulates, such as between the teeth and close to gingival margins, and in pits and fissures. Brown stain can be caused by stannous fluoride tooth pastes (**Figure 10.126**) and other substances.

Black stain (**Figure 10.127**) is of unknown aetiology and is unusual in that it seems to be associated, by an unknown mechanism, with caries-resistance. It is seen in clean mouths. Black-staining of teeth is carried out deliberately for cosmetic reasons in some communities.

Green stain is more common, especially in children with poor oral hygiene, and may result from breakdown of blood pigment after gingival haemorrhage, or from chromogenic bacteria.

'Nicotine' stain (**Figure 10.128**) is caused by cigarette smoking, or tobacco chewing, especially in a person with poor oral hygiene. Dentine, exposed in this case by attrition, also stains dark brown. Tobacco use predisposes to oral keratoses and cancer. Staining can also be produced by chewing habits such as use of betel or khat (*see* **Figure 17.30**).

Chlorhexidine stain is seen in **Figure 10.129**. Chlorhexidine is an effective oral antiseptic and binds to dental pellicle where it can produce discoloration, especially in drinkers of tea or coffee.

(Contd)

188

EXTRINSIC TOOTH STAINING
(Contd)

Iron stain (**Figure 10.130**) may result from iron preparations taken orally.

Finally, lead stain may be seen (**Figure 10.131**). Lead-induced pigmentation is rare and usually follows accidental or occupational exposure. Deposits of lead sulphide in the gingival margin may produce a black 'lead line', especially where oral hygiene is poor.

MATERIA ALBA

Figure 10.132 is an extreme example of poor oral hygiene — a mentally handicapped patient whose teeth were virtually never cleaned. The teeth are covered with calculus, plaque and debris from food.

DENTAL CALCULUS

If plaque is not removed it readily calcifies to produce calculus (tartar), especially in sites close to salivary duct orifices, lingual to the lower incisors (**Figure 10.133**) and buccal to upper molars.

Before oral cleansing (**Figure 10.134**) the calculus is covered with plaque, cannot be removed by toothbrushing, and is associated with periodontal disease. After professional cleansing (**Figure 10.135**), the extent of periodontal destruction and consequent recession is clearly seen.

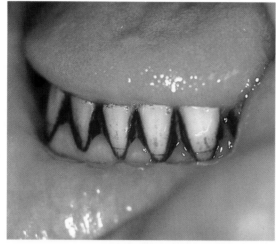

10.130

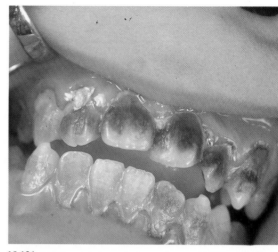

10.131

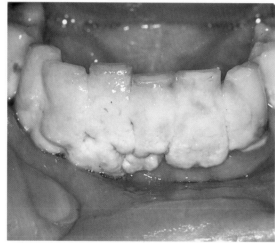

10.132

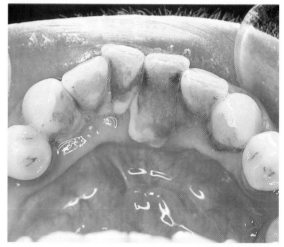

10.133

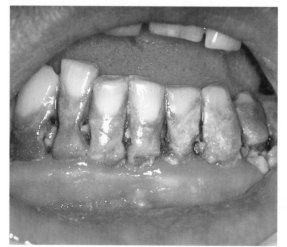

10.134

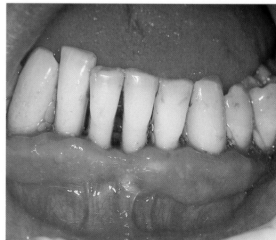

10.135

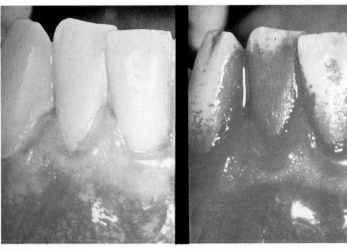

10.136

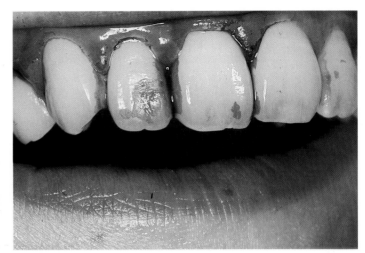

10.137

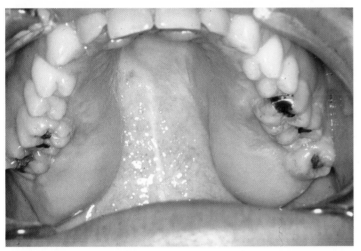

10.138

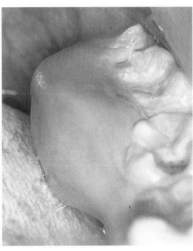

10.139

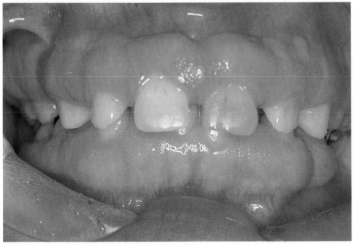

10.140

DENTAL BACTERIAL PLAQUE

Plaque is not especially obvious clinically (**Figure 10.136**), although teeth covered with plaque lack the lustre of clear teeth. Various solutions can be used to disclose the plaque (**Figures 10.136** and **10.137**).

Even after thorough toothbrushing, plaque often remains between the teeth unless they are flossed.

GINGIVAL FIBROMATOSIS

Enlarged maxillary tuberosities are a localized form of gingival fibromatosis (**Figure 10.138**).

Occasionally fibromatosis is found in the posterior mandibular region (**Figure 10.139**).

Hereditary gingival fibromatosis is a familial condition, in which generalized gingival fibromatosis (**Figure 10.140**) is often associated with hirsutism. Hereditary gingival fibromatosis usually becomes most apparent at the time teeth are erupting. Rarely, the fibromatosis is one feature of a multisystem syndrome (*see* pages 15 and 300).

TRAUMATIC OCCLUSION

Trauma can damage the periodontium, often through excessive occlusal stresses and sometimes through direct damage. In **Figure 10.141** both upper and lower incisors are retroclined and the upper incisors are traumatizing the lower labial gingiva (class II division 2 malocclusion) (**Figure 10.142**).

There is stripping of the periodontium labial to the lower incisors. The upper incisor periodontium may also be traumatized palatally by the lower incisors.

GINGIVAL CYST

Gingival cysts are rare in adults (**Figure 10.143**) They are often solitary and found typically in the mandibular canine or premolar region as a small, painless swelling of the attached or free gingiva, especially near the interdental papilla.

GIANT CELL GRANULOMA (*Giant cell epulis*)

This is a non-neoplastic swelling of proliferating fibroblasts in a highly vascular stroma containing many multinucleate giant cells. It is most common in children (**Figure 10.144**) after tooth extraction.

Giant cell epulides are usually deep red or purple in colour (**Figure 10.145**). Kaposi's sarcoma and epithelioid angiomatosis may have a similar appearance.

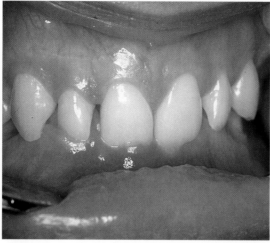

10.141

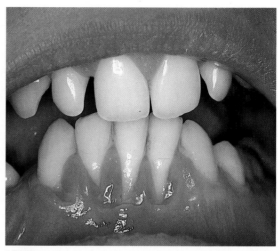

10.142

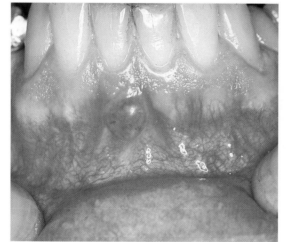

10.143

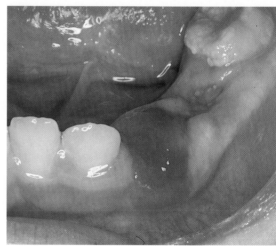

10.144

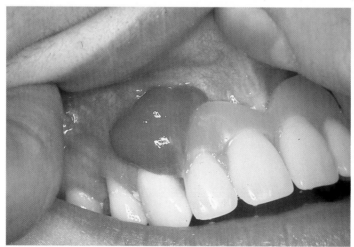

10.145

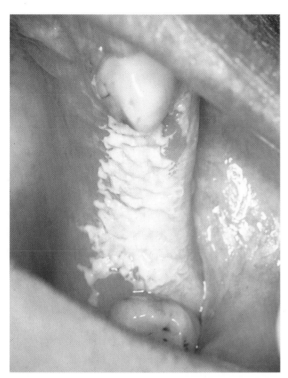

10.146

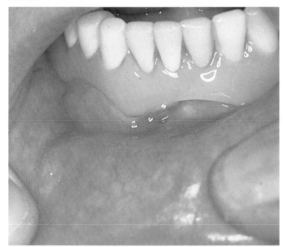

10.148

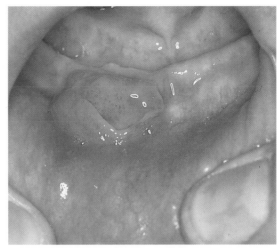

10.147

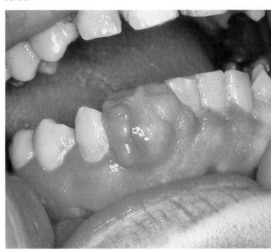

10.149

KERATOSIS
(*Leukoplakia*)

Keratosis (hyperkeratinization) is fairly common on edentulous ridges (**Figure 10.146**) and often produced by friction from chewing on the ridge, by smoking or by tobacco-chewing, but some cases are idiopathic.

DENTURE-INDUCED HYPERPLASIA
(*Epulis fissuratum*)

A denture margin (flange) may cause ulceration of the vestibule, and chronic irritation may produce hyperplasia (**Figure 10.147**).

In **Figure 10.148** the denture fits neatly into the groove between the hyperplastic leaves of tissue (same patient as **Figure 10.147**). This condition is quite benign but, very occasionally, hyperplasia results from a lesion proliferating beneath and impinging on a denture flange.

FIBROUS EPULIS

An epulis is a discrete gingival swelling. Low grade gingival irritation can produce a fibrous epulis — a benign process (**Figure 10.149**).

Most epulides are seen in the anterior part of the mouth and most are fibrous epulides.

192

MALOCCLUSION

Figure 10.150 shows the typical bird face of mandibular retrusion.

Maxillary protrusion is seen in **Figure 10.151**. This type of malocclusion is class II division I — compare with that in **Figures 10.141** and **10.142**.

Figure 10.152 is a case of mandibular protrusion (class III malocclusion): the Hapsburg chin of a prognathic mandible. In mandibular protrusion, the teeth often show reverse overjet with the upper incisors occluding lingual to the lowers (**Figure 10.153**).

Another form of malocclusion is open bite (**Figure 10.154**). The posterior teeth are in occlusion but the incisors fail to meet. Anterior open bites may be caused by increased height of the lower face; tongue posture; dentoalveolar factors; trauma, or thumb-sucking. The upper lateral incisors are also congenitally absent in this patient.

(Contd)

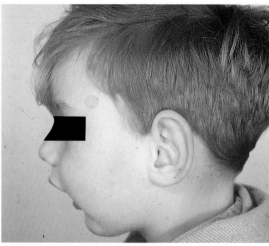
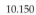

10.150

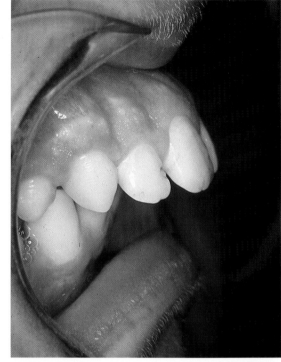

10.151

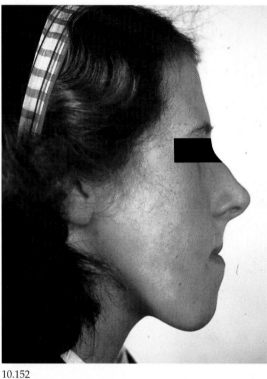

10.152

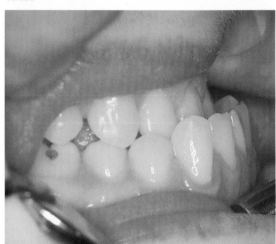

10.153

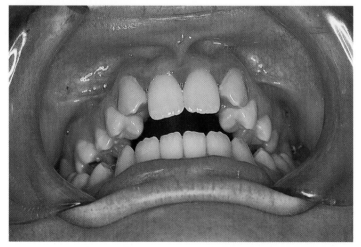

10.154

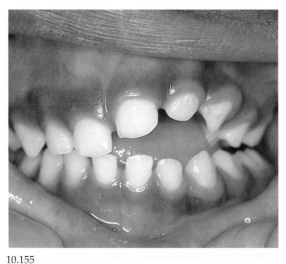

10.155

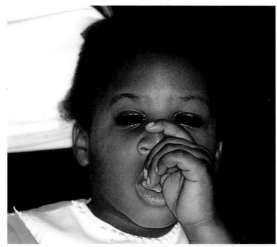

10.156

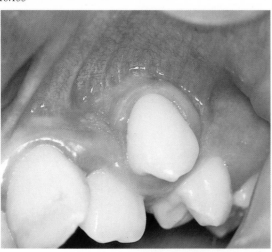

10.157

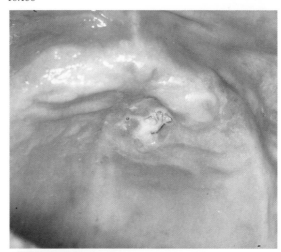

10.158

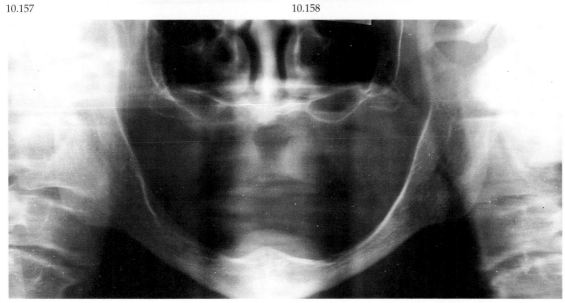

10.159

Obvious malocclusion and anterior open bite can be caused by thumb-sucking (**Figures 10.155** and **10.156**).

Finally, the permanent canine normally erupts slightly later than the premolar and lateral incisor and, if there is lack of space in the dental arch (dentoalveolar disproportion), it is crowded out (**Figure 10.157**). Second premolars and third molars are the other teeth that may suffer this fate. Any of these teeth, especially lower third molars, may then impact.

RETAINED ROOT

Retained roots are often asymptomatic but may 'erupt' under a denture (**Figure 10.158**), or may give rise to a periapical abscess, or cyst.

ALVEOLAR ATROPHY

The alveolar bone of the jaw normally bears the teeth. When teeth are removed, or exfoliate in periodontitis, the alveolar bone atrophies and the jaw occasionally becomes so thin (**Figure 10.159**) that denture retention is difficult and, in extreme cases, the mandible fractures under relatively little stress.

Osteoporosis may affect the jaws as other bones and is seen particularly in post menopausal women and patients taking systemic corticosteroids. It is also seen in the short-bowel syndrome (*see* page 228).

ERUPTION CYST

A cyst often presents clinically as a smooth, rounded swelling with a bluish appearance if there is no overlying bone (**Figure 10.160**). Eruption cysts often break down spontaneously as the tooth erupts. The eruption cyst is a type of dentigerous cyst; that is, it surrounds the crown of the tooth.

Removal of the operculum (and incidental papilloma) from the cyst in **Figure 10.161** reveals an erupting upper first molar (**Figure 10.162**).

ODONTOGENIC KERATOCYST (*Primordial cyst*)

Odontogenic cysts are often asymptomatic but may produce an intraoral swelling and occasionally an extraoral swelling (**Figures 10.163** and **10.164**). Odontogenic keratocysts are typically seen in young persons and especially in the mandibular molar region.

The odontogenic keratocyst has a tendency to recur after removal. Usually seen in isolation, multiple cysts are a feature of Gorlin's syndrome (*see* page 294).

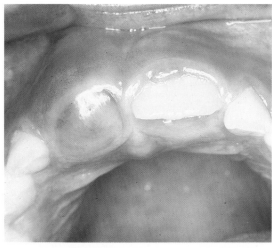

10.160

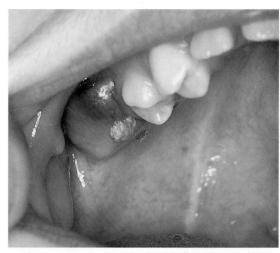

10.161

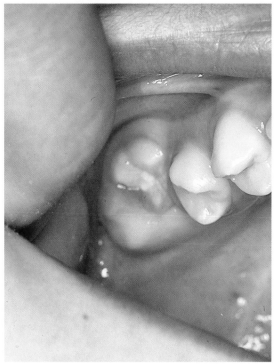

10.162

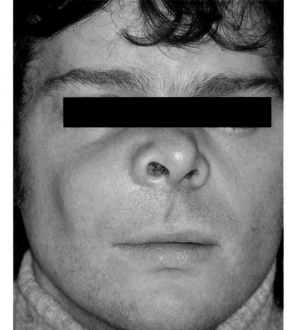

10.163

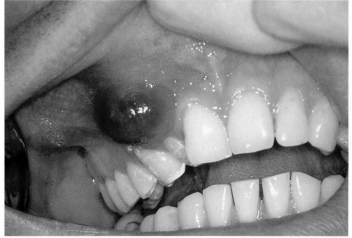

10.164

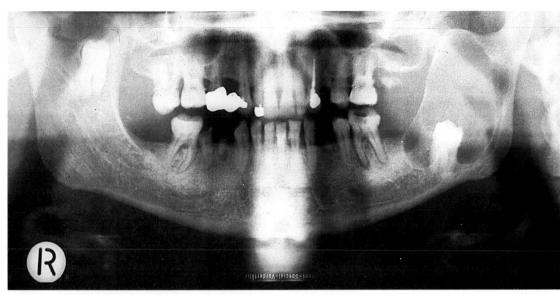

10.165

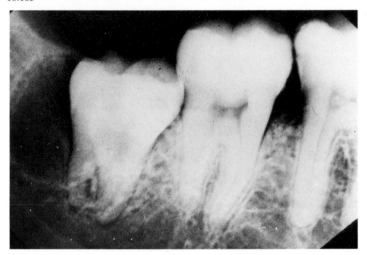

10.166

DENTIGEROUS CYST (*Follicular cyst*)

A dentigerous cyst envelops the crown of a tooth and is attached to its neck. Most involve third molars or canine teeth. In **Figure 10.165** the left ramus of mandible is occupied by a dentigerous cyst related to a molar, probably the third molar. The other lower third molar is ectopic.

Multiple dentigerous cysts can be a feature of cleidocranial dysplasia (*see* page 278).

LATERAL PERIODONTAL CYST

A lateral periodontal cyst may be follicular in origin; may arise from remnants of the dental lamina; or may be associated with a lateral pulp canal in a non-vital tooth. The cyst in **Figure 10.166** closely resembles a dentigerous cyst.

GLOBULO-MAXILLARY CYST

A probable misnomer, most cysts in the upper lateral incisor canine region (**Figure 10.167**) prove to be odontogenic rather than developmental (non-odontogenic, fissural) cysts. This cyst has displaced the maxillary right canine and lateral incisor teeth.

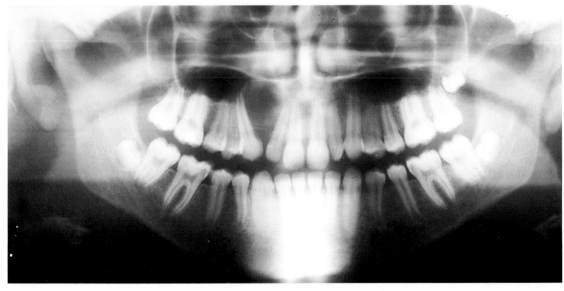

10.167

196

NASOPALATINE DUCT CYST
(*Incisive canal cyst*)

Epithelial remnants related to the nasopalatine canal may give rise to a cyst. Most nasopalatine cysts are seen in adult males from the age of 40. If large, the cyst may produce a swelling beneath the upper lip and anterior nares (**Figure 10.168**).

The swelling may extend to the nasal floor and palatal vault (**Figure 10.169**), and may discharge a salty fluid.

Dental cysts related to non-vital incisors can be confused with the nasopalatine cyst. Furthermore, the normal incisive canal can be difficult to distinguish radiographically from a cyst, although it is generally accepted that a radiolucency greater than 6 mm in diameter is probably a cyst (**Figure 10.170**).

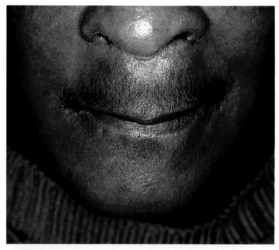

10.168

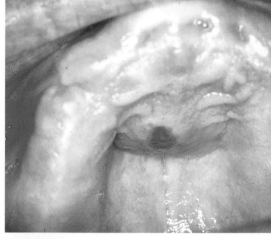

10.169

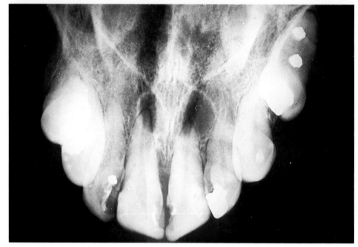

10.170

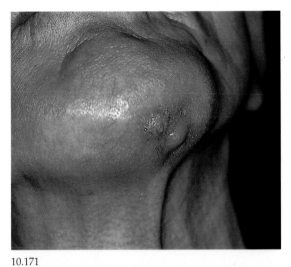

10.171

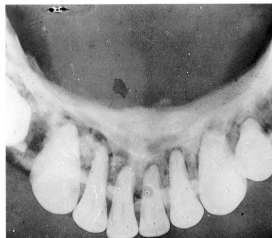

10.172

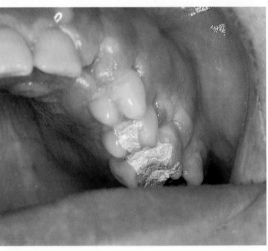

10.173

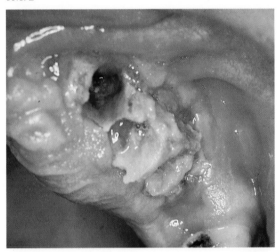

10.174

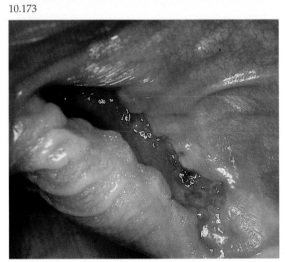

10.175

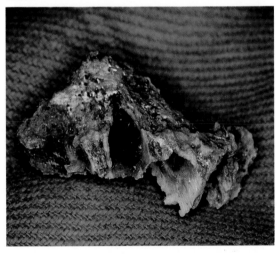

10.176

ACUTE OSTEOMYELITIS

Osteomyelitis is an infection of the bone, rare in the jaws. Acute osteomyelitis is seen mainly in the mandible, the infection usually originating from odontogenic infection or trauma. Extreme pain, swelling, labial anaesthesia, tenderness on biting and eventual discharge of pus (**Figure 10.171**) are the main features.

Radiological signs take some weeks to develop but the bone eventually becomes 'moth-eaten' (**Figure 10.172**).

Figures 10.173–10.176 show a sequence from a patient with rare maxillary osteomyelitis. At the early stage (**Figure 10.173**) there is pain and swelling by the upper second premolar and first molar which were then extracted.

Two months later, a sequestrum appeared (**Figure 10.174**).

After a further 2 weeks the necrotic bone sequestrates (**Figure 10.175**). The sequestrum is shown in **Figure 10.176**.

Osteomyelitis is predisposed by various immune defects, diabetes mellitus, Paget's disease, osteopetrosis, irradiation or local factors, such as foreign bodies.

(Contd)

ACUTE OSTEOMYELITIS
(*Contd*)

Acute osteomyelitis is very rare in the maxilla and, when seen, is usually in neonates (**Figure 10.177**). It is possible that *Staphylococcus aureus* infects the maxilla, either haematogenously or entering via an oral wound.

CHRONIC OSTEOMYELITIS

Proliferative periostitis is an uncommon chronic low grade infection, seen usually in the lower molar region (**Figure 10.178**). There are several clinical patterns of chronic osteomyelitis.

OSTEORADIO-NECROSIS

Endarteritis obliterans, following irradiation of the jaws, predisposes to infection after tooth extraction (**Figure 10.179**). Here there is a chronic submandibular sinus.

This was a not uncommon problem in the past but, with the advent of plesiotherapy and other improved radiotherapeutic techniques and a better understanding by dental surgeons, it is now less common.

In **Figure 10.180**, a sequestrum is forming slowly. Radiation-scarring with telangiectasia is also evident in the floor of the mouth.

Radiography shows the 'moth-eaten' appearance of the mandible and a pathological fracture (**Figure 10.181**).

Jaw necrosis was also caused in the past by occupational exposure to red phosphorus, or exposure to heavy metals, and occasionally follows the use of toxic endodontic materials, severe herpes zoster or other infections.

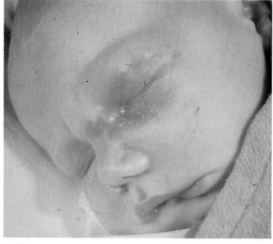

10.177

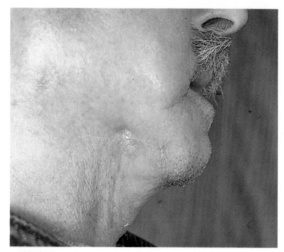

10.179

10.181

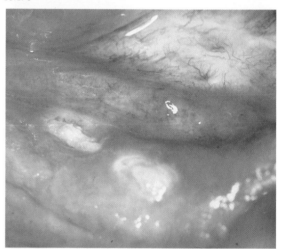

10.178

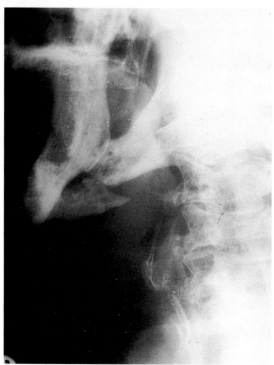

10.180

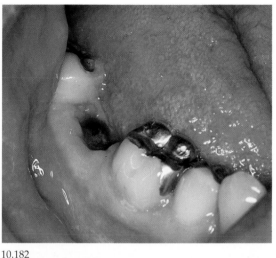

10.182

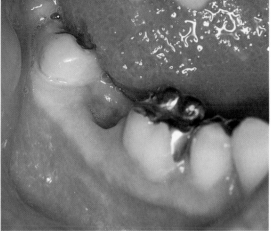

10.183

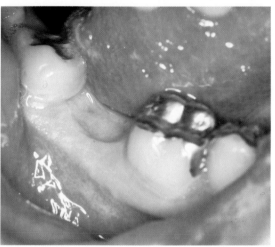

10.184

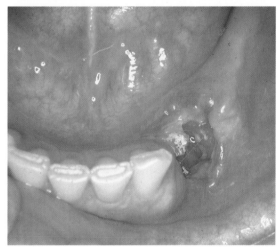

10.185

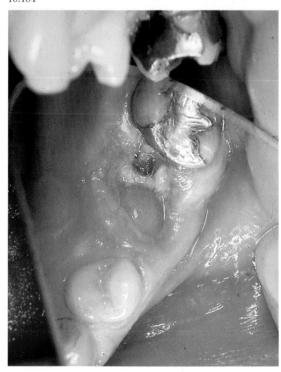

10.186

HEALING EXTRACTION SOCKET

An extraction socket rapidly fills with blood which normally clots and remains *in situ* (**Figure 10.182**). Later post-extraction haemorrhage is usually from mucosal rather than bony vessels.

After a few days (**Figure 10.183**) the wound contracts. The clot begins to organize.

By a month (**Figure 10.184**) the socket is epithelializing and the area will soon appear healed clinically, although radiographically it will still be evident several months later. There will be some remodelling of the alveolar bone.

DRY SOCKET (*Alveolar osteitis*)

If the blood clot in an extraction socket breaks down, presumably from the action of fibrinolysins, then the socket is 'dry'. Dry socket manifests with the onset of fairly severe pain 2–4 days after extraction, bad taste in the mouth, and halitosis. The socket has no clot and the surrounding mucosa is inflamed (**Figure 10.185**).

Dry socket is typically seen after extractions in young persons; in the mandible; in the molar region; after extractions under local anaesthesia; and after traumatic extractions. Oral contraceptive use predisposes to dry socket. Healing is aided if debris (such as in **Figure 10.86**) is irrigated away and the socket dressed.

TORUS MANDIBULARIS

Mandibular tori are uni- or bilateral bony lumps lingual to the lower premolars (**Figures 10.187** and **10.188**). They are of developmental origin and benign.

Tori are fairly common (about 60% of the population) but are especially seen in Mongoloid races.

TORUS PALATINUS

Palatal tori are common bony lumps (seen in up to 20% of the population) typically in the midline vault of palate (**Figures 10.189** and **10.190**)

Palatal tori are most common in Mongoloid races and can sometimes be quite protrusive. Again, they are benign.

EXOSTOSES

It is fairly common to see exostoses buccal to the maxillary posterior teeth (**Figure 10.191**).

GARDNER'S SYNDROME

Multiple jaw osteomas are occasionally a feature of Gardner's syndrome, which is an autosomal dominant trait characterized by colonic polyps (often pre-malignant), epidermoid cysts, desmoid tumours, pigmented ocular fundic lesions and impacted supernumerary teeth. These patients may also develop extra-colonic neoplasms.

Mandibular osteomas are more prevalent in sporadic colonic adenocarcinoma and may be regarded as a marker.

STAFNE BONE CAVITY (*Latent bone cyst*)

A Stafne 'cyst' is not a cyst at all but a well-demarcated radiolucency at the lower border of the mandible, always below the inferior alveolar canal (**Figure 10.192**). It contains some normal submandibular salivary gland tissue. It is a developmental defect.

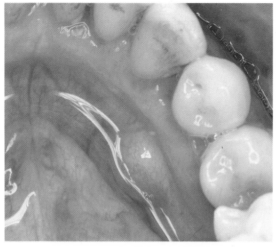

10.187

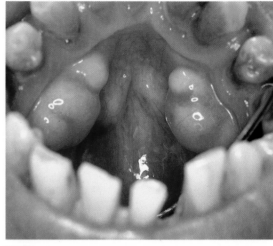

10.188

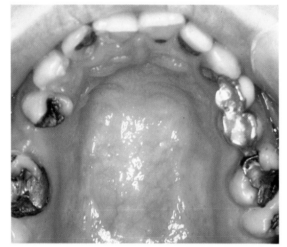

10.189

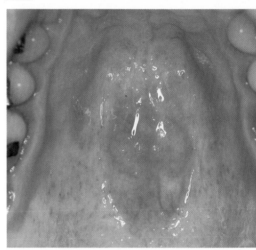

10.190

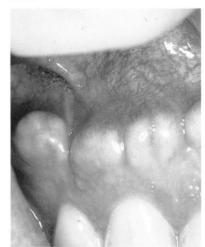

10.191

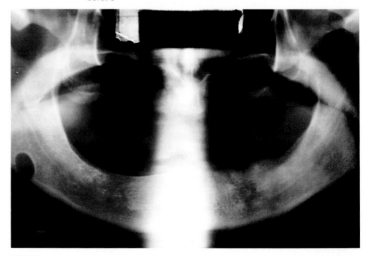

10.192

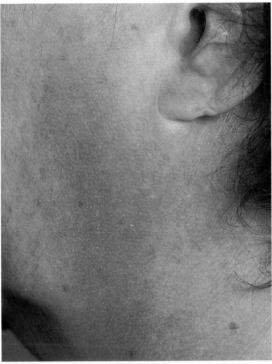

10.193

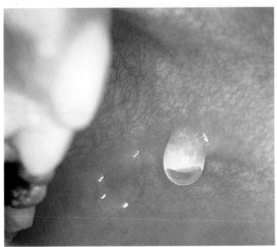

10.195

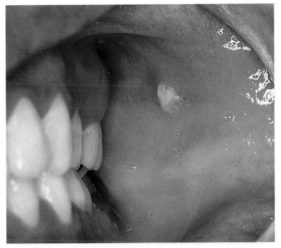

10.194

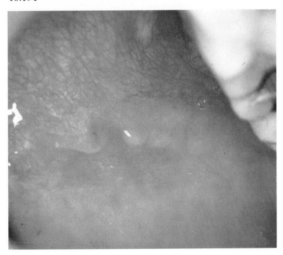

10.196

ACUTE BACTERIAL SIALADENITIS

This is almost invariably a mixed infection, often including penicillin-resistant *Staphylococcus aureus* that ascends the duct because of xerostomia or a ductal anomaly. There is severe pain over the gland and often trismus if the parotid is affected. There is erythema and swelling over the gland (**Figure 10.193**) which is tender to palpation.

Enteric Gram-negative rods have a high oropharyngeal colonization in hospitalized persons and these rods and pseudomonads have been implicated in a few cases of sialadenitis.

Purulent saliva (**Figure 10.194**) or frank pus may be expressed from the duct of the affected gland — in this case the parotid.

In children, there is a rare form of recurrent parotitis that is of uncertain aetiology mainly seen in boys. It is characterized by recurrent painful swelling, usually unilaterally. Peak incidence is between ages 3–6 years. The condition resolves spontaneously at puberty in most cases.

NORMAL PAROTID SALIVATION

Figure 10.195, shown here for comparison with **Figure 10.194**, shows clear, watery, normal parotid saliva flowing from Stensen's duct.

SALIVARY FISTULA

Internal fistulae (**Figure 10.196**) may be of congenital origin or acquired. They are inconsequential.

External fistulae usually follow trauma in an accident, assault, or after surgery, and are disconcerting and unpleasant for the patient.

SUBMANDIBULAR SIALOLITHIASIS

Salivary calculi are not uncommon and usually affect the submandibular duct. Sometimes asymptomatic, the typical presentation is pain in, and swelling of, the gland around mealtimes (**Figure 10.197**).

Calculi are usually yellow or white and can sometimes be seen in the duct (**Figure 10.198**) (which has ulcerated in this case), or may be palpable. Not all are radio-opaque. Quite large submandibular calculi (**Figure 10.199**) can form, and calculi may be multiple. Chronic sialadenitis may develop if a salivary obstruction is not removed.

PAROTID OBSTRUCTIVE SIALADENITIS

Stones are less common in the parotid and less often radio-opaque, but obstruction (**Figure 10.200**) can also be caused by mucus plugs, strictures, or the oedema associated with ulcer-ation of the parotid papilla. Rarely, salivary obstruction has other aetiologies.

SIALOLITH IN MINOR SALIVARY GLAND

Occasionally a stone forms in one of the minor salivary glands (**Figure 10.201**).

ADENOMATOID HYPERPLASIA

This is a rare idiopathic non-inflammatory, non-neoplastic and benign lesion of minor salivary glands, that typically presents with a tumour-like mass in the palate (**Figure 10.202**). The lesion is usually a painless, sessile, firm or soft swelling of normal colour, of indeterminate duration, located in the hard palate, although other intra-oral sites have occasionally been reported. Most have been in males, usually middle-aged or older. The aetiology is quite unclear though most patients are smokers.

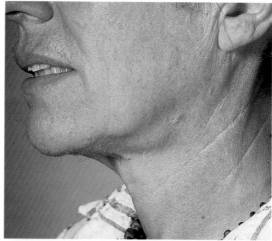

10.197

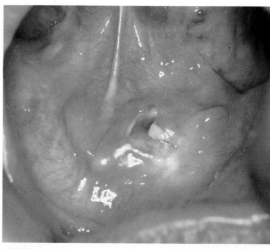

10.198

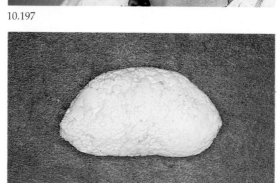

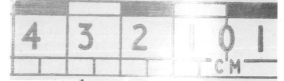

10.199

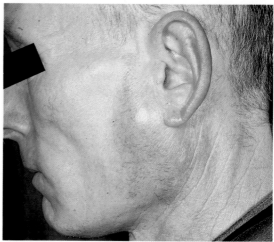

10.200

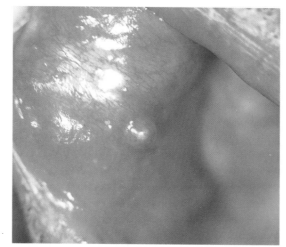

10.201

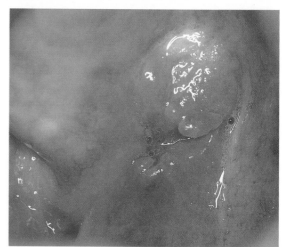

10.202

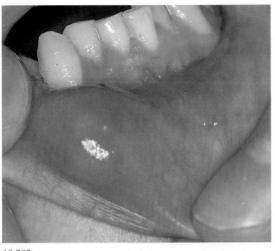

10.203

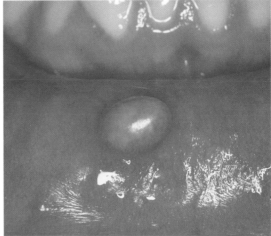

10.204

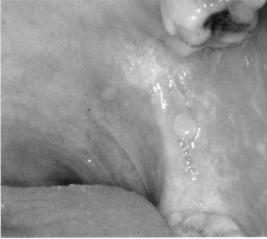

10.205

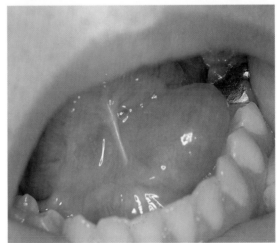

10.206

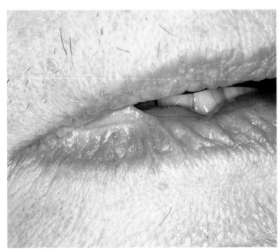

10.207

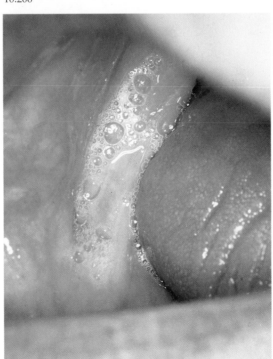

10.208

MUCOCELES

Most mucoceles are caused by saliva extravasating into the tissues from a damaged salivary duct. They are most common in the lower labial (**Figure 10.203**) and ventral lingual mucosa. Occasional mucoceles are retention cysts.

The mucocele is a dome-shaped, fluctuant, bluish, non-tender, submucosal swelling with a normal overlying mucosa (**Figure 10.204**).

Cysts may occasionally develop within salivary neoplasms.

In the case of a superficial mucocele, intraepithelial or occasionally sub-epithelial vesiculation may be caused by small extravasation mucoceles. Seen typically in females of middle or later age, this is often in the palate (**Figure 10.205**) or buccal mucosae, and frequently in patients with oral lichen planus.

Extravasation mucoceles arising from the sublingual gland are termed ranulas, because of their resemblance to a frog's belly (**Figure 10.206**). Rarely, a ranula extends through the mylohyoid muscle — a plunging ranula.

XEROSTOMIA

Many patients complain of a dry mouth and yet lack objective evidence of xerostomia. In true xerostomia the dry mucosa may become tacky and the lips can adhere one to another (**Figure 10.207**). An examining dental mirror may often stick to the mucosa.

There may be lack of salivary pooling in the floor of the mouth: any saliva present tends to be viscous and appear frothy (**Figure 10.208**) and saliva flows poorly, if at all, from the ducts of the major glands on stimulation or palpation.

The main causes of dry mouth are drugs (those with anticholinergic or sympathomimetic activity), irradiation of the salivary glands, Sjögren's syndrome (*see* page 262), HIV disease, sarcoidosis and dehydration.

SIALOSIS
(*Sialadenosis*)

Painless bilateral chronic swelling of the salivary glands, typically the parotids (**Figures 10.209** and **10.210**) without xerostomia, characterizes sialosis. There appears to be serous cell hypertrophy and striated duct atrophy.

Although sialosis is benign and usually idiopathic, it is important to exclude underlying causes such as drugs (eg, methyldopa), endocrinopathies (eg, diabetes mellitus and acromegaly), alcoholic liver cirrhosis or malnutrition such as in bulimia.

Salivary glands, especially the submandibular, may also swell in cystic fibrosis and most affected children also have antral polyps.

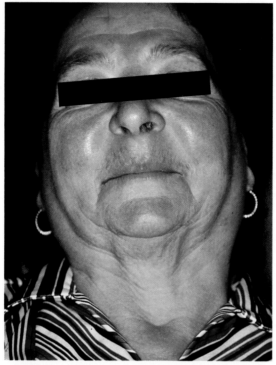

10.209

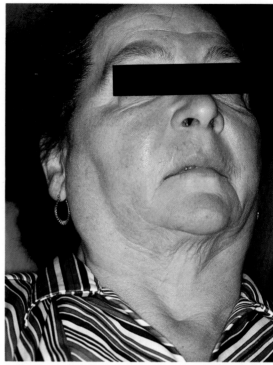

10.210

NECROTIZING SIALOMETAPLASIA

Necrotizing sialometaplasia is a rare ulcerative lesion of unknown aetiology, seen especially in the hard palate in adult males. It may resemble a neoplasm clinically and histologically.

Figures 10.211 and **10.212** show a chronic swelling of the palate which ulcerated and then healed slowly over 1–2 months.

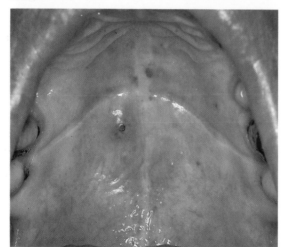

10.211

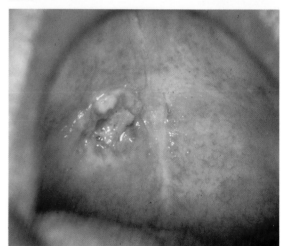

10.212

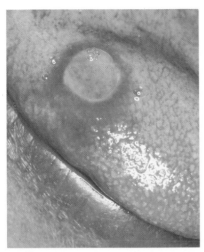

10.213

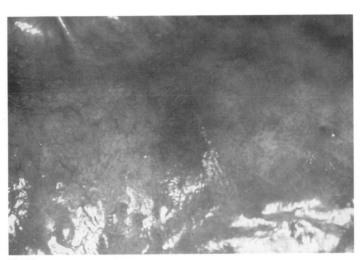

10.214

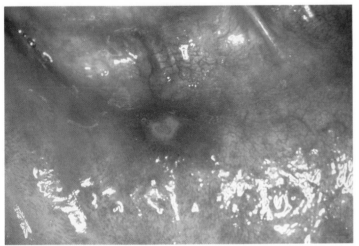

10.215

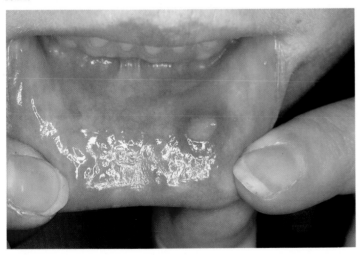

10.216

RECURRENT APHTHAE (*Recurrent aphthous stomatitis, RAS*)

Recurrent aphthae are typically ovoid or round ulcers with a yellow floor and pronounced inflammatory halo (**Figure 10.213**). Episodes begin usually in childhood and the natural history is of spontaneous remission after some years. The aetiology is unknown.

Minor aphthae (Mikulicz aphthae) are small, 2–4 mm in diameter (**Figure 10.214**), last 7–10 days, tend not to be seen on gingiva, palate or dorsum of tongue, and heal with no obvious scarring. This is an early lesion.

Figure 10.215 shows the same patient as **Figure 10.214** 24 hours later, showing an obvious ulcer. Most patients develop not more than six ulcers at any single episode.

Figure 10.216 is a typical minor aphthous ulcer in a common site in a teenager.

Most patients with RAS are otherwise apparently well, but a significant proportion of those referred to a hospital clinic prove to be deficient in a haematinic such as iron, folate or vitamin B_{12}; 2–3 per cent have coeliac disease; and there are also occasional associations with menstruation, stress, food allergy and immuno-deficiencies. Most patients with aphthae are non-smokers and others may develop aphthae for the first time on ceasing smoking.

Aphthae may occasionally be a manifestation of Behçet's syndrome (*see* page 207) or Sweet's syndrome.

Aphthous-like ulcers may occasionally be a manifestation of cyclic or chronic neutropenia, or a similar recently-described syndrome with periodic fever and pharyngitis, but with no neutropenia.

(*Contd*)

RECURRENT APHTHAE
(*Contd*)

Major aphthae are recurrent, often ovoid ulcers with an inflammatory halo, but are less common, much larger (**Figure 10.217**), more persistent than minor aphthae, and can affect the dorsum of tongue and soft palate as well as other sites.

Sometimes termed Sutton's ulcers or periadenitis mucosa necrotica recurrens (PMNR), major aphthae can be well over 1 cm in diameter and can take several months to heal. At any one episode there are usually fewer than six ulcers present. In **Figure 10.218** the ulcer is beginning to epithelialize.

In **Figure 10.219**, the major aphtha has almost healed. Major aphthae may leave obvious scars on healing (**Figure 10.220**).

Herpetiform aphthae are so termed because the patients have a myriad of small ulcers that clinically resemble those of herpetic stomatitis (**Figure 10.221**). It is, however, a distinct entity, lacking the associated fever, gingivitis and lymph node involvement of primary herpetic stomatitis.

Pinpoint herpetiform aphthae (Cooke's aphthae) enlarge and fuse to produce irregular ulcers (**Figure 10.222**). These aphthae affect females more than males, present at a slightly later age (often from 30 years of age) than other forms of RAS, and affect any site in the mouth.

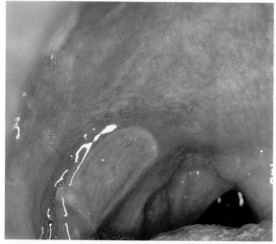

10.217

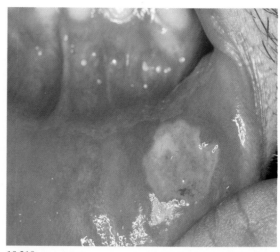

10.218

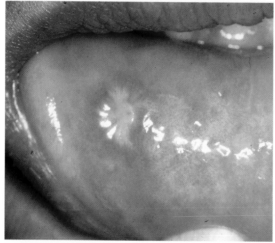

10.219

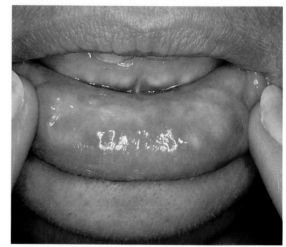

10.220

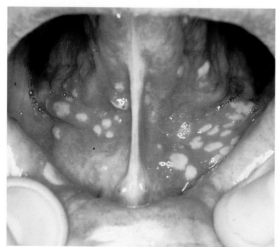

10.221

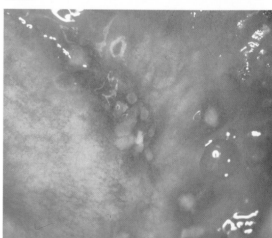

10.222

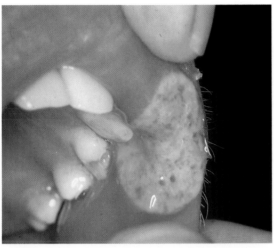

10.223

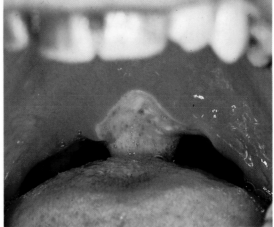

10.224

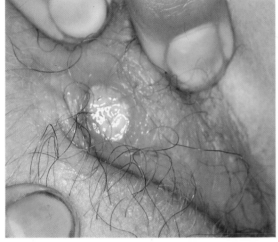

10.225

BEHÇET'S SYNDROME (*Behçet's disease*)

Aphthae of any of the types previously described usually occur in isolation in apparently healthy persons. A minority are a manifestation of Behçet's syndrome (**Figure 10.223**), where aphthae are associated with genital ulcers and uveitis.

Behçet's syndrome is a multisystem disease affecting the mouth in most cases: **Figure 10.224** shows a major aphtha. Genital ulcers in Behçet's syndrome often closely resemble oral aphthae (**Figure 10.225**). Other sites commonly affected are eyes, skin and joints; but Behçet's syndrome is not the only cause of this constellation of lesions. Other causes, such as ulcerative colitis, Crohn's disease, mixed connective tissue disease, lupus erythematosus and Reiter's syndrome, should be excluded.

Behçet's syndrome is most common in Japan, China, Korea and the Middle East.

(Contd)

BEHÇET'S SYNDROME
(*Contd*)

Uveitis (posterior uveitis (**Figure 10.226**): retinal vasculitis) is one of the more important ocular lesions of Behçet's syndrome but anterior uveitis and other changes occur. The left pupil in **Figure 10.226** has been dilated for fundoscopy. Ocular and arthritic symptoms are more common in males. Neurological involvement may cause headache, psychiatric, motor or sensory manifestations.

Erythema nodosum can be a feature of Behçet's syndrome (**Figure 10.227**), particularly in females.

Of the various rashes seen in Behçet's syndrome, an acneiform pustular rash (**Figure 10.228**) is most common.

Patients with Behçet's syndrome may develop pustules at the site of vene-puncture (pathergy) but this feature is uncommon in British patients.

Although large joint arthropathy is not uncommon in Behçet's syndrome, an overlap syndrome with relapsing polychondritis has also been described (mouth and genital ulcers with inflamed cartilage (MAGIC) syndrome).

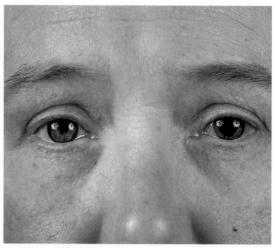

10.226

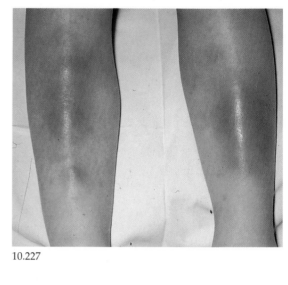

10.227

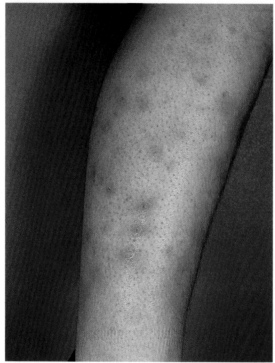

10.228

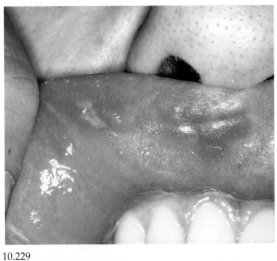

10.229

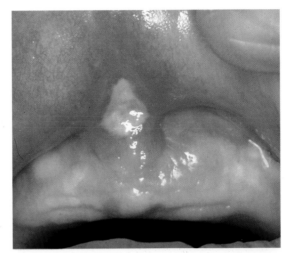

10.230

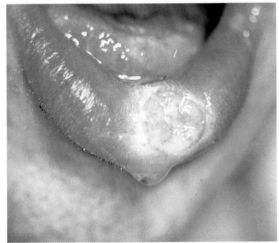

10.231

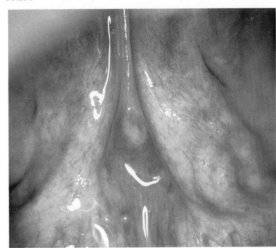

10.232

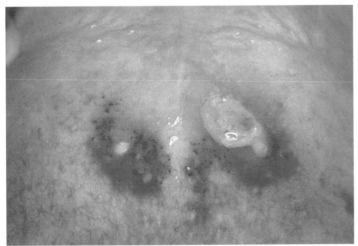

10.233

TRAUMATIC ULCERS

Traumatic ulcers are common, usually caused by accidental biting, hard foods, appliances such as dentures or orthodontic appliances, or following dental treatment. Less common causes are shown in the figures. **Figure 10.229** shows small bruises and ulcers which have followed a blow on the lip.

In child abuse syndrome (non-accidental injury) the mouth is often traumatized. Bruised and swollen lips, lacerated fraenum (**Figure 10.230**) and even subluxed teeth or fractured mandible can be features.

Chronic self-induced traumatic ulcers (**Figure 10.231**) may be seen in self-mutilation in a mentally handicapped or disturbed patient. This is a chronic ulcer with surrounding keratosis.

The lingual fraenum can be traumatized by repeated rubbing over the lower incisor teeth (cunnilingus tongue is shown in **Figure 10.232**). A similar lesion can be seen in children with recurrent bouts of coughing as in whooping cough, termed Riga–Fedes disease.

Traumatic ulceration of the soft palate is fairly uncommon. Trauma from an erect penis together with oral suction can produce ulceration, bruising and petechiae (fellatio palate is shown in **Figure 10.233**).

Neonates occasionally develop an ulcer at a similar site (Bednar's ulcer) which it is thought may be caused by trauma from the examining finger of the paediatrician.

DERMOID CYST

Dermoid cyst is an uncommon midline entity, often presenting with a slowly growing swelling beneath the chin (**Figure 10.234**).

Found in the floor of the mouth, the dermoid cyst sometimes resembles a ranula (**Figure 10.235**).

GINGIVAL CYSTS IN NEONATES

Small white nodules are extremely common on the alveolar ridge (**Figure 10.236**) and midline palate of the newborn. Sometimes termed Epstein's pearls or Bohn's nodules, they usually disappear spontaneously by rupturing or involution within a month or so.

There may be an association of gingival cysts with milia (superficial epidermal inclusion cysts). **Figure 10.237** shows the same infant as in **Figure 10.236**.

Oral cysts are otherwise rare in neonates, although cysts may rarely be present at the base of the tongue where they can cause stridor.

LYMPHOEPITHELIAL CYST

The lymphoepithelial cyst is a rare lesion associated with lymphoid tissue, usually seen as an asymptomatic small yellowish movable cystic swelling in the floor of the mouth or ventrum of tongue (**Figure 10.238**), and may represent simple oral lymphoid tissue.

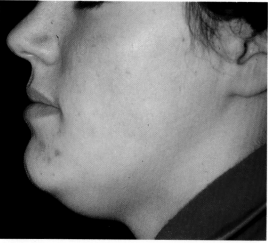

10.234

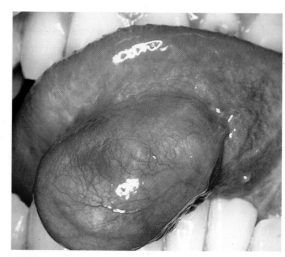

10.235

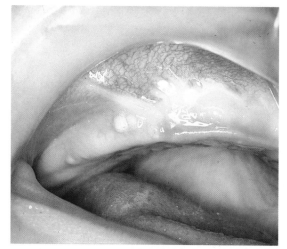

10.236

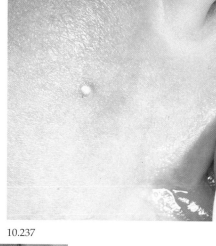

10.237

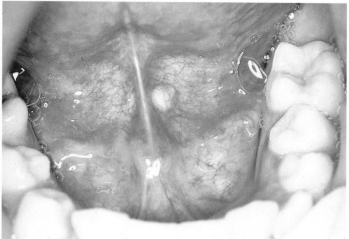

10.238

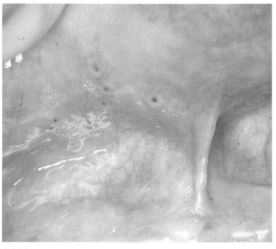

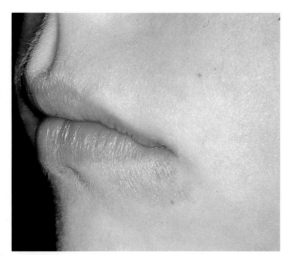

10.239

10.240

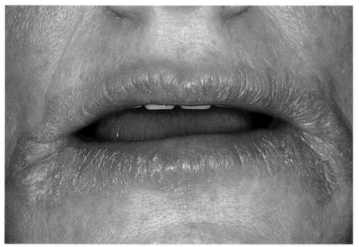

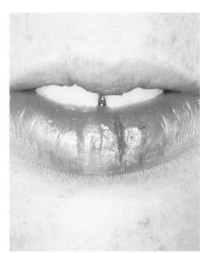

10.241

10.242

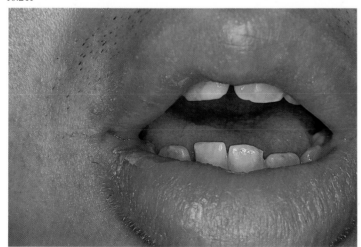

10.243

CHEILITIS

Cheilitis glandularis is shown in **Figure 10.239**. The black puncta in this case, inside the upper lip, were associated with swelling and a thick mucinous exudate from the minor salivary glands. This lesion, of unknown aetiology, may be premalignant and usually affects the lower lip.

Cheilitis is also caused by lip-licking: children in particular may develop a habit of licking the lip and adjacent skin, leading to erythematous lesions (**Figure 10.240**). Candidosis may infect some of these lesions.

PERIORAL DERMATITIS

Perioral dermatitis is seen mainly in females and related to the use of cosmetics (**Figure 10.241**), corticosteroid creams or ointments, or retinoids.

Allergic reactions may follow contact with a variety of topical agents (especially essential oils); with various vegetables (especially artichokes and asparagus); with medicaments or dental materials (*see* pages 243 and 307).

LIP FISSURE

A fissure may develop in the lip where a patient, typically a child, is mouth-breathing (**Figure 10.242**). Lip fissures are common in Down's syndrome. In others there may be a hereditary predisposition for weakness in the first branchial arch fusion. The lips may also crack in this way if swollen, for example in oral Crohn's disease.

EXFOLIATIVE CHEILITIS

Persistent scaling of the vermilion of the lips is seen mainly in adolescent or young adult females (**Figure 10.243**). It may have a somewhat cyclical nature but is of unknown, possibly factitious, aetiology. The lips scale and peel and can be covered with a shaggy yellowish coating.

212

KERATOSIS
(*Leukoplakia*)

Hyperkeratosis in the mouth can present as a white lesion (**Figure 10.244**). Most keratoses are flat and smooth-surfaced (homogeneous), and benign.

In **Figure 10.245** the homogeneous leukoplakia of the lower lip was seen in a heavy smoker. Smoking and tobacco-related habits are, with friction, the most common identifiable causes of keratoses.

Figure 10.246 shows homogeneous keratosis in the buccal mucosa, a common site. Keratoses may be extremely pronounced (**Figure 10.247**).

In **Figure 10.248** the keratosis of the palate has two components: a diffuse overall keratosis with a more verrucous area centrally. Verrucous or nodular keratoses have a low premalignant potential but higher than that of homogeneous keratoses.

A recently described variant termed proliferative verrucous leukoplakia is seen especially in the buccal mucosa in older women and about one half develop carcinoma.

In **Figure 10.249**, the lesion in the anterior part is somewhat nodular and developed into a carcinoma.

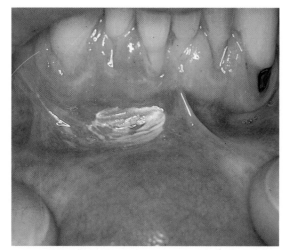

10.244

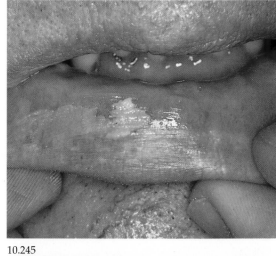

10.245

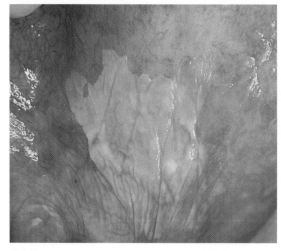

10.246

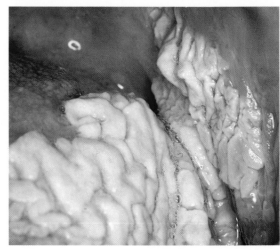

10.247

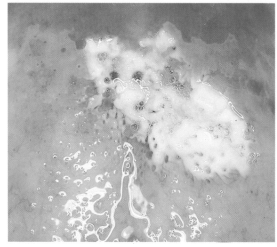

10.248

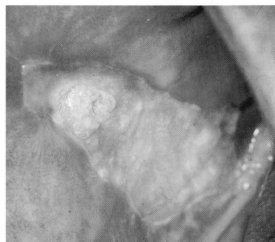

10.249

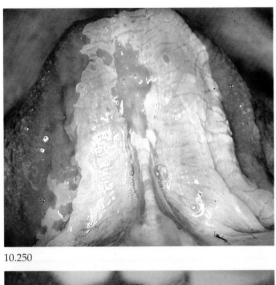

10.250

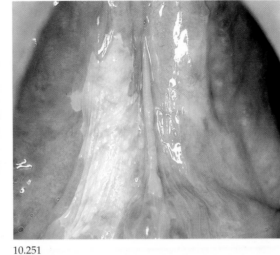

10.251

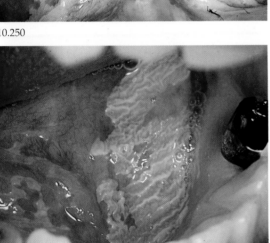

10.252

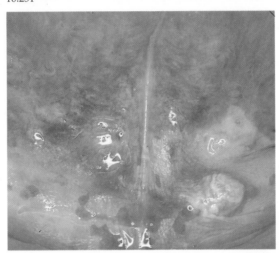

10.253

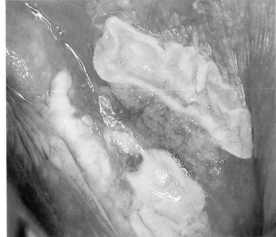

10.254

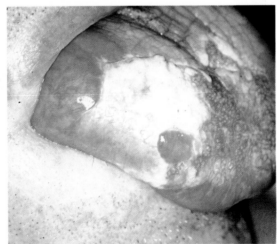

10.255

Keratosis on the ventrum of the tongue and floor of the mouth has a higher premalignant potential than similar lesions elsewhere (**Figures 10.250** to **10.253**).

Seen especially in middle-aged or older women, the sublingual keratosis is usually bilateral, but not invariably (**Figure 10.251**).

The surface may have a so-called 'ebbing tide' appearance, resembling the appearance of sand on the beach as the tide ebbs (**Figure 10.252**), and the lesion may be a mixture of white and red lesions: a speckled leukoplakia (**Figure 10.253**). The red areas are most sinister.

Keratoses must be examined clinically with care and biopsied: the white lesions in **Figure 10.254** flanked a carcinoma.

Although the most obvious lesions on the tongue in **Figure 10.255** are white, the more sinister is the red lesion (erythroplasia) on the lateral margin which showed severe epithelial dysplasia on histology. The patient had already had a carcinoma of the buccal mucosa excised and skin-grafted: he has widespread 'field changes' and may well develop another oral carcinoma.

Leukoplakia and glossitis on the dorsum of the tongue may sometimes have a syphilitic origin.

(Contd)

KERATOSIS
(Contd)

Speckled leukoplakias have the highest premalignant potential of the keratoses. Keratoses such as these (**Figure 10.256**) may have a candidal association, although these are typically located at the commissures.

ERYTHROPLASIA
(Erythroplakia)

Less common than leukoplakia, erythroplasia (**Figure 10.257**) is characterized by epithelial atrophy and pronounced dysplasia. Erythroplasia is seen mainly in elderly males, in the buccal mucosa or palate.

STOMATITIS NICOTINA
(Smoker's palate)

Stomatitis nicotina is a fairly common lesion, seen typically in middle-aged or elderly pipe smokers. The palate is diffusely white and the orifices of the minor salivary glands are obvious as red spots (**Figure 10.258**).

In **Figure 10.259**, a close-up view shows the typical features and the heavily tobacco-stained teeth. Smoker's keratosis is usually a benign lesion that regresses if smoking is stopped.

If a denture is worn, the mucosa is protected by the denture and appears normal in contrast to the non-denture bearing area (**Figure 10.260**). The obvious red area proved, however, to be dysplastic.

PAPILLOMATOSIS

Papillomatous lesions in the vault of the palate may occasionally result from obstructed ducts of minor salivary glands (**Figure 10.261**).

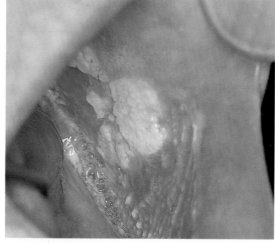
10.256

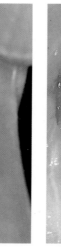
10.257

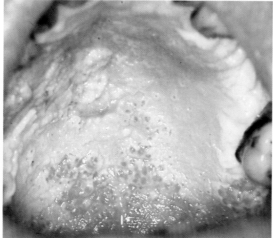
10.258

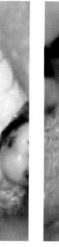
10.259

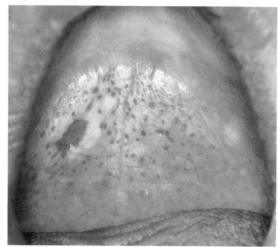
10.260

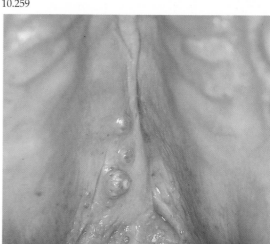
10.261

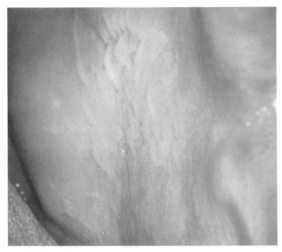

10.262

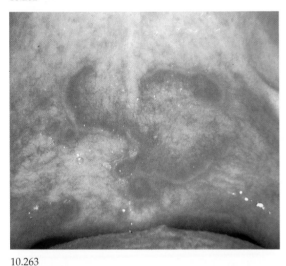

10.263

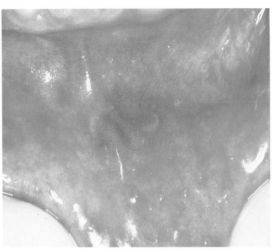

10.264

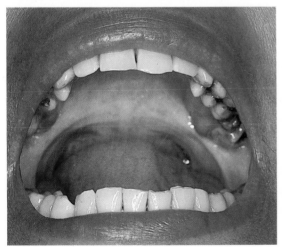

10.265

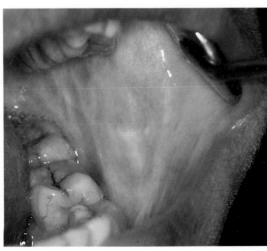

10.266

LEUKOEDEMA

Leukoedema is the term given to the clinical appearance of a milky whitish wrinkled film in the buccal mucosa (**Figure 10.262**). It is a normal variant. It disappears if the mucosa is stretched when the cheek is pushed in from outside (as demonstrated posteriorly here).

ERYTHEMA MIGRANS (*Geographic or migratory stomatitis*)

Erythema migrans is common on the tongue but uncommon elsewhere. Often asymptomatic, the lesions are characterized by a somewhat serpiginous yellow-white lesion with surrounding erythema, which can simulate snailtrack ulcers (**Figure 10.263**) (*see also* pages 89 and 228).

Figure 10.264 shows a less pronounced lesion of erythema migrans. The lesions change in shape and site and are totally benign. They may represent a variant of psoriasis.

ORAL SUBMUCOUS FIBROSIS

Oral submucous fibrosis (OSMF) is a chronic disorder affecting the oral and sometimes pharyngeal mucosa, characterized by pain and the development of epithelial atrophy and fibrosis leading to stiffening of the mucosa and restricted mouth-opening (**Figures 10.265** and **10.266**).

The mucosa is pale, tight, with vertical submucosal fibrous bands and may develop carcinoma. Seen in persons who use betel (*Areca catechu*) nuts, the lesions of OSMF appear to be due to constituents such as alkaloids, tannin and catechin. OSMF is seen mainly in Asians. There appears to be a genetic predisposition.

216

FIBROUS LUMP (*Fibroepithelial polyp*)

Fibrous lumps may be related to irritation, but this is not always evident (**Figure 10.267**).

In **Figure 10.268**, the lesion in **Figure 10.267** is a so-called 'leaf fibroma', although it is not actually a true fibroma. It is totally benign.

Fibrous lumps on the margin of the tongue may also be benign, although biopsy is prudent (**Figure 10.269**).

PAPILLARY HYPERPLASIA

Papillary hyperplasia of the palate is a benign condition of unknown aetiology (**Figure 10.270**), but is often more obvious where a denture is worn and where there is denture-induced stomatitis.

Papillary hyperplasia can also appear in the absence of dentures (**Figure 10.271**).

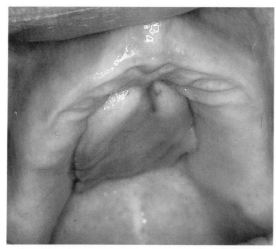
10.267

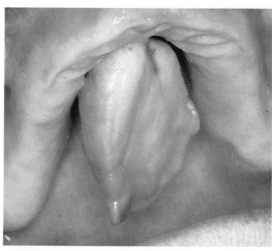
10.268

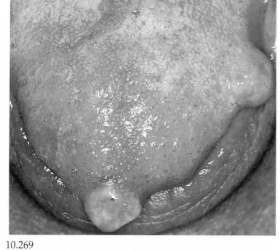
10.269

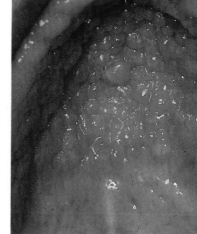
10.270

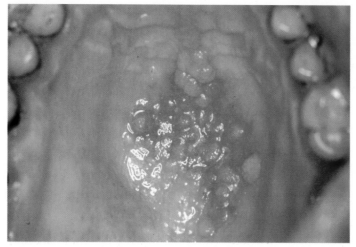
10.271

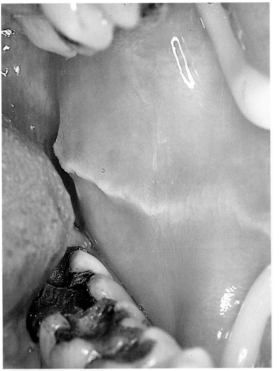

10.272

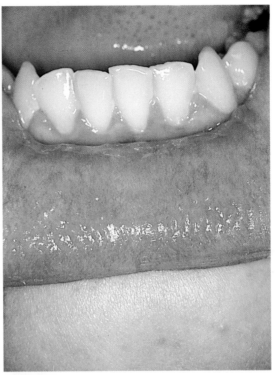

10.273

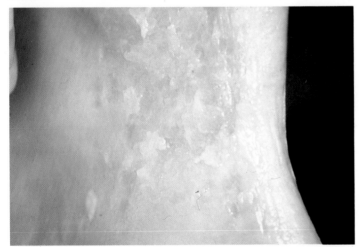

10.274

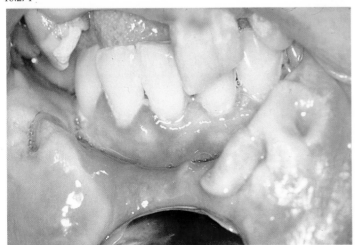

10.275

LINEA ALBA
(*Occlusal line*)

A horizontal whitish line at the level where the teeth occlude (**Figure 10.272**) is a common benign lesion, more obvious in patients with parafunctional habits such as jaw clenching or tooth-grinding, and in those with temporomandibular pain–dysfunction syndrome.

LIP-BITING
(*Morsicatio buccarum*)

Lip-biting is a common habit (**Figure 10.273**), particularly in anxiety states, and may be associated with a few traumatic petechiae.

CHEEK-CHEWING

The mucosa in cheek-chewing is shredded with a shaggy white appearance similar to that of white sponge naevus (*see* page 277) but restricted to areas close to the occlusal line (**Figure 10.274**).

Figure 10.275 shows an extreme example of self-induced lesions. This may be seen in disturbed psychiatric or mentally-handicapped patients.

PYOGENIC GRANULOMA

Pyogenic granulomas are an exaggerated response to minor trauma. They tend to be soft, fleshy, rough-surfaced vascular lesions that bleed readily (**Figure 10.276**).

The gingiva is the most common site, the granuloma often arising on the buccal aspect from the interdental papilla (**Figure 10.277**) and especially where there is a slight malocclusion leading to plaque accumulation (**Figure 10.278**).

Most pyogenic granulomas are seen in the maxilla, anteriorly.

EOSINOPHILIC ULCER (*Eosinophilic granuloma of oral mucosa*)

Eosinophilic granuloma of the oral mucosa is a rare chronic lesion found typically on the tongue of males (**Figure 10.279**), and supposed to have a traumatic aetiology. Numerous eosinophils are seen on biopsy examination, though a T-lymphocyte aetiology is now suspected.

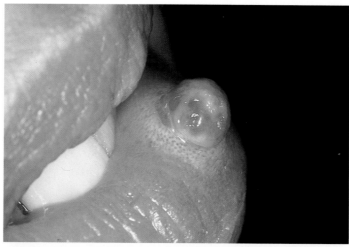

10.276

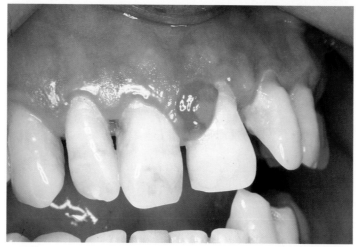

10.277

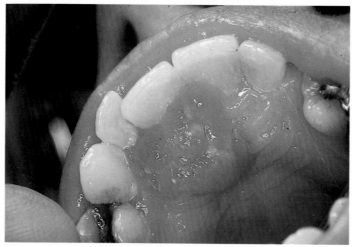

10.278

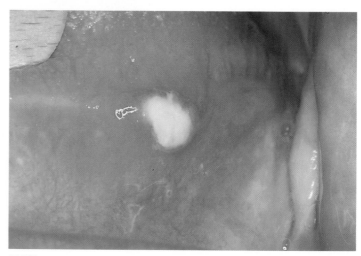

10.279

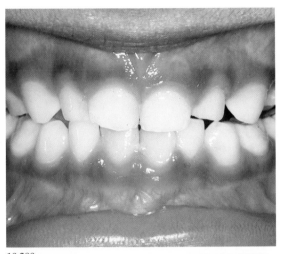

10.280

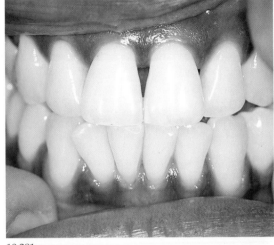

10.281

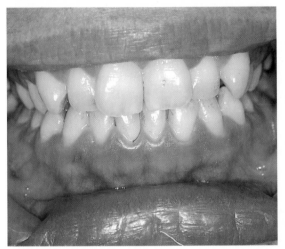

10.282

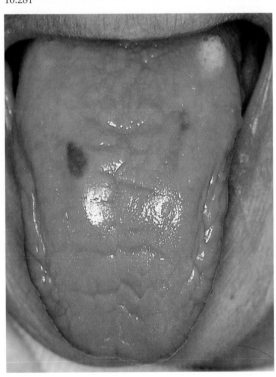

10.283

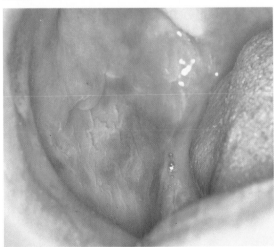

10.284

RACIAL PIGMENTATION

There is no direct correlation between skin colour and gingival pigmentation. **Figures 10.280–10.282** show the range of racial pigmentation that may be seen. In **Figure 10.280**, pigmentation is clearly visible on the attached gingiva in this Asian child.

Figure 10.281 shows an adult negro with racial pigmentation on the gingiva and **Figure 10.282** shows racial pigmentation in a patient of southern European descent.

MELANOTIC MACULES

Oral melanotic macules are brown or black macules (**Figure 10.283**), seen typically on the lips and especially in females. They are benign and are unrelated to racial pigmentation. Other oral pigmented naevi include the intramucosal naevus and blue naevus.

Naevi of Ota, seen mainly in young female Japanese, affect the first or second divisions of the trigeminal nerve with pigmentation of the choroid and iris (oculodermal melanocytosis).

PIGMENTARY INCONTINENCE

Pigmentary incontinence may rarely be seen in lichen planus and can persist after the lichen planus has resolved (**Figure 10.284**) (*see also* **Figure 10.288**).

220

TATTOO

Foreign body tattoo (**Figure 10.285**): pigmentation after foreign material (metal) was left in the lip after an accident.

'Cosmetic tattoo' (**Figure 10.286**): tattooing of the upper gingiva as a tribal custom.

Deliberate tattoo (**Figure 10.287**): tattooing of the lower labial mucosa, perhaps as a tribal custom.

MELANOSIS IN SMOKERS

Figure 10.288 shows melanosis in a smoker (who also has keratosis) caused by pigmentary incontinence following chronic irritation.

Pigmentation of the soft palate may be seen in conditions with ectopic production of adrenocorticotrophic hormone, for example, bronchogenic carcinoma.

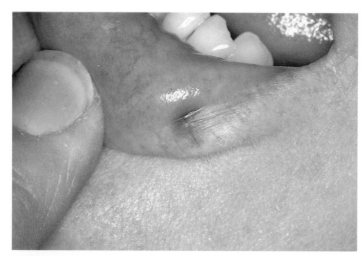

10.285

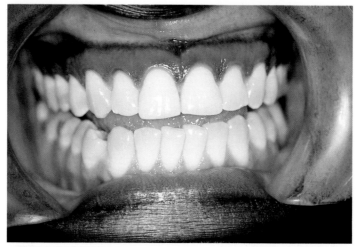

10.286

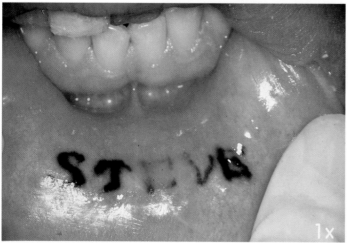

10.287

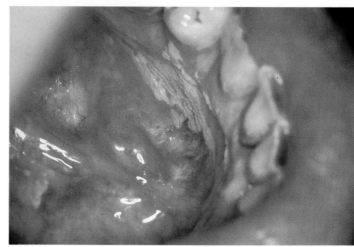

10.288

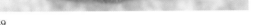

10.289

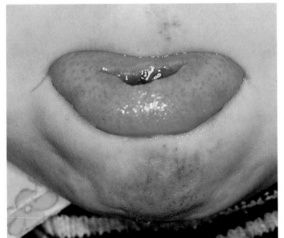

10.291

10.290

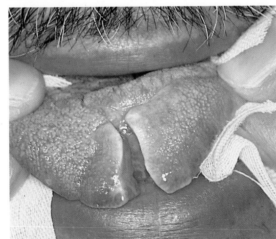

10.292

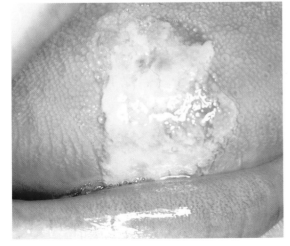

10.293

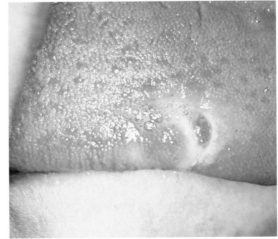

10.294

LINGUAL ABSCESS

Lingual abscesses are uncommon but may follow a penetrating injury (**Figure 10.289**), or infection of a lesion such as a neoplasm, cyst or haematoma.

LINGUAL HAEMATOMA

Trauma to the tongue, especially in a patient with a bleeding tendency (**Figure 10.290**), may produce a haematoma.

LINGUAL LACERATION

Figure 10.291 shows a laceration of the tongue by the teeth of a child who fell on his chin.

Figure 10.292 shows a laceration that was not sutured has resulted in the appearance of a false bifid tongue.

LINGUAL TRAUMATIC ULCER, SELF-INDUCED

Figure 10.293 shows an unusual ulcer on the tongue in a child that was self-induced.

Figure 10.294 is the same patient after 2 weeks.

ERYTHEMA MIGRANS
(*Geographic tongue, benign migratory glossitis*)

Erythema migrans is an extremely common benign condition, of unknown aetiology, in which the filiform papillae desquamate in irregular demarcated areas. Patients with a fissured (scrotal) tongue often have erythema migrans. Most patients with erythema migrans are otherwise healthy, but it may be a forme fruste of psoriasis and may be seen in some patients with cyanotic cardiac disease.

Figures 10.295 and **10.296** show the same patient at first presentation and on the following day, showing the appearance of a second area of depapillation and changed configuration of the initial lesion. On the third day the lesions seen in **Figures 10.295** and **10.296** have enlarged and coalesced (**Figure 10.297**).

In **Figure 10.298**, a different patient, the yellowish serpiginous borders are more obvious than the areas of depapillation.

Figure 10.299 is an example which shows a single depapillated patch with yellowish margin.

If the tongue is furred, the lesions of erythema migrans appear quite pronounced (**Figure s 10.295–10.297** and **10.300**).

(Contd)

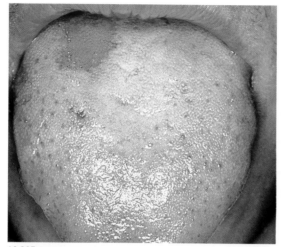

10.295

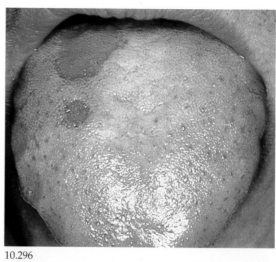

10.296

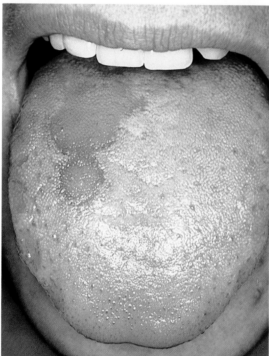

10.297

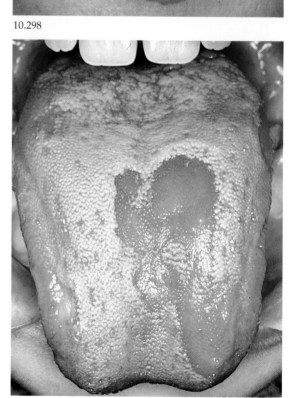

10.298

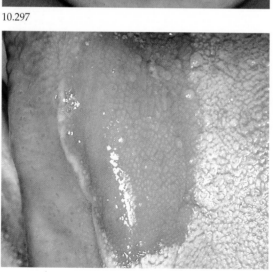

10.299

10.300

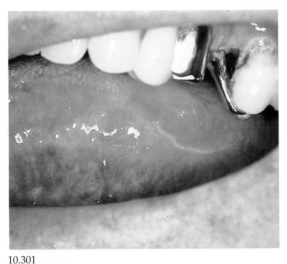

10.301

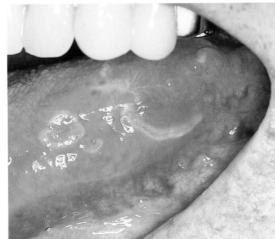

10.302

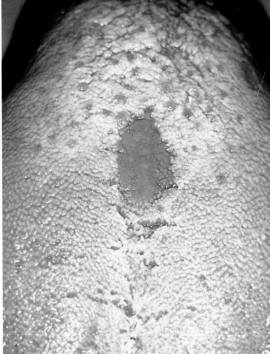

10.303

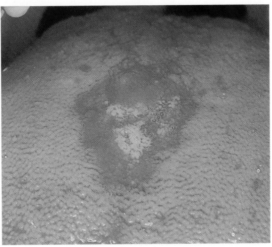

10.304

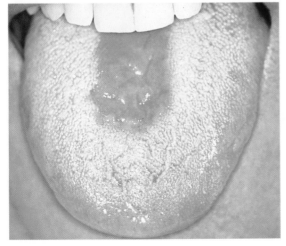

10.305

Though the configuration of the lesions can change over a few hours, there are rare examples where the lesion is persistent and unchanging (erythema migrans perstans is the rather inappropriate term used) (**Figure 10.301**).

The patient seen in **Figure 10.302** (same patient as **Figure 10.301**) has had a virtually identical lesion over 4 years: biopsy has confirmed this is erythema migrans.

MEDIAN RHOMBOID GLOSSITIS (*Central papillary atrophy*)

Median rhomboid glossitis is a rhomboidal red depapillated area in the midline of the dorsum of tongue, just anterior to the circumvallate papillae (**Figure 10.303**).

Median rhomboid glossitis was thought to be a development anomaly owing to persistence of the tuberculum impar, but is now thought to be related to localized candidosis, predisposed by smoking, the wearing of dentures, diabetes and HIV disease. Occasionally, it is a mixed red and white lesion (**Figure 10.304**).

Median rhomboid glossitis is usually asymptomatic though it may cause slight discomfort. Some lesions may appear somewhat sinister (**Figure 10.305**). The finding of candida-induced pseudoepitheliomatous hyperplasia has caused some of these lesions to be misdiagnosed as carcinomas. Oral carcinoma is rare at this site.

A report of the isolation of *Neisseria gonorrhoeae* from tongue lesions resembling median rhomboid glossitis may be coincidental, since the mouth can be a reservoir for this organism.

FURRED TONGUE

The tongue is rarely furred in a healthy child but may be lightly furred in a healthy adult, especially if the oral hygiene is poor, the patient smokes, wears full dentures, or the diet is soft. Any febrile illness (**Figure 10.306**) may cause a furred tongue.

BROWN HAIRY TONGUE

Although often idiopathic, a brown hairy tongue (**Figure 10.307**) may be seen for any of the reasons discussed above. Mouthwashes, antibiotics, smoking, or gastrointestinal disease may predispose.

White or coloured lesions of the tongue are also sometimes seen in immunocompromised patients. It is now evident that any of a range of microorganisms may become opportunistic pathogens in such patients. For example, a soil saprophytic fungus *Ramichloridium schulzeri* has been described as causing a 'golden' tongue.

BLACK HAIRY TONGUE

Overgrowth of the filiform papillae, with proliferation of chromogenic bacteria may cause a black hairy tongue (**Figure 10.308**). This patient also incidentally has a cleft lip and palate.

FOLIATE PAPILLITIS

The size and shape of the foliate papillae are variable and occasionally they swell if irritated mechanically or if there is an upper respiratory infection (**Figure 10.309**). Located at a site of high predilection for lingual carcinoma, they may give rise to anxiety about cancer.

Inflammation of the lingual tonsils may also give rise to concern as it may present with pain and dysphagia.

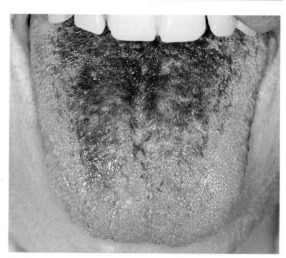

10.307

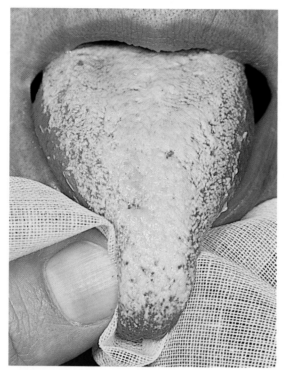

10.306

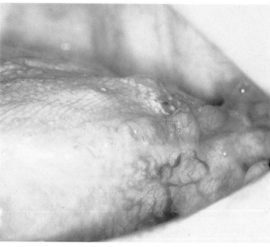

10.309

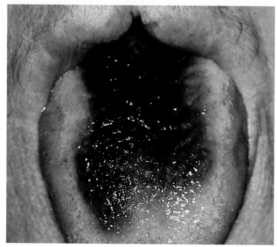

10.308

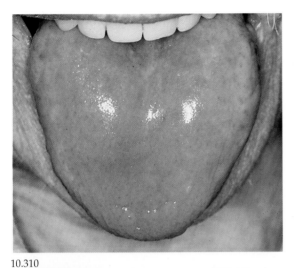

10.310

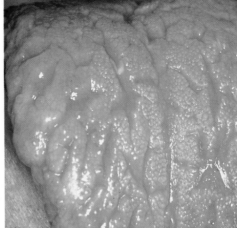

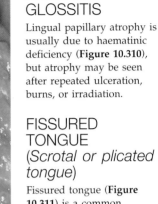

10.311

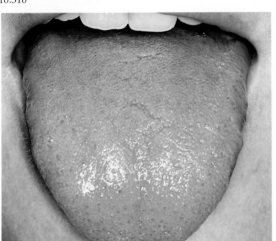

10.312

10.313

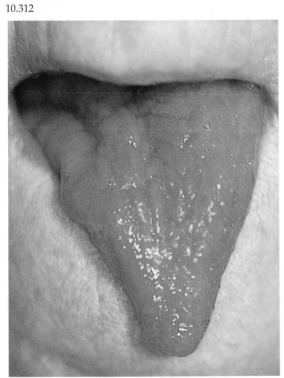

10.314

ATROPHIC GLOSSITIS

Lingual papillary atrophy is usually due to haematinic deficiency (**Figure 10.310**), but atrophy may be seen after repeated ulceration, burns, or irradiation.

FISSURED TONGUE (*Scrotal or plicated tongue*)

Fissured tongue (**Figure 10.311**) is a common developmental anomaly (affecting up to 15% of the population) that may appear after puberty. It is of little significance, though often (20%) associated with erythema migrans. Fissured tongue is one feature of Melkersson–Rosenthal syndrome (*see* page 227) and is found more frequently than normal in Down's syndrome (*see* page 290) and psoriasis.

GLOSSODYNIA (*Glossopyrosis*)

Most patients with glossodynia have no identifiable organic lesion of the tongue (**Figure 10.312**) and the discomfort has a psychogenic basis (*see also* page 144).

LINGUAL HEMIHYPERTROPHY

Hypertrophy of the right side of the tongue (**Figure 10.313**).

The whitish lines on the tongue are caused by strands of saliva, as this patient also has xerostomia.

LINGUAL HEMIATROPHY

A lower motor neurone hypoglossal nerve lesion (**Figure 10.314**) can cause atrophy.

CROHN'S DISEASE

Crohn's disease is a chronic inflammatory bowel disease of unknown aetiology, affecting mainly the ileum although any part of the gastrointestinal tract can be involved, including, in up to 10%, the mouth. Non-caseating granulomas are also seen in sarcoid and it is possible that oral Crohn's disease is actually a similar but distinct condition. Some use the term 'orofacial granulomatosis'. Swelling of the lips and angular stomatitis are common (**Figures 10.315** and **10.316**). Biopsy of the lip shows lymphoedema and granulomas.

Facial swelling (**Figure 10.317**) may occur and gingival swelling may be a feature (**Figure 10.318**).

Persistent irregular ulcers (**Figure 10.319** and **10.320**) or classic aphthae, are common features. Pyostomatitis vegetans (*see* page 228) may also be seen, but is usually associated with ulcerative colitis.

The majority of patients with 'oral Crohn's disease' do not have identifiable gastro-intestinal lesions and some seem to have lesions as a consequence of food or food additive 'allergy'.

(*Contd*)

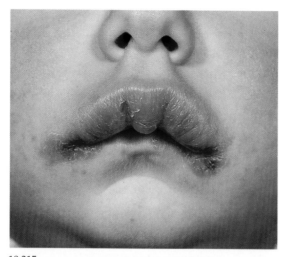

10.315

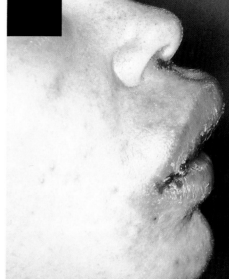

10.316

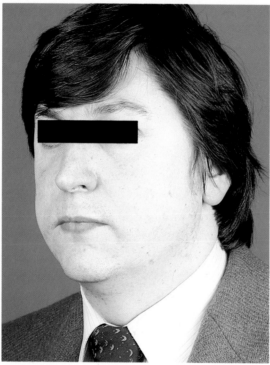

10.317

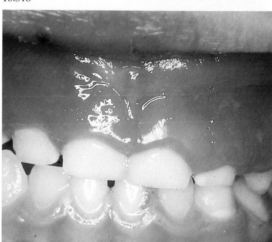

10.318

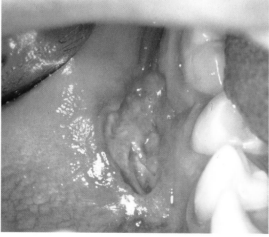

10.319

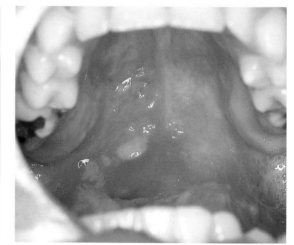

10.320

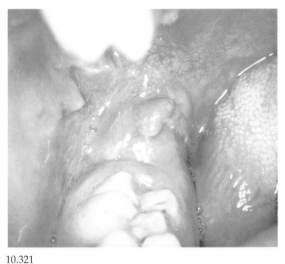

10.321

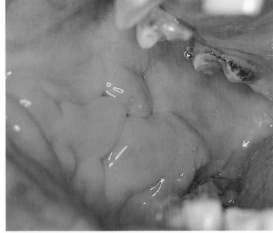

10.322

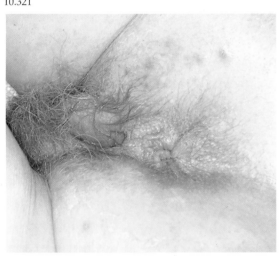

10.323

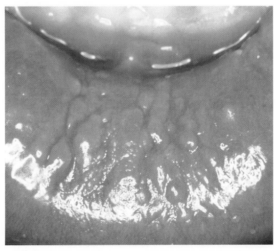

10.324

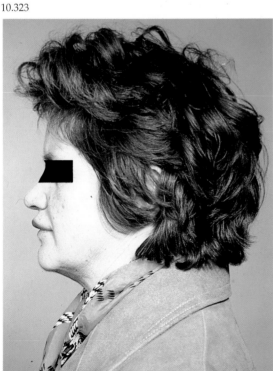

10.325

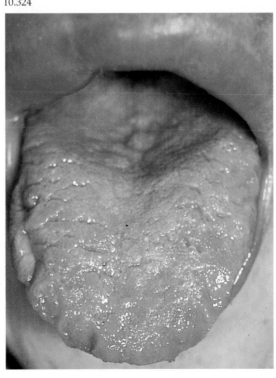

10.326

Mucosal tags are a feature in some patients (**Figure 10.321**) and folding of the oral mucosa may lead to a 'cobblestone' appearance (**Figure 10.322**).

Perianal tags are also seen in Crohn's disease (**Figure 10.323**).

OROFACIAL GRANULOMATOSIS

The clinical features seen in Crohn's disease may be present in the absence of identifiable intestinal disease. The patient in **Figure 10.324**, for example, who had a somewhat swollen lower lip with a cobblestoned mucosa, proved to be reacting to cinnamon.

MELKERSSON– ROSENTHAL SYNDROME

Melkersson–Rosenthal syndrome is the association of orofacial swelling, fissured tongue (30%) and unilateral lower motor neurone facial palsy (**Figures 10.325** and **10.326**). It appears to be related to cheilitis granulomatosa, oral Crohn's disease, sarcoidosis and orofacial granulomatosis.

The swelling is non-tender and will not pit on pressure. Intraorally, swellings may involve the buccal mucosa and gingiva and there may be ulceration.

Partial forms of the syndrome are not infrequent.

ULCERATIVE COLITIS

Oral lesions in ulcerative colitis include ulcers and pustules (pyostomatitis vegetans) which may also be found in Crohn's disease or overlap syndromes (**Figure 10.327**).

Ulceration (**Figure 10.327**) may be widespread and produce an unusual type of desquamative gingivitis (**Figure 10.328**). The tongue is only rarely ulcerated in ulcerative colitis.

Multiple small pustules (**Figure 10.329**) and irregular ulceration may clinically resemble a 'snailtrack' ulcer, resulting from fusion of the ulcerated pustules (**Figure 10.330**).

An aphthous type of ulcer may be a manifestation of pyostomatitis gangrenosum (**Figure 10.331**).

GLUTEN-SENSITIVE ENTEROPATHY (*Coeliac disease*)

Coeliac disease is commonly associated with enamel defects which can also be seen in healthy first-degree relatives. Up to 3 per cent of patients seen as out-patients with aphthae prove to have coeliac disease (**Figure 10.332**).

Patients with dermatitis herpetiformis often also suffer from coeliac disease. (*See also* page 244).

Peutz–Jegher's syndrome (*see* page 296) and Gardner's syndrome (*see* page 200) also have oral manifestations and the short-bowel syndrome may be associated with alveolar bone loss.

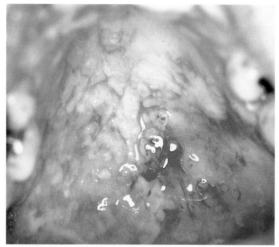

10.327

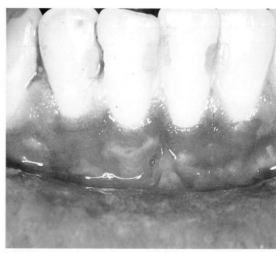

10.328

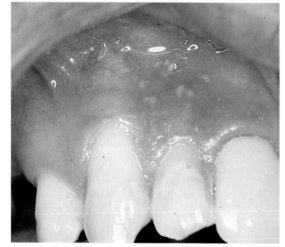

10.329

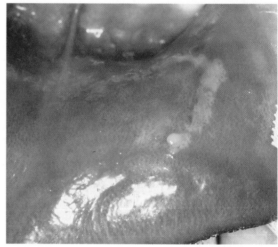

10.330

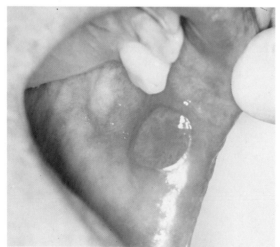

10.331

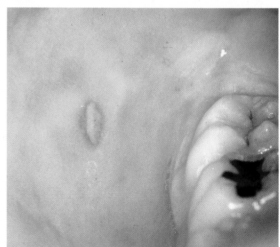

10.332

11 DISEASES OF THE LIVER

BILIARY ATRESIA

Oral manifestations have seldom been reported in patients with biliary atresia, but there may be enamel hypoplasia, delayed tooth eruption and green teeth (**Figure 11.1**) (*see also* **Figure 10.61**) or gingival discoloration.

Immunosuppressant agents in liver transplant patients may be associated with oral adverse effects such as herpetic (**Figure 11.2**) or candidal infections, gingival hyperplasia, vesiculo-bullous lesions and hairy leukoplakia.

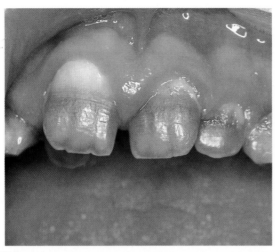

11.1

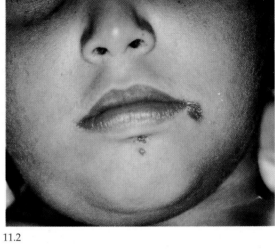

11.2

ALCOHOLIC CIRRHOSIS

Sialosis (**Figure 11.3**), and tooth erosion from gastric acid regurgitation are fairly common oral features of alcoholism, and alcohol use predisposes to oral cancer. Hyperpigmentation may be seen.

Liver failure may cause hepatic fetor with pronounced halitosis.

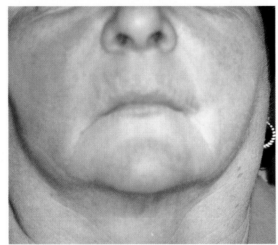

11.3

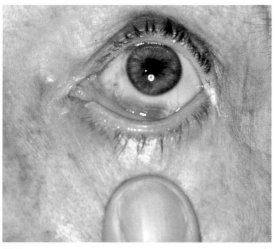

11.4

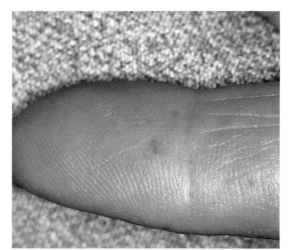

11.5

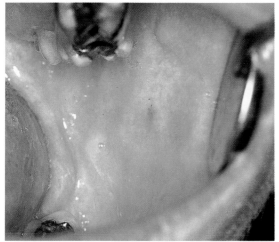

11.6

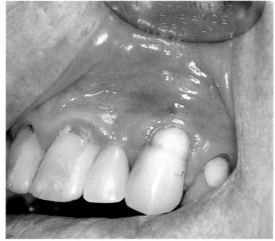

11.7

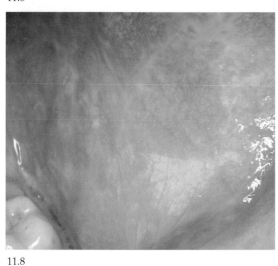

11.8

PRIMARY BILIARY CIRRHOSIS

Icterus and telangiectasia (**Figure 11.4**) are common features of primary biliary cirrhosis (PBC), an autoimmune chronic destructive non-suppurative cholangitis characterized by progressive inflammatory destruction of intrahepatic bile ducts. Over 90% of patients are female. PBC may be associated with a variety of other autoimmune disorders such as scleroderma, CRST syndrome (calcinosis cutis, Raynaud's phenomenon, sclerodactyly and telangiectasia), CREST syndrome (CRST syndrome plus oesophageal dysmotility) or rheumatoid arthritis. Over 90% of PBC patients have serum antimitochondrial antibodies, and some also express antibodies directed against ribosomal, smooth muscle, nuclear, double-stranded deoxyribonucleic acid and thyroid components.

Telangiectasia may be seen on the skin (**Figure 11.5**) and intra-orally (**Figure 11.6**).

A connection exists between PBC and a sicca syndrome of dry mouth (**Figure 11.7**) and dry eyes. Other oral conditions that may be associated with PBC include lichenoid lesions, gingival xanthomatosis, green staining of teeth and mucosa and enamel hypoplasia.

CHRONIC ACTIVE HEPATITIS

Lichen planus can also be seen in chronic active hepatitis (**Figure 11.8**). In some patients, particularly those of southern European extraction, there often appears to be an association between oral lichen planus and infection with hepatitis C virus or hepatitis B virus.

12 DISEASES OF THE GENITO-URINARY SYSTEM

CHRONIC RENAL FAILURE, DIALYSIS AND TRANSPLANTATION

White lesions of the tongue (**Figure 12.1**), or hyperpigmentation of the mucosa, may be seen in uraemia. After renal dialysis, the lesions may resolve (**Figure 12.2**).

The immunosuppression following renal transplantation also predisposes to oral candidosis (**Figure 12.3**), hairy leukoplakia, Kaposi's sarcoma and carcinoma of the lip, while gingival hyperplasia may be related to cyclosporin or calcium-channel blocker use (**Figure 12.4**).

An unpleasant taste, halitosis and dry mouth are common in chronic renal failure; other oral lesions may include ulcers and mixed bacterial plaques (**Figure 12.5**), keratosis, candidosis and purpura.

Skeletal changes, which seem especially to affect the jaws in patients on haemodialysis, include changes in trabecular pattern and localized radiolucencies. The dental pulp chambers tend to narrow.

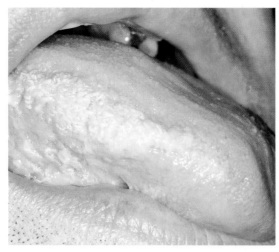

12.1

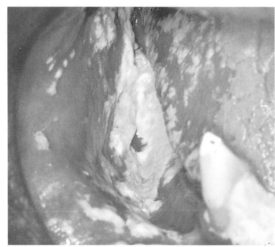

12.3

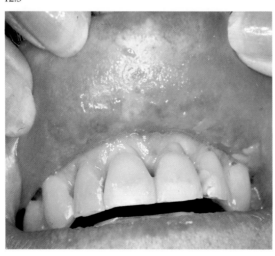

12.5

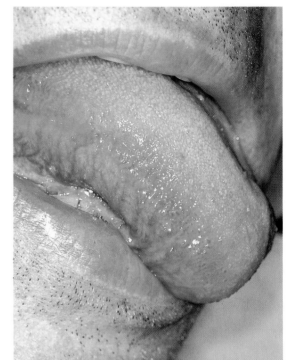

12.2

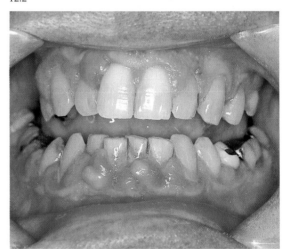

12.4

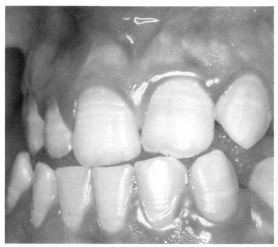

12.6

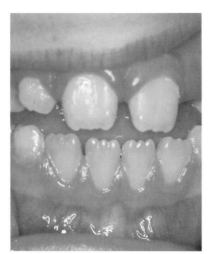

12.7

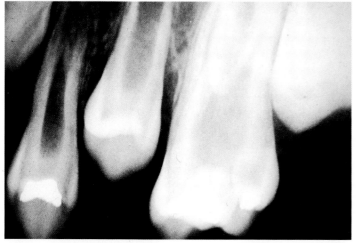

12.8

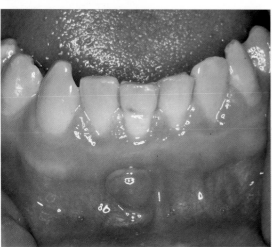

12.9

HYPO-PHOSPHATAEMIA (*Vitamin D-resistant rickets, renal rickets*)

This is a sex-linked disorder characterized by a renal tubular defect of phosphate resorption due to end-organ resistance to vitamin D. Teeth may be hypoplastic (**Figure 12.6**; incidentally, the upper lateral incisor is absent).

The condition may be genetically linked: **Figure 12.7** is the brother of the patient in **Figure 12.6**.

The teeth may be hypoplastic and eruption retarded. The teeth have large pulp chambers and abnormal dentine calcification (**Figure 12.8**). Even minimal caries or attrition can produce pulpitis: periapical abscesses are thus common (**Figure 12.9**).

13 COMPLICATIONS OF PREGNANCY, CHILDBIRTH AND THE PUERPERIUM

GINGIVITIS DURING MENSTRUATION

Where there is gingivitis, for example where plaque accumulates on the crowded teeth (**Figure 13.1**), there may be an exacerbation premenstrually.

PREGNANCY GINGIVITIS

Gingivitis is most prevalent in pregnancy if oral hygiene is poor. A highly vascular marginal gingivitis (**Figure 13.2**) appears at the second month of pregnancy, reaches a maximum intensity by the eighth month, and then regresses.

CHLOASMA

Facial pigmentation may be seen in pregnancy (**Figure 13.3**). Hyperpigmented patches may be seen over the cheeks, temples, or forehead. They tend to resolve after parturition.

Similar changes may be seen after use of petroleum jelly or some photosensitising facial creams (chloasma cosmeticum).

Facial telangiectasia may appear in pregnancy or in those on synthetic oestrogens.

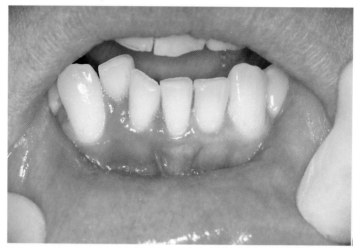

13.1

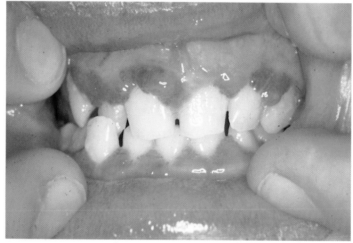

13.2

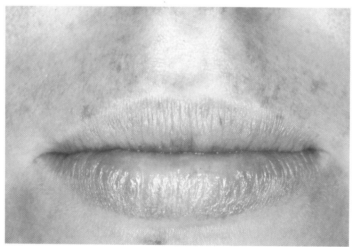

13.3

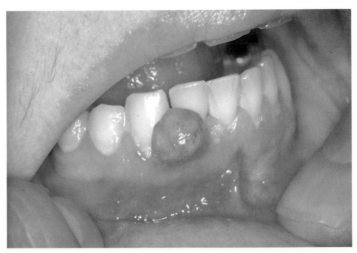

13.4

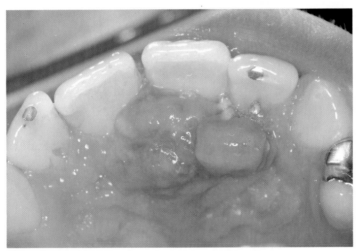

13.5

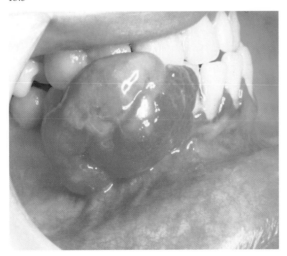

13.6

PREGNANCY EPULIS
(*Pregnancy granuloma*)

Pyogenic granulomas are common in pregnancy (**Figures 13.4** to **13.6**). They may bleed or be asymptomatic. They are benign.

14 DISEASES OF THE SKIN AND SUBCUTANEOUS TISSUES

242

CARBUNCLE

Carbuncles are not seen in the mouth but may rarely affect the lip with tender red swelling and eventual suppuration (**Figures 14.1** and **14.2**).

An extreme example of a carbuncle of the lower lip is shown in **Figure 14.3**.

LUDWIG'S ANGINA

Ludwig's angina is infection of the sublingual and submandibular fascial spaces, usually of odontogenic origin. It manifests with pain, submandibular swelling (**Figure 14.4**), dysphagia and fever and may be a hazard to the airway.

NECROTIZING FASCIITIS

Necrotizing fasciitis is due to Group A streptococci or a mixture of other bacteria, and is seen most commonly on the head and neck (**Figures 14.5** and **14.6**) or the limbs.

The portal of entry is a cut or surgical wound. The patients usually present with a hot, tender area of swelling which is erythematous, or dusky. Bullae and necrosis of underlying tissue may intervene, the overlying skin may become anaesthetic and the lesion spreads rapidly.

The patient is usually severely ill and toxic and there is a mortality of over 45% reported in some series. Similar conditions include: (1) progressive bacterial synergistic gangrene and (2) gangrenous cellulitis due to other pathogens such as *Pseudomonas* species or zygomycete fungi (mucormycosis) mainly seen in the immunocompromised patient.

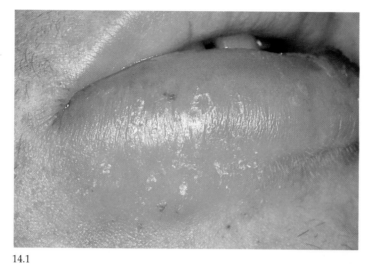

14.1

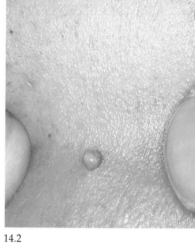

14.2

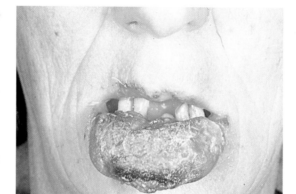

14.3

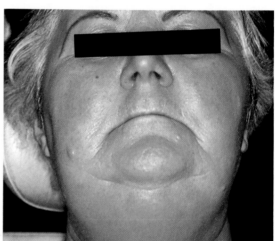

14.4

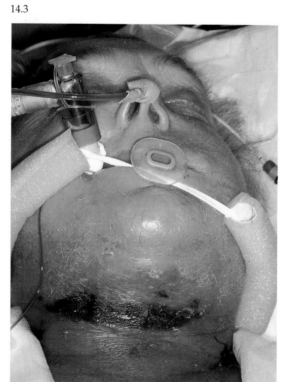

14.5

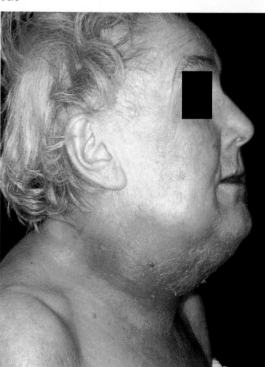

14.6

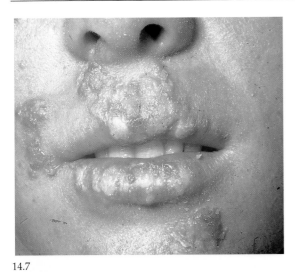

14.7

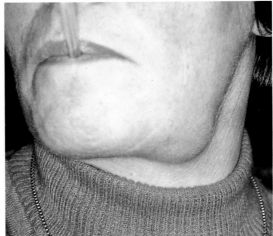

14.8

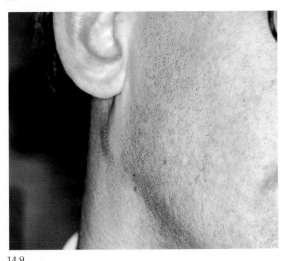

14.9

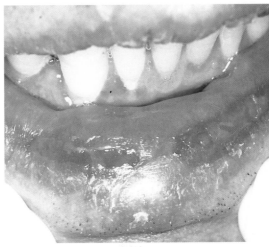

14.10

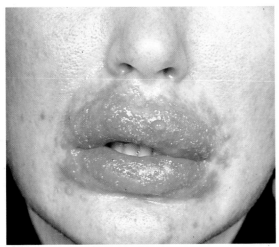

14.11

IMPETIGO

Perioral lesions such as herpes labialis or chickenpox may be secondarily infected with *staphylococci* or *streptococci*, resulting in impetigo (**Figure 14.7**). Alternatively, there may be a primary infection or spread of impetigo from elsewhere.

ACUTE LYMPHADENITIS

Lymphadenitis is usually a consequence of spread of infection from a focus in the drainage area. Occasionally a facial node (**Figure 14.8**), submandibular or other node is infected but the source unidentified. Such idiopathic submandibular abscesses are usually seen in pre-school children who are apparently healthy. *Staphylococcus aureus* is usually implicated and it is presumed that a small lesion in the nose or mouth is the focus.

Parotid lymph nodes may occasionally become infected (**Figure 14.9**), typically from a cutaneous lesion.

Cervical lymph nodes may also be enlarged in the absence of an identifiable local infective lesion; in some systemic infections; in malignant disease; in connective tissue diseases; in sarcoid; and for other reasons (*see* page 18).

ACTINIC CHEILITIS (*Solar elastosis*)

Outdoor workers, and others chronically exposed to sunlight, may develop ulcers and crusting, especially of the lower lip (**Figure 14.10**). Ultraviolet light appears to cause change of collagen into an elastic-like material. Actinic cheilitis may sometimes be followed by carcinoma.

ALLERGIC CHEILITIS

An allergic reaction to lipstick or other cosmetics is not uncommon. Swelling and sometimes blistering of the lips is seen (**Figure 14.11**).

DERMATITIS HERPETIFORMIS (*Duhring's disease*)

Dermatitis herpetiformis (DH) is an uncommon skin disease, often associated with gluten-sensitive enteropathy, and most common in adult males.

Oral lesions, seen in up to 10%, start as vesicles that rupture to leave non-specific ulcers (**Figure 14.12**).

Some patients also have desquamative gingivitis or hyperkeratotic areas (**Figure 14.13**). Coeliac-disease type enamel hypoplasia may be seen.

The typical rash is very itchy and consists of multiple, tense, vesicles on the elbows, shoulders and other extensor surfaces (**Figure 14.14**). Granular deposits of IgA are seen in the epithelial basement membrane zone. Iodine allergy is common.

LINEAR IgA DISEASE

Linear IgA disease is a variant of DH in which the IgA deposits are linear rather than granular at the epithelial basement membrane zone. Oral vesicles or ulcers may be seen (**Figure 14.15**).

Desquamative gingivitis may also be seen in linear IgA disease (**Figure 14.16**).

Chronic bullous dermatosis of childhood is a rare related disorder, seen in young children, which may produce similar oral lesions.

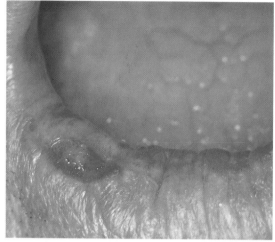

14.12

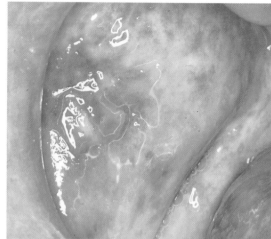

14.13

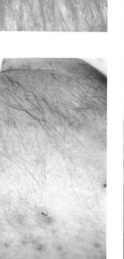

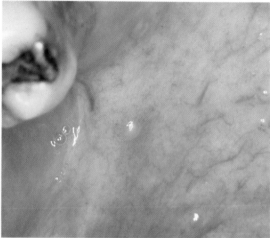

14.14

14.15

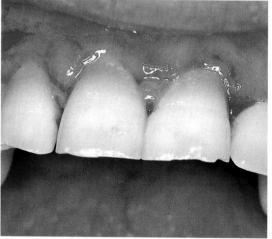

14.16

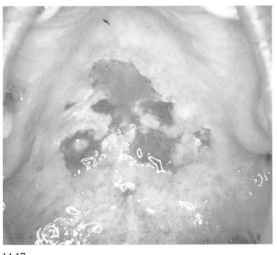

14.17

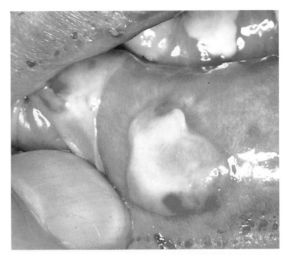

14.18

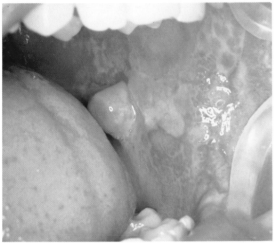

14.19

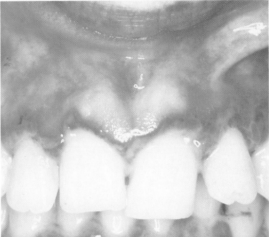

14.20

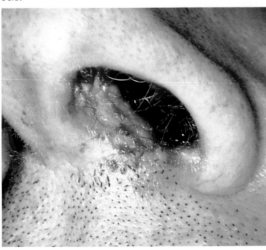

14.21

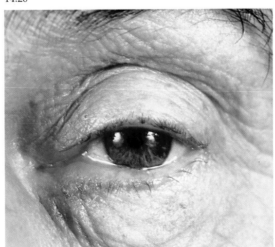

14.22

PEMPHIGUS

Pemphigus is a potentially lethal disorder characterized by autoantibodies (mainly IgG) directed against intercellular substance of stratified squamous epithelium, and seen especially in the middle-aged or elderly. Oral lesions often precede skin manifestations.

Pemphigus vulgaris is the most common type of pemphigus involving the mouth, although still an uncommon disease. Pemphigus vegetans may involve the mouth but oral lesions of the foliaceus and erythematosus types of pemphigus are very rare.

Occasional cases of pemphigus are drug-related (for example, to penicillamine or rifampicin) or para-neoplastic.

Vesicles or blisters are rarely seen intact in the mouth as they break down rapidly to superficial irregular ulcers as in **Figures 14.17** and **14.18**. The ulcers may be covered with a fibrin slough.

Widespread erosions may be seen, especially where the mucosa is traumatized in the buccal mucosa (**Figure 14.19**), palate or gingiva.

Gingival involvement leads to one form of desquamative gingivitis (**Figure 14.20**).

Pemphigus can affect any other stratified squamous epithelium such as the anterior nasal mucosa (**Figure 14.21**) or conjunctivae (**Figure 14.22**).

(Contd)

PEMPHIGUS
(Contd)

Skin blisters tend to be flaccid, and appear at sites of trauma (Nikolsky sign) (**Figure 14.23**; these lesions, on the anterior chest wall, were produced by the edge of a brassière). The skin blisters break down to leave extensive scabbed lesions (**Figure 14.24**).

The axilla and groin are other lesion sites (**Figure 14.25**). Rarely, the nail beds are involved (**Figure 14.26**).

PEMPHIGUS VEGETANS

Pemphigus vegetans often presents initially in the mouth or at the commissures and, even in those with initial skin lesions, the mouth is usually eventually involved. White serpiginous lesions or sometimes vegetations (**Figure 14.27**) are the main manifestations.

The Neumann type follows a similar course to pemphigus vulgaris, whereas the Hallopeau type is more benign. Oral lesions are, however, virtually invariable in both types.

The commissures are the sites most commonly affected and the tongue may be affected with white serpiginous lesions, and sometimes described as a 'cerebriform tongue' (**Figure 14.28**).

BENIGN PEMPHIGUS (*Hailey–Hailey disease*)

Oral lesions are rare and indistinguishable clinically from those of pemphigus vulgaris.

INTRA-EPIDERMAL IgA PUSTULOSIS

Oral blisters and erosions have been described in a few patients with this recently described disease in which there is acantholysis with intercellular IgA deposits.

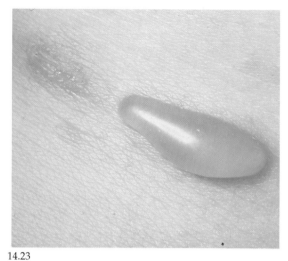

14.23

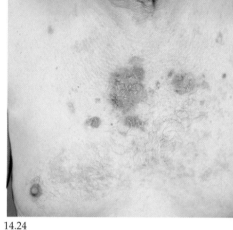

14.24

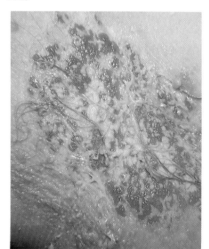

14.25

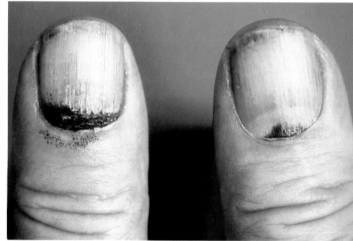

14.26

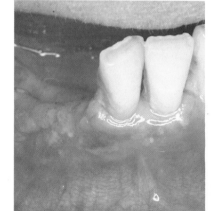

14.27

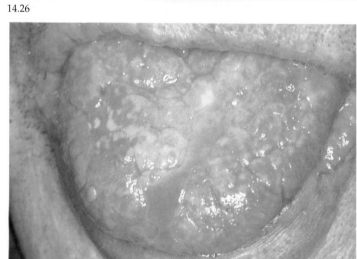

14.28

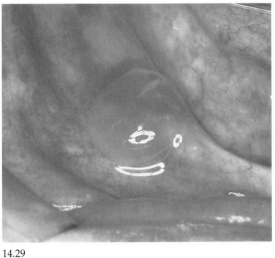

14.29

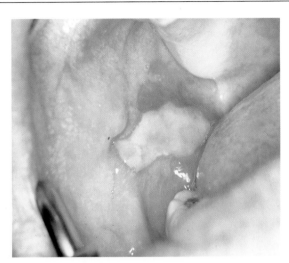

14.30

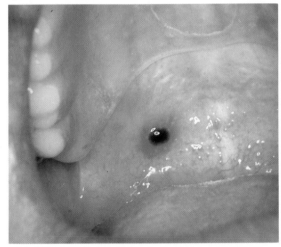

14.31

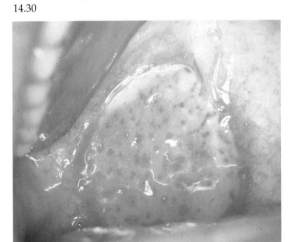

14.32

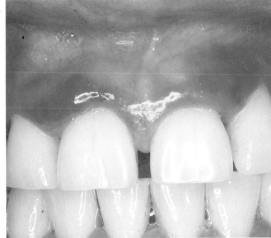

14.33

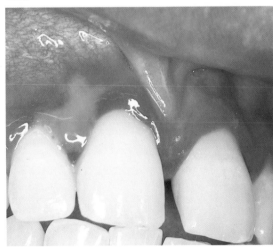

14.34

MUCOUS MEMBRANE PEMPHIGOID (*Cicatricial pemphigoid*)

Mucous membrane pemphigoid is a disorder of stratified squamous epithelia in which there are usually IgG autoantibodies against epithelial basement membrane zone.

Mucous membrane pemphigoid often causes oral lesions: bullous pemphigoid rarely involves the mouth.

Although intact vesicles or bullae may be seen (**Figure 14.29**), they eventually break down to leave irregular ulcers (**Figure 14.30**).

Lesions typically affect the buccal mucosa, palate, and gingiva. Blisters are sometimes blood-filled (**Figure 14.31**).

Figure 14.32 shows the lesion in **Figure 14.31** which enlarged dramatically and broke down to leave an ulcer.

Mucous membrane pemphigoid is a frequent cause of desquamative gingivitis. Desquamation leads to patches of sore erythema (**Figure 14.33**). In contrast to marginal gingivitis, the interdental papillae and gingival margins may appear normal.

Occasionally there is frank gingival ulceration (**Figure 14.34**) as well as superficial gingival desquamation.

(Contd)

MUCOUS MEMBRANE PEMPHIGOID
(Contd)

Conjunctivae and other squamous epithelia may be involved. Scarring may lead to symblepharon (**Figure 14.35**) or, in the larynx, to stenosis. Skin lesions are uncommon.

Ocular involvement is potentially serious since it may culminate in blindness. The eyes are dry and the cornea becomes opaque (**Figure 14.36**).

BULLOUS PEMPHIGOID

Skin lesions are far more common than oral lesions in bullous pemphigoid. Oral vesicles, bullae and erosions may, however, be seen (**Figure 14.37**).

The skin vesicles and bullae of pemphigoid tend to be more tense than those of pemphigus and are seen most often on the abdomen, groin, axillae and flexures (**Figure 14.38**). Bullous pemphigoid is occasionally drug-induced, or secondary to ultraviolet light exposure. Brunsting–Perry disease is a mild variant of bullous pemphigoid.

LOCALIZED ORAL PURPURA
(Angina bullosa haemorrhagica)

Localized oral purpura is a common condition that mimics pemphigoid, although it is unassociated with an immunopathogenesis. Patients present with blood blisters, typically on the soft palate, often after eating (**Figure 14.39**). There is subepithelial vesiculation and an ulcer eventually forms. This type of ulcer has been described as a 'sunburst ulcer' (**Figure 14.40**).

This condition must be differentiated from pemphigoid, and acquired epidermolysis bullosa in particular (*see* Box 1, page 3).

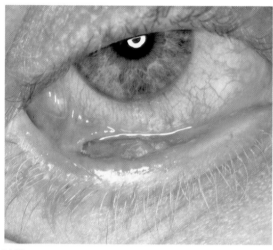

14.35

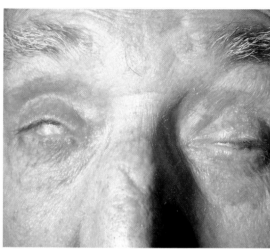

14.36

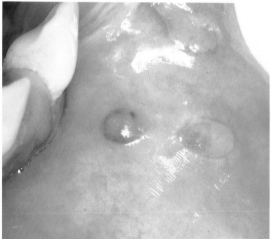

14.37

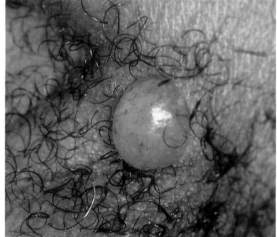

14.38

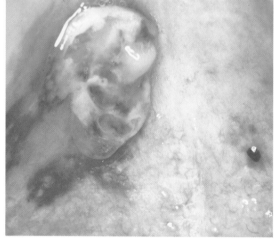

14.39

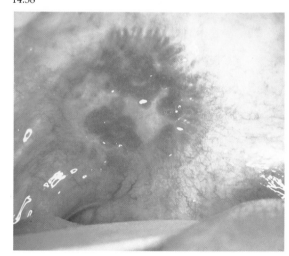

14.40

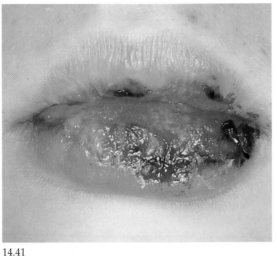

14.41

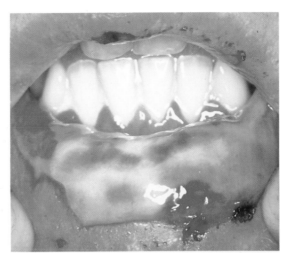

14.42

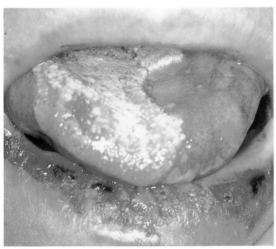

14.43

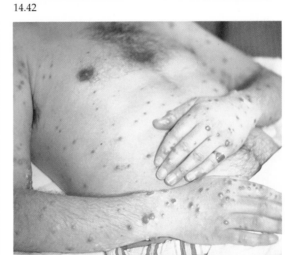

14.44

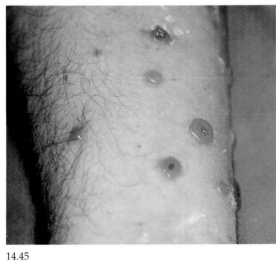

14.45

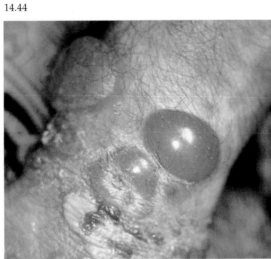

14.46

ERYTHEMA MULTIFORME

Erythema multiforme minor affects typically the back and palms and sometimes the anterior oral mucosa. Erythema multiforme major (Stevens–Johnson syndrome) affects any mucosae, skin and other sites.

The virtually pathognomonic feature of erythema multiforme is swollen, blood-stained or crusted lips (**Figure 14.41**). Oral lesions progress through macules to blisters and ulceration, typically most pronounced in the anterior parts of the mouth (**Figure 14.42**). Extensive oral ulceration may be seen (**Figure 14.43**).

Although the aetiology is unclear in most patients, in some the disorder is precipitated by infections (such as herpes simplex or mycoplasma), by drugs (sulphonamides, barbiturates, hydantoins and others) or by a range of other triggers, even HIV and menstruation. Most patients are males, typically adolescents or young adults, and there are periods of remission from the disease.

Most patients have oral lesions only but, in some, other squamous epithelia are involved. Rashes of various types (hence 'erythema multiforme') are seen (**Figure 14.44**).

Figure 14.45 shows a close-up of the same patient as in **Figure 14.44** showing a vesiculo-bullous rash: the blisters are collapsed and scabbed centrally.

More pronounced blisters in erythema multiforme may resemble pemphigoid (**Figure 14.46**).

(Contd)

ERYTHEMA MULTIFORME
(Contd)

The characteristic rash consists of 'target' or 'iris' lesions in which the central lesion has a surrounding ring of erythema (**Figure 14.47**).

Figure 14.48 shows a later stage of target lesions showing darkening and loss of distinction.

STEVENS–JOHNSON SYNDROME
(Erythema multiforme exudativum)

Conjunctivitis, stomatitis, fever and rash constitute the Stevens–Johnson syndrome (**Figure 14.49**). The ocular changes resemble those of mucous membrane pemphigoid: dry eyes and symblepharon may result.

Figure 14.50 shows the patient shown in **Figure 14.49** upon recovery.

Oral lesions (stomatitis) may be seen with conjunctivitis, genital and cutaneous lesions. Balanitis (**Figure 14.51**), urethritis and vulval ulcers are the typical genital lesions. Broncho-pulmonary and renal involvement may also be seen.

TOXIC EPIDERMAL NECROLYSIS (TEN)

TEN is a variant of erythema multiforme in children sometimes known as staphylococcal scalded skin syndrome (Lyell's disease) which may also produce oral ulceration.

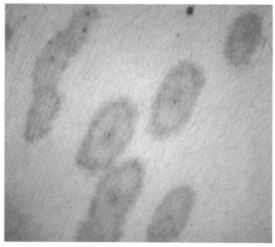

14.47

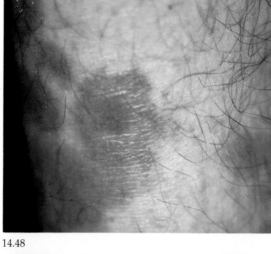

14.48

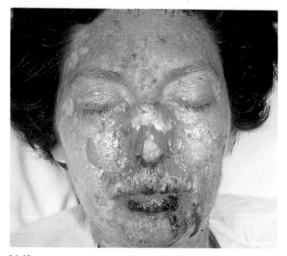

14.49

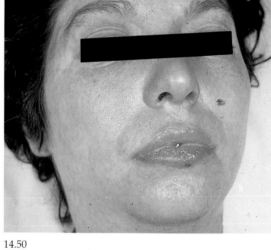

14.50

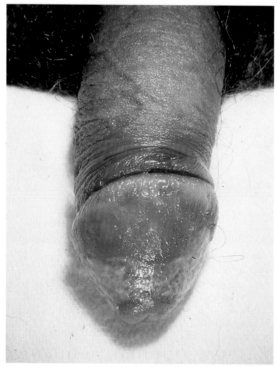

14.51

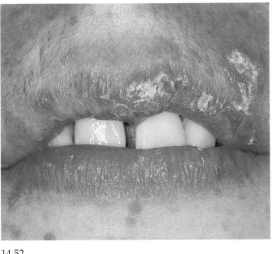

14.52

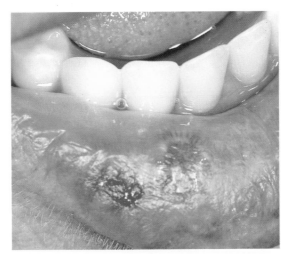

14.53

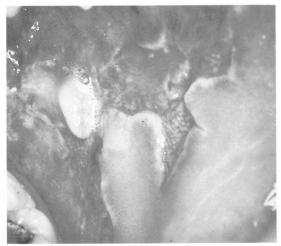

14.54

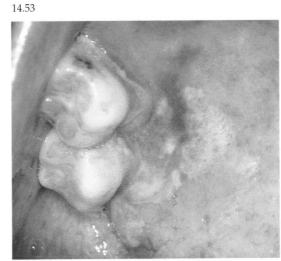

14.55

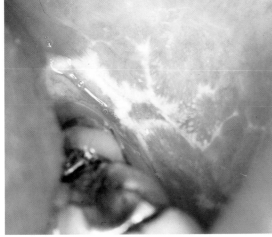

14.56

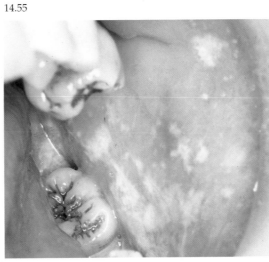

14.57

DISCOID LUPUS ERYTHEMATOSUS

Discoid lupus erythematosus is an immunologically-mediated disorder characterized by a rash on face, scalp, ears and hands, consisting of red patches with scaling and follicular plugging. There may be scaly lesions on the vermilion and perioral skin (**Figure 14.52**; the pigmented lesions (freckles) are unrelated).

The lesions may ulcerate (**Figure 14.53**). and there is a premalignant predisposition, especially in males with lesions on the lip.

The typical oral lesions, seen in up to 25%, are found in the buccal mucosa mainly and have an irregular white border with telangiectasia, surrounding a central atrophic area in which there are small white papules (**Figure 14.54**).

Palatal lesions are far more common in lupus erythematosus (**Figure 14.55**) than in lichen planus — the oral lesions of which can be difficult to differentiate clinically from lupus erythematosus.

LICHEN PLANUS

White lesions in the mouth are the typical feature of lichen planus (**Figure 14.56**) and although often distinct from lupus erythematosus are by no means invariably so.

Oral lichen planus (LP) is common, mostly idiopathic and often asymptomatic. Of the many types described on the following pages, papular LP is the most common (**Figure 14.57**). White papules are seen typically in the buccal mucosa bilaterally.

(Contd)

LICHEN PLANUS
(Contd)

Lichen planus lesions are typically bilateral. Circinate types (**Figure 14.58**), reticular types (**Figure 14.59**) and mixed papular and reticular types (**Figure 14.60**) may be seen.

Plaque type (**Figure 14.61**) lichen planus, especially in smokers, can give rise to confluent white patches difficult to distinguish clinically from keratoses (leukoplakia).

Although the buccal mucosa is the common site for LP, lesions may also involve the dorsum and lateral margins of the tongue (**Figure 14.62**).

Figure 14.63 shows plaque and atrophic types: the white lesion on the left side of the tongue is LP. On the right side is an atrophic depapillated lesion of LP.

Oral lesions of LP are often persistent and patients typically have lesions for many years.

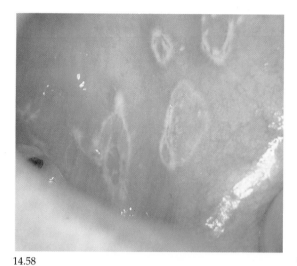

14.58

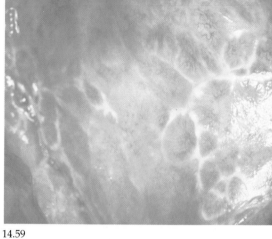

14.59

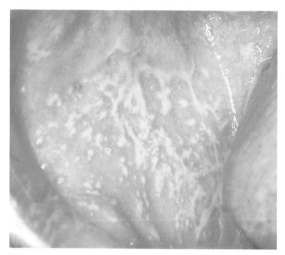

14.60

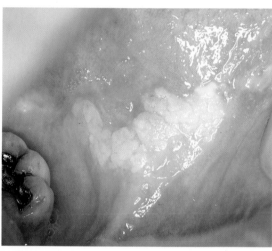

14.61

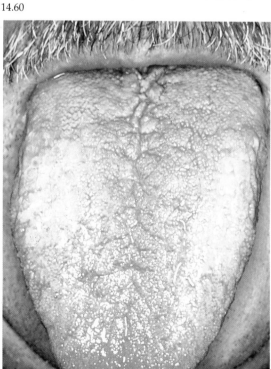

14.62

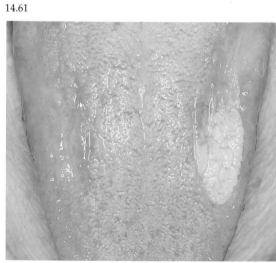

14.63

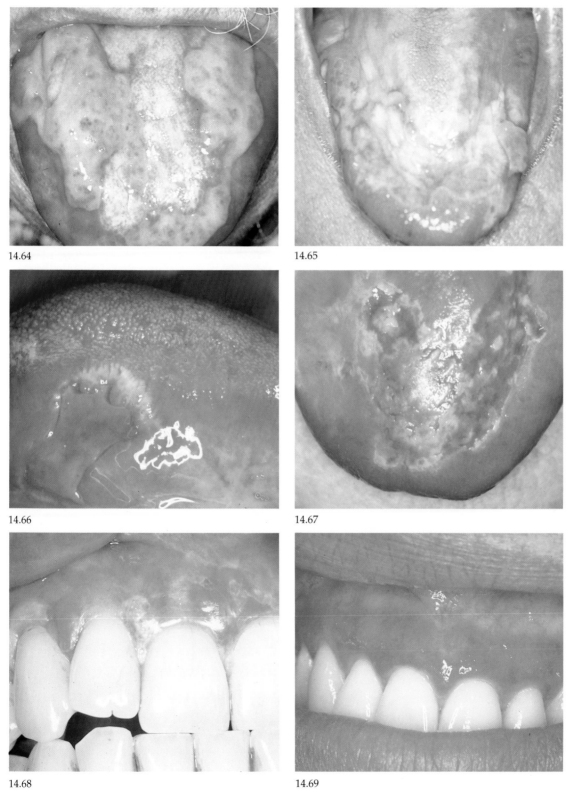

14.64

14.65

14.66

14.67

14.68

14.69

Erosive LP (**Figure 14.64**) can cause pronounced discomfort. Erosions are irregular, often widespread, in the buccal and lingual mucosa, and persistent.

Erosive (**Figure 14.65**) and atrophic forms of LP may be premalignant in less than 3 per cent of cases though these may represent associated lichenoid dysplasia or erythroplasia.

The erosions may be irregular, often shaped like the leaf of a holly tree, and there may be associated white lesions (**Figure 14.66**).

Atrophic erythroplastic lesions may precede the development of squamous carcinoma (**Figure 14.67**).

Lichen planus is also a fairly common cause of desquamative gingivitis (**Figures 14.68** and **14.69**).

(Contd)

LICHEN PLANUS
(Contd)

Lesions that resemble LP clinically (**Figure 14.70**) and histologically may be induced by various identifiable factors. These lichenoid lesions may be caused by antihypertensives, oral hypoglycaemics, non-steroidal anti-inflammatory agents and a range of other drugs.

Lichenoid lesions may also appear in relation to metal restorative materials used in dentistry, or in relation to HIV disease or hepatitis C, and are a frequent complication of graft-versus-host disease.

Lichen planus has occasional overlaps with other disorders such as pemphigoid, lichen sclerosus or lupus erythematosus, and occasional associations with other diseases, especially with diabetes mellitus and autoimmune disorders, and possibly other hepatitis viruses.

Pigmentary incontinence resulting in hyper-pigmentation may be seen in older lesions of oral LP (**Figure 14.71**) but not as frequently as in cutaneous LP.

Cutaneous lesions of LP if present are typically purple, polygonal, pruritic, papules on the flexor surfaces of the wrists (**Figure 14.72**). White striae may be seen on the surfaces of the papules (**Figures 14.73** and **14.74**) (Wickham's striae).

Cutaneous lesions may be widespread (**Figure 14.75**) and cause extreme itching.

(Contd)

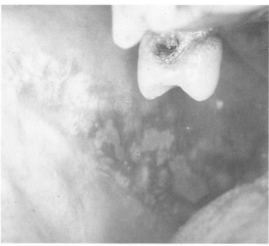

14.70

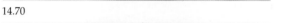

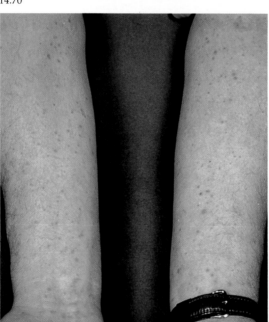

14.72

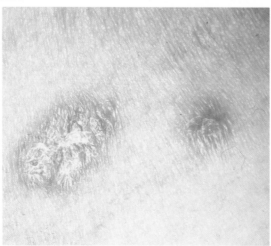

14.74

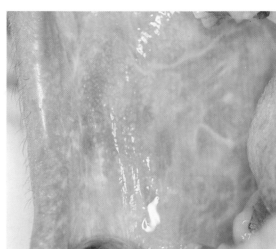

14.71

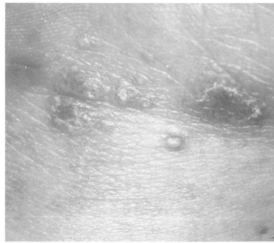

14.73

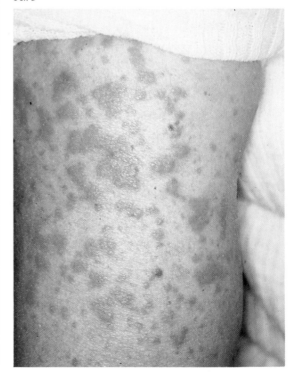

14.75

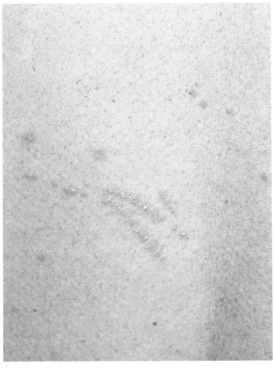

14.76

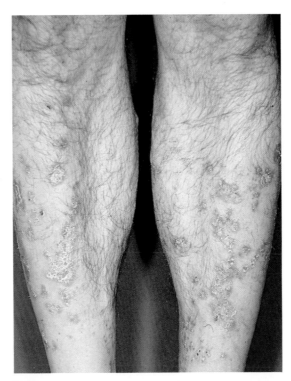

14.77

Rubbing or scratching the skin may produce a row of lesions, termed the Koebner phenomenon (**Figure 14.76**).

Lesions are also common over the shins (**Figure 14.77**) and may also be seen elsewhere (**Figure 14.78**), but are rare on the face. Alopecia may be seen and nail involvement may produce longitudinal ridging (**Figure 14.79**) and other changes.

CHRONIC ULCERATIVE STOMATITIS

Some lesions that appear clinically as erosive lichen planus prove, on immunostaining, to be associated with stratified squamous epithelium specific anti-nuclear antibodies.

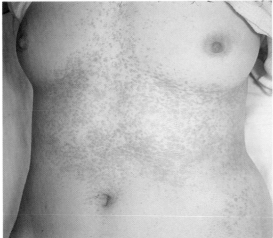

14.78

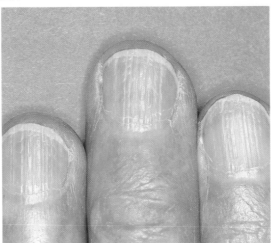

14.79

256

ACANTHOSIS NIGRICANS

Acanthosis nigricans is a rare disorder characterized by hyperkeratosis and pigmentation. The so-called 'malignant type' precedes, accompanies, or follows the detection of an internal malignancy, especially gastric adenocarcinoma.

Acanthosis nigricans is characterized by grey–brown pigmentation, hyperkeratosis and subsequent exaggeration of skin-fold markings of the axillae, neck (**Figure 14.80**), anogenital areas, groin, flexures and submammary sites. In addition, there may be symmetrical velvety papulomatous plaques of the same sites.

Mucosal involvement is variable, but in up to 40% there can be oral manifestations such as velvet-like oedematous mucosae, papillomatous proliferation of the lips (**Figure 14.81**) and tongue and occasionally diffuse hyperpigmentation.

The lips and tongue are most frequently involved. Thickening of the mucosa with a papilliferous surface (**Figures 14.82** and **14.83**) characterizes acanthosis nigricans.

Acanthosis nigricans can be inherited (autosomal dominant), drug-induced (diethylstilboestrol, nicotinic acid), or associated with insulin-resistance and other endocrinopathies or various other rare disorders such as Prader–Willi syndrome, Crouzon syndrome or Bloom syndrome.

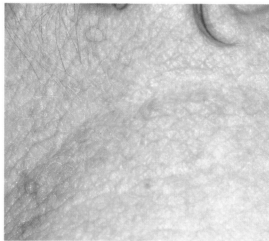

14.80

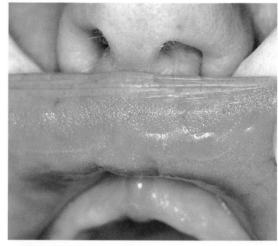

14.81

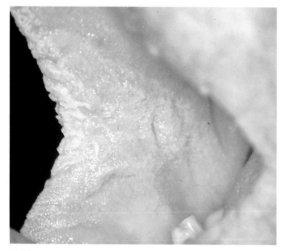

14.82

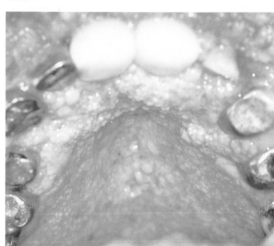

14.83

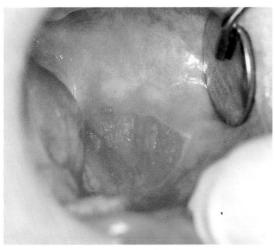

14.84

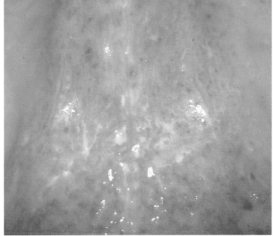

14.85

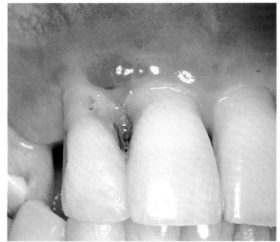

14.86

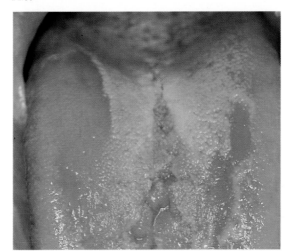

14.87

LICHEN SCLEROSUS

Lichen sclerosus et atrophicus (LSA) is a relatively rare idiopathic dermatosis characterized by white, macular lesions on the skin, and is usually associated with an atrophic mucosa (**Figure 14.84**) with or without concurrent genital or skin lesions. There are some patients who have an overlap syndrome with lichen planus.

PIGMENTED PURPURIC STOMATITIS

The pigmented purpuric dermatoses are a group of disorders in which there is chronic capillaritis, with pigmented purpuric lesions predominantly on the lower limbs. Chronic oral lesions in keeping with the purpuric lichenoid dermatitis of Gougerot and Bloom syndrome are seen rarely (**Figure 14.85**).

EPIDERMOLYSIS BULLOSA ACQUISITA

Epidermolysis bullosa is rarely acquired (**Figure 14.86**).

PSORIASIS

Erythema migrans is regarded by some as a minor variant of psoriasis (**Figure 14.87**). Classical psoriasis affects the elbows, knees, scalp and nails, and may cause an arthropathy. Pustular psoriasis may occasionally involve the mouth with pustules in the palate or elsewhere.

15 DISEASES OF THE MUSCULOSKELETAL SYSTEM AND CONNECTIVE TISSUE

CONNECTIVE-TISSUE DISORDERS

Raynaud's phenomenon, in which there is exceptional vasoconstriction in the digits in response to cold (**Figure 15.1**) is common in many of the connective-tissue disorders.

Sjögren's syndrome (dry eyes and dry mouth) is an inflammatory autoimmune exocrinopathy, common in many of the connective-tissue disorders (*see* page 262). The salivary glands, particularly the parotid glands, may enlarge (**Figure 15.2**).

SYSTEMIC LUPUS ERYTHEMATOSUS

Systemic lupus erythematosus (SLE) is a multisystem immune complex-mediated disorder affecting in particular the skin, blood and kidneys. The classic rash is over the bridge of nose and cheeks ('butterfly' or 'malar' rash) (**Figure 15.3**). SLE is also associated with photosensitivity, arthritis, serositis, anaemia, leukopenia and multiple autoantibodies, especially antibodies to double-stranded DNA, as well as non-specific features such as malaise or fever.

Oral lesions include petechiae and persistent irregular red lesions, sometimes with keratosis. The palate is a common site (**Figure 15.4**). Sjögren's syndrome may be associated.

SYSTEMIC SCLEROSIS (*Scleroderma*)

Systemic sclerosis is an immunologically-mediated multisystem disorder. The most common manifestation is Raynaud's phenomenon. The skin becomes tight, waxy and eventually hidebound, and the face smooth with a 'Mona Lisa' appearance (**Figure 15.5**). Skin pigmentation is also increased. The lips tighten with radiating furrows — the so-called 'tobacco pouch' mouth (**Figure 15.6**) — and

(*Contd*)

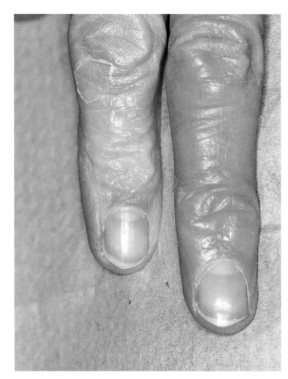

15.1

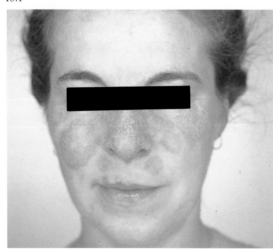

15.3

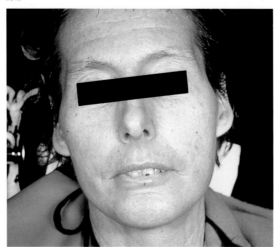

15.5

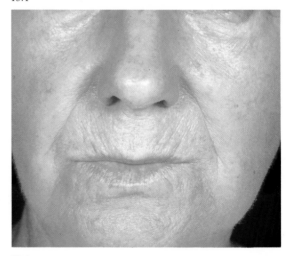

15.2

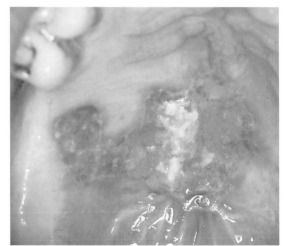

15.4

15.6

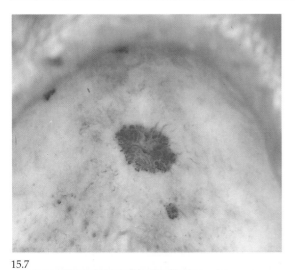

15.7

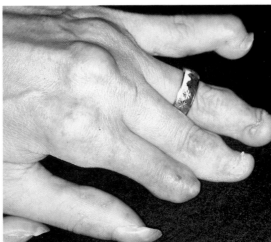

15.8

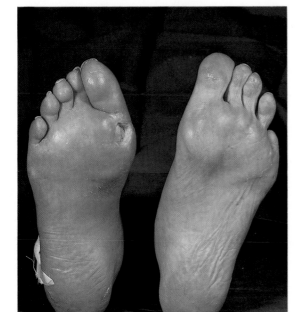

15.9

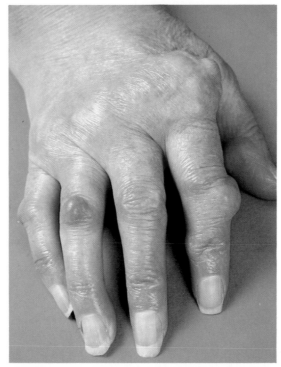

15.10

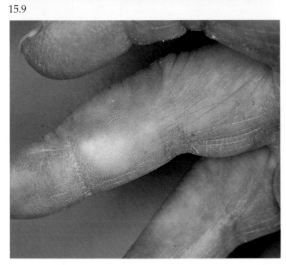

15.11

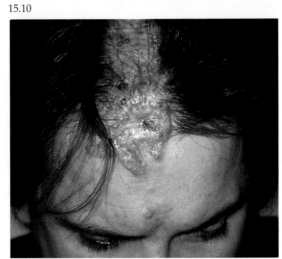

15.12

oral opening is restricted not only by the tight skin but also by pseudoankylosis of the temporomandibular joint. The mandibular condyles, coronoids or zygomatic arches are, rarely, resorbed.

Telangiectasia may appear in the mouth and periorally, especially in the CRST variant (**Figure 15.7**). Widening of the periodontal ligament is seen radiographically in some patients. Sjögren's syndrome may be associated.

Raynaud's phenomenon is common in systemic sclerosis and can lead to digital wasting and necrosis (**Figure 15.8**), or ulceration (**Figure 15.9**).

Systemic manifestations of systemic sclerosis include pulmonary fibrosis in most patients, hypomobile gastrointestinal tract, pulmonary hypertension, pleurisy and pericarditis.

Rare cases are drug-induced (bleomycin, tryptophan or carbidopa), associated with graft-versus-host disease or occupational (polyvinyl chloride, silicosis).

CRST OR CREST SYNDROME

Calcinosis (**Figure 15.10**) may be associated with Raynaud's phenomenon, scleroderma, oesophageal immobility and telangiectasia (**Figure 15.7**) in the CRST or CREST syndrome.

The calcific deposits are most evident in the fingers (**Figure 15.11**) but there may also be widespread calcification of internal organs.

LOCALIZED SCLERODERMA (*Morphoea*)

The lesions are typically a perpendicular groove paramedially running from the forehead to the hairline, or on the chin giving a 'coup de sabre' appearance (**Figure 15.12**).

SJÖGREN'S SYNDROME

Sjögren's syndrome is the association of dry eyes (keratoconjunctivitis sicca) with dry mouth (xerostomia: **Figure 15.13**). Alone these are termed primary Sjögren's syndrome (SS-1), but if a connective tissue disorder such as rheumatoid arthritis is present, the condition is termed secondary Sjögren's syndrome (SS-2).

Dry eyes (leading to keratoconjunctivitis, **Figure 15.14**) and rheumatoid arthritis (**Figure 15.15**) are the most common features.

There are frequent associations with primary biliary cirrhosis, rheumatoid arthritis, systemic lupus erythematosus, systemic sclerosis, and other disorders.

Dry mouth predisposes to oral infections, especially candidosis, and caries (**Figure 15.16**; incidentally, the black lesion in the lower vestibule is an amalgam tattoo after a previous apicetomy).

The salivary glands swell in up to one-third of patients with Sjögren's syndrome. The parotid glands most commonly enlarge (**Figure 15.17**).

Acute bacterial sialadenitis may be a complication in Sjögren's syndrome (**Figure 15.18**).

Sjögren's syndrome is a multisystem disorder affecting many exocrine glands. Respiratory, vaginal, and gastrointestinal secretions are impaired. There may also be neuropathy, renal tubular acidosis and interstitial pneumonitis. Rare complications of Sjögren's syndrome include lymphomas and other lymphoproliferative disorders.

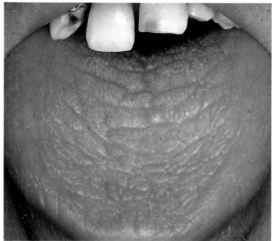

15.13

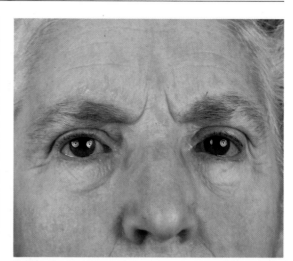

15.14

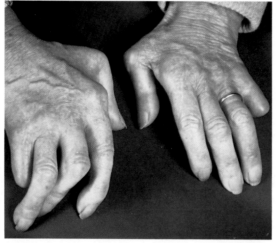

15.15

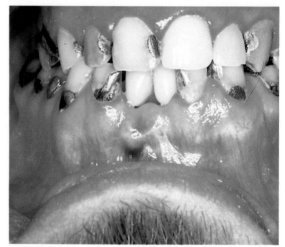

15.16

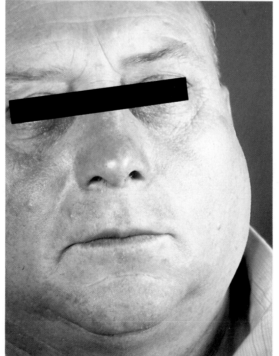

15.17

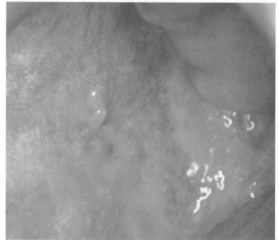

15.18

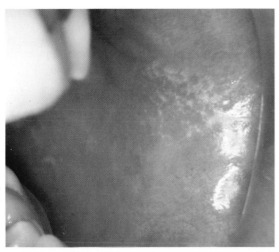

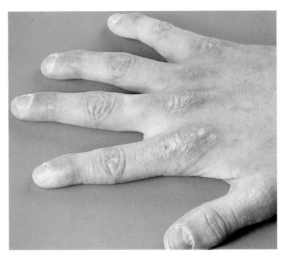

15.19

15.20

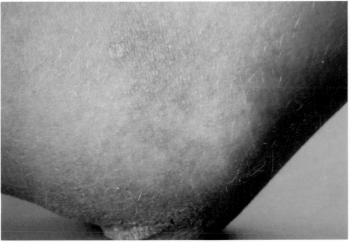

15.21

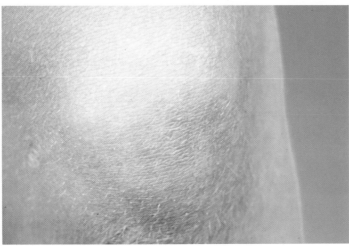

15.22

DERMATOMYOSITIS

Dermatomyositis and polymyositis are part of a group of immunologically-mediated inflammatory disorders of skeletal muscle. All have symmetric weakness of proximal muscles. Primary idiopathic dermatomyositis presents mainly in the middle-aged or elderly, with difficulty in climbing stairs, getting out of a chair or raising the head from the pillow.

Oral lesions may resemble lichen planus (**Figure 15.19**), or may show a dark red or bluish colour. There is also oedema of the gingiva.

Sjögren's syndrome, or other connective tissue disorders such as SLE, may be seen in some patients with dermatomyositis.

Dermatomyositis is characterized by localized or diffuse erythema of the skin, maculopapular rash, eczematoid dermatitis, or an almost pathognomonic lilac-coloured (heliotrope) change, especially over the eyelids, midface, around the nails and over the knuckles (**Figure 15.20**), the elbow (**Figure 15.21**) or the knee (**Figure 15.22**). Skin changes precede, accompany or follow a proximal muscle weakness resembling polymyositis.

Dermatomyositis is occasionally (up to 20 per cent) associated with internal malignancy (lung, ovary, breast or stomach) or may be induced by drugs such as penicillamine or by Coxsackie viruses.

Childhood dermatomyositis is distinguished by vasculitis, arthritis, Raynaud's phenomenon and calcinosis.

MIXED CONNECTIVE-TISSUE DISEASE

Mixed connective-tissue disease (MCTD) is an uncommon multisystem disorder with two or more of the following: SLE, scleroderma or polymyositis. Sjögren's syndrome is the main complication of dental interest.

Presenting features include polyarthropathy, sclerodactyly, myositis, oesophageal hypomotility and Raynaud's phenomenon. Patients have antibodies to nuclear ribonuclear protein.

Oral features, apart from Sjögren's syndrome, include weakness of the tongue and occasionally petechiae (**Figure 15.23**) and gingival lesions (**Figure 15.24**), as well as ulceration neuralgia, neuropathy and lymphadenopathy.

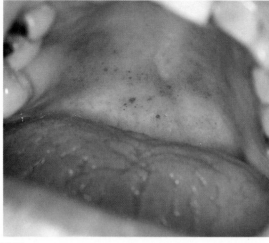

15.23

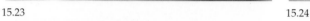

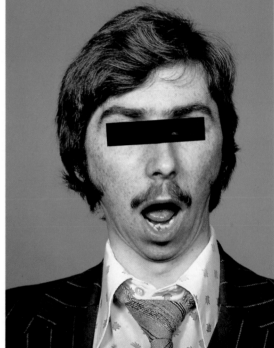

15.24

PYOGENIC ARTHRITIS

Pyogenic arthritis of the temporomandibular joint (TMJ) is rare but may follow a penetrating injury; may result from contiguous infection; or may be haematogenous, for example, gonococcal. Infection may result in micrognathia and ankylosis (**Figure 15.25**).

RHEUMATOID ARTHRITIS

Rheumatoid arthritis (RA) is a chronic relapsing inflammatory arthritis. It usually affects many diathrodial joints and is characterized by morning stiffness of the joints which, in advanced disease, become severely deformed.

Juvenile rheumatoid arthritis (20 per cent of which is Still's syndrome, with systemic disease) may interfere with mandibular growth (**Figure 15.26**) and cause ankylosis. Sjögren's syndrome, however, is the most common oral complication of rheumatoid arthritis.

(Contd)

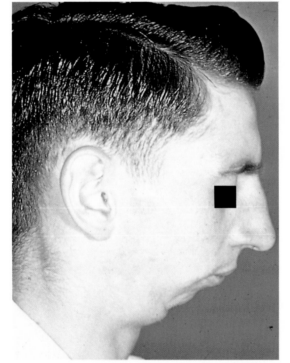

15.25

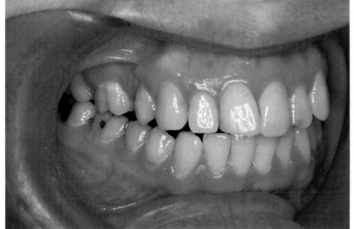

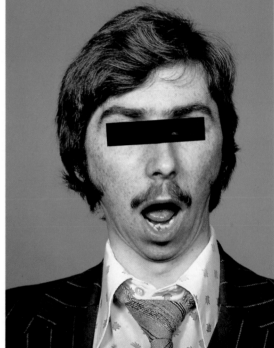

15.26

15.27

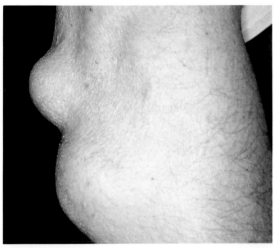

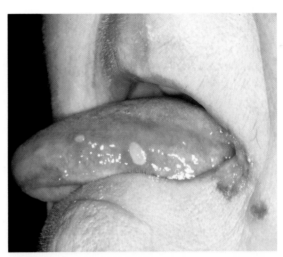

15.28

15.29

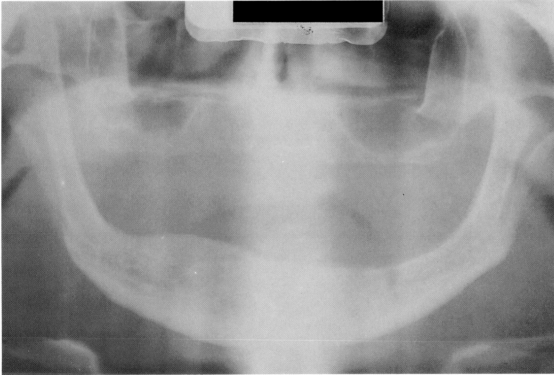

15.30

Involvement of the TMJ is common in rheumatoid arthritis but symptoms are rare. Osteoporosis, flattening of the mandibular condyle, marginal irregularities and limited movement may be seen. There may be restricted oral opening. The condyle may necrose in a patient on corticosteroids, leading to a slight anterior open bite (**Figure 15.27**).

Extra-articular features of RA include subcutaneous nodules (**Figure 15.28**), nail-bed vascular loops, pleurisy, pulmonary fibrosis, pericarditis, scleritis and episcleritis, nerve entrapment syndromes and vasculitic skin ulcers.

FELTY'S SYNDROME

Felty's syndrome is the association of rheumatoid arthritis with splenomegaly and neutropenia, manifesting with recurrent infections. Patients with Felty's syndrome have a higher incidence of episcleritis, leg ulcers, pleurisy and neuropathy than do those with classical RA. Oral ulceration may be seen, either herpetic or non-specific (**Figure 15.29**).

POLYVINYL CHLORIDE ACRO-OSTEOLYSIS

Occupational exposure to polyvinyl chloride may rarely cause a scleroderma-like disorder, sometimes with destruction of the mandibular condyle (**Figure 15.30**) or resorption of the zygomatic arches.

OSTEOARTHROSIS

Osteoarthrosis may also affect the TMJ but, unlike RA, virtually never causes ankylosis.

MASSETERIC HYPERTROPHY

The masseter hypertrophies especially where there are parafunctional habits such as jaw-clenching (**Figure 15.31**).

A computed tomography scan shows the thickened masseters (**Figure 15.32**).

TEMPORO-MANDIBULAR JOINT SUBLUXATION

Some patients are able to sublux their TMJ deliberately (**Figure 15.33**). Subluxation is especially liable to occur in hypermobility syndromes, such as Ehlers–Danlos syndrome (*see* page 286).

TEMPORO-MANDIBULAR PAIN–DYSFUNCTION SYNDROME (*Facial arthromyalgia*)

A common complaint is of discomfort, and/or clicking and/or locking of the TMJ. Seen predominantly in young adult females the aetiology is unclear but may include psychogenic and/or occlusal factors. Clinical features include normal radiographic findings but discomfort on palpation of the TMJ and masticatory muscles, sometimes crepitus, and limitation of mandibular movements. **Figure 15.34** shows a girl who has caused erythema on the face by repeatedly rubbing the painful area.

Pain–dysfunction syndrome of the TMJ may be associated with other disorders which have a psychogenic element.

TEMPORO-MANDIBULAR JOINT ARTHRITIDES

Apart from rheumatoid arthritis and osteoarthritis, psoriatic arthritis and, rarely, infective arthritides may be encountered.

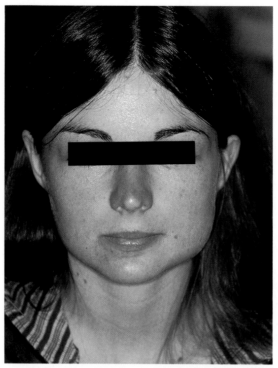

15.31

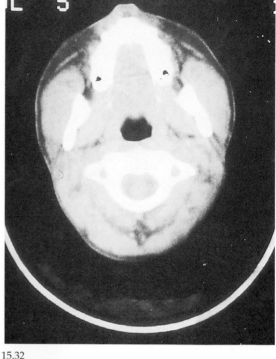

15.32

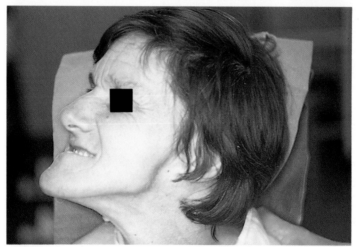

15.33

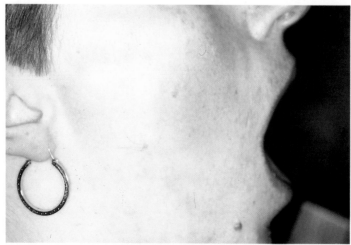

15.34

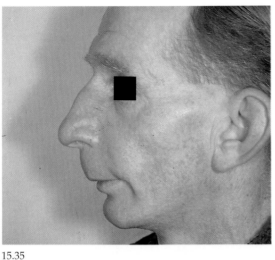

15.35

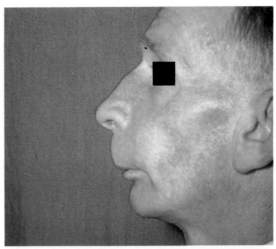

15.36

PAGET'S DISEASE
(*Osteitis deformans*)

Paget's disease of bone is common in Western countries, particularly the United Kingdom, in males aged over 50 years. Of unknown aetiology, possibly viral, the disease usually presents with swelling, often of skull bones. The calvarium thickens in about one-half of the patients with clinical Paget's disease.

Swelling of the maxilla (leontiasis ossea) may be seen in Paget's disease (**Figure 15.35**; **Figure 15.36** shows the same patient after 4 years, showing the increase in maxillary swelling).

Apart from the maxillary swelling, the teeth may become spaced (**Figure 15.37**).

The skull bones thicken and show a 'cotton wool' appearance on radiography (**Figures 15.38** and **15.39**). There may be overgrowth at the base.

Hypercementosis is a common feature of Paget's disease affecting the jaws (**Figure 15.40**).

(Contd)

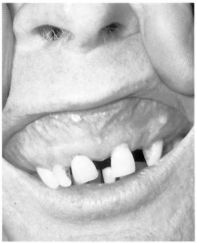

15.37

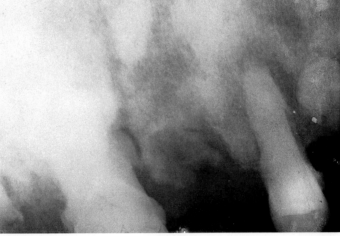

15.38

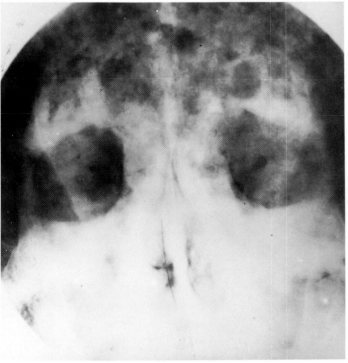

15.39

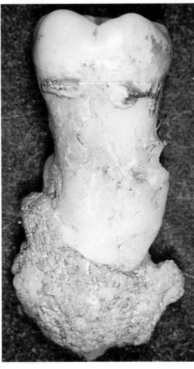

15.40

PAGET'S DISEASE
(*Contd*)

The sacral and lumbar vertebrae, pelvis, tibiae and femur are commonly involved. The affected bones soften and bend (**Figure 15.41**).

Lytic areas are seen in long bones in the early phase of Paget's disease (**Figure 15.42**). The bone shows an irregularly widened cortex and sometimes perpendicular radiolucent lines (cortical infractions), or fractures.

Pelvic changes include bone resorption and new bone formation and a thickening of the pelvic brim (**Figure 15.43**; here there is mainly innominate and ilial involvement).

Osteosarcoma (**Figure 15.44**) is a rare complication of Paget's disease and is particularly unusual in the jaws.

Other complications of Paget's disease include pathological fractures, spinal compression, arteriovenous shunts that may lead to high-output cardiac failure, calcific aortic valve disease, cranial nerve palsies and post-extraction haemorrhage or infection.

HYPEROSTOSIS CORTICALIS DEFORMANS JUVENILIS

This is a rare disorder that may be a juvenile form of Paget's disease with skull and maxillary enlargement and bowing of the legs.

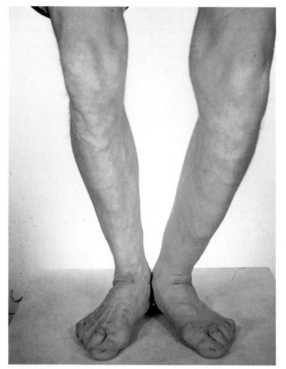

15.41

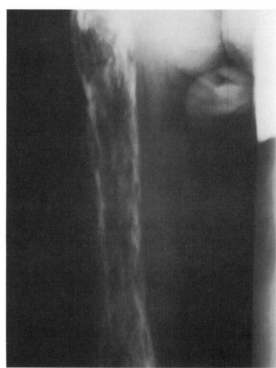

15.42

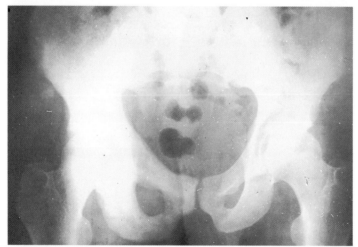

15.43

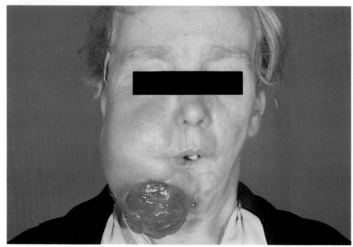

15.44

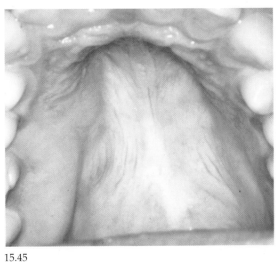

15.45

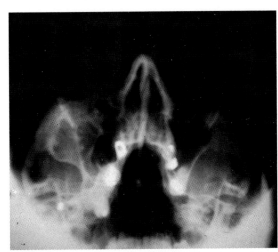

15.46

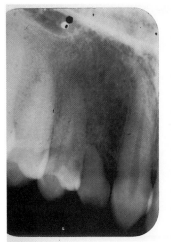
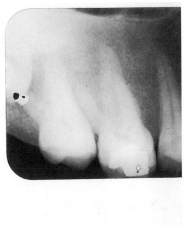

15.47

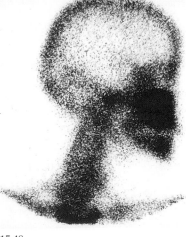

15.48

FIBROUS DYSPLASIA

Fibrous dysplasia is an uncommon benign fibro-osseous lesion, of unknown aetiology, often affecting one bone (Jaffe–Lichtenstein syndrome, **Figure 15.45**). The swelling is painless and typically ceases to grow at the time of skeletal maturity.

Four subgroups of fibrous dysplasia have been described: monostotic, polyostotic, polyostotic fibrous dysplasia of Albright's syndrome and a form confined to the craniofacial complex (craniofacial fibrous dysplasia).

In **Figure 15.46**, radiography shows fibrous dysplasia on the right maxilla alone in monostotic fibrous dysplasia.

The typical appearance on radiography is of a 'ground glass' pattern (**Figure 15.47**).

A bone scan using technetium diphosphonate shows increased uptake of radionuclide in fibrous dysplasia (**Figure 15.48**).

Several bones may be affected (**Figure 15.49**; here the humerus is involved).

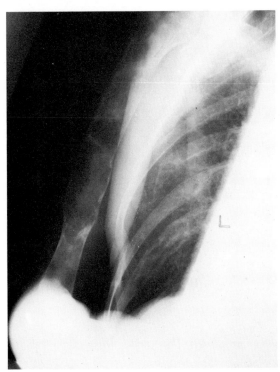

15.49

ALBRIGHT'S SYNDROME (*McCune–Albright syndrome*)

Albright's syndrome is the association of polyostotic fibrous dysplasia with cutaneous hyperpigmentation (**Figure 15.50**), precocious puberty and occasionally other endocrine disorders.

Oral hyperpigmentation is occasionally a feature of Albright's syndrome (**Figure 15.51**).

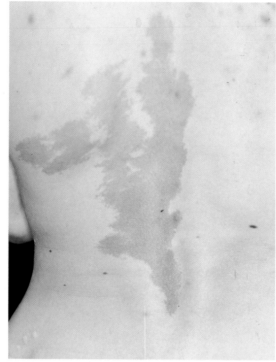

15.50

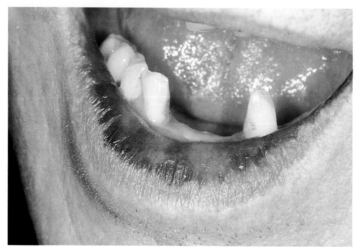

15.51

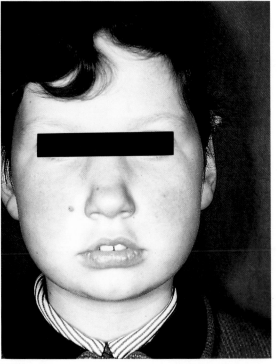

15.52

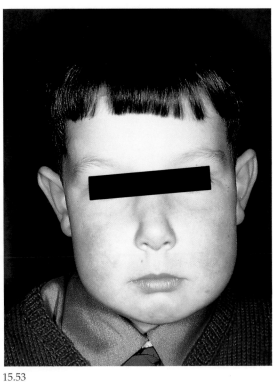

15.53

CHERUBISM
(*Familial fibrous dysplasia*)

Cherubism is the term given to a familial type of fibrous dysplasia which typically affects the angles of the mandible to produce a cherubic appearance (**Figure 15.52**).

Cherubism is an autosomal dominant trait (**Figure 15.53** is the brother of the patient shown in **Figure 15.52**). Cherubism is seen especially in males and presents usually after the age of 4–5 years.

The radiograph shows multilocular mandibular radiolucencies, expansion of the mandible and absent second molar (**Figure 15.54**), features common to cherubism.

The swellings increase in size and then usually regress, at least partially, at puberty. Occasionally the maxillae are involved.

Rarely, cherubism may be associated with Noonan's syndrome (short stature, neck webbing, cubitus valgus and often cardiac anomalies).

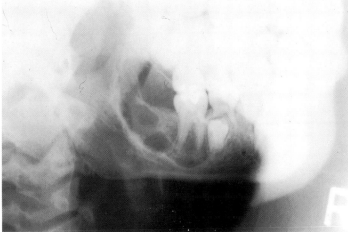

15.54

16 CONGENITAL AND DEVELOPMENTAL ANOMALIES

BRANCHIAL CYST

A branchial cyst is a painless, developmental fluctuant swelling on the lateral aspect of the neck (**Figure 16.1**).

CYSTIC HYGROMA

Cervical cystic hygroma is a lymphangioma extending from the tongue down into the neck (**Figure 16.2**). A developmental anomaly, cystic hygroma usually presents at birth and virtually always in the first 2 years of life. Some cause dysphagia or respiratory embarrassment. A minority extend into the base of the tongue and some extend into the mediastinum.

TETRALOGY OF FALLOT

Tetralogy of Fallot is one of the most frequent of the cyanotic congenital heart diseases. Ventricular septal defect, pulmonary stenosis, right ventricular hypertrophy and an aorta that overrides both ventricles are the features of the tetralogy. Central cyanosis is seen in lips (**Figure 16.3**), tongue and other mucosae (**Figure 16.4**) and the teeth are milky white in contrast. There is an increased prevalence of fissured and geographic tongue in children with cyanotic heart disease (*see also* **Figure 8.13**).

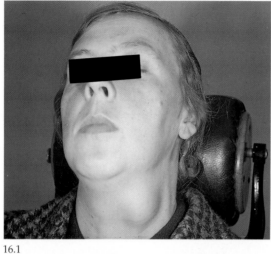

16.1

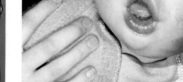

16.2

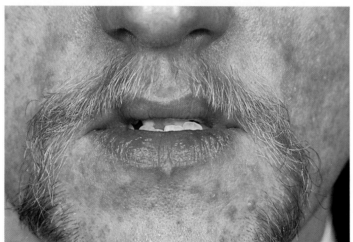

16.3

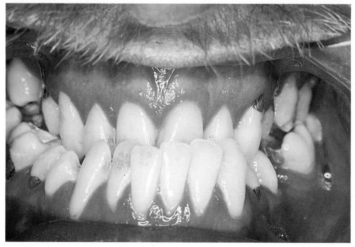

16.4

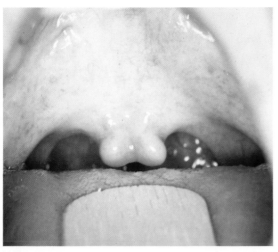

16.5

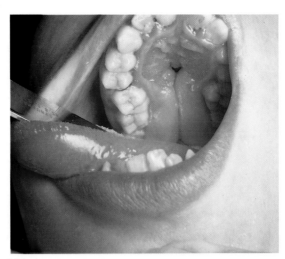

16.6

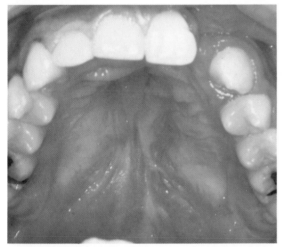

16.7

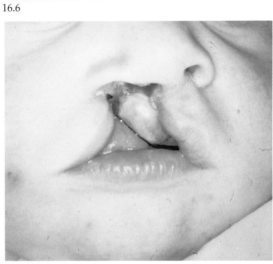

16.8

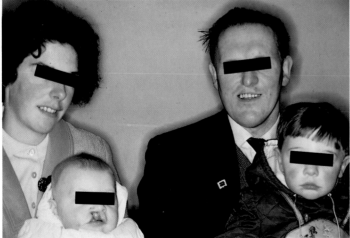

16.9

BIFID UVULA
(*Cleft uvula*)

Bifid or cleft uvula (**Figure 16.5**) is a fairly common minor manifestation of cleft palate but of little consequence apart from sometimes signifying a submucous cleft.

CLEFT PALATE

Figure 16.6 shows a cleft of the secondary palate.

Figure 16.7 shows a complete unilateral cleft palate and lip after repair.

CLEFT LIP AND PALATE

Cleft lip and palate are more common together than is cleft lip alone. The cleft is on the left in over 60 per cent of patients, although the lip in **Figure 16.8** is cleft on the right. The cleft may be bilateral.

There is a familial tendency (**Figure 16.9**). When one parent is affected, the risk to a child is about 10 per cent.

Cleft lip and palate are, in about 20 per cent of cases, associated with anomalies of head and neck, extremities, genitalia or heart. There are occasional associations with conditions such as orofacial–digital syndromes.

Isolated cleft palate is especially associated with Down's syndrome, Pierre Robin sequence, Treacher Collins' syndrome and Klippel–Feil syndrome.

TONGUE-TIE (*Ankyloglossia*)

Ankyloglossia (**Figure 16.10**) is usually a congenital anomaly of little consequence. There is no evidence that ankyloglossia interferes with speech.

The main consequence of ankyloglossia is difficulty in using the tongue to cleanse food away from the teeth and vestibules (**Figure 16.11**).

Associations reported with deviation of the epiglottis and larynx remain to be confirmed.

LIP PIT

Commissural lip pits are blind epithelial-lined developmental anomalies of no consequence (**Figure 16.12**).

Pits may also be paramedian on the vermilion and may exude mucus.

FORDYCE SPOTS

Fordyce spots are sebaceous glands in the vermilion of the lip (mainly the upper lip), and in the oral mucosa, especially in the anterior buccal mucosa (**Figure 16.13**). The retromolar region is often affected (**Figure 16.14**).

Often few in number, Fordyce spots are rare in children but found in about 80 per cent of the adult population and become increasingly obvious with age.

Fordyce spots are common in the upper lip (**Figure 16.15**) and may cause the patient to complain because of their appearance. They are of no consequence, but appear to be increased in patients with rheumatic disorders, especially Reiter's syndrome.

Intraoral sebaceous hyperplasia occurs when a lesion, judged to require biopsy has histologic features of one or more well-differentiated sebaceous glands that exhibit no fewer than 15 lobules per gland. Sebaceous glands with fewer than 15 lobules that form an apparently distinct clinical lesion on the buccal mucosa are considered normal, whereas similar lesions of other intraoral sites are considered ectopic sebaceous glands.

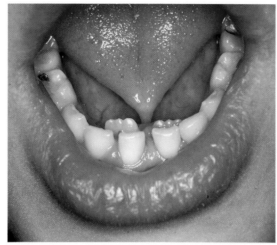

16.10

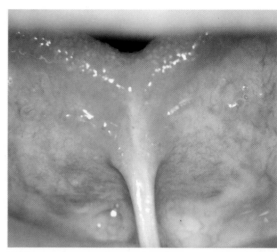

16.11

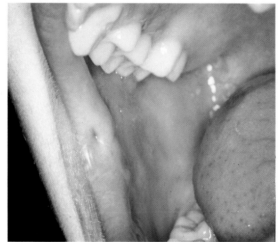

16.12

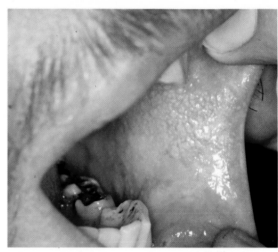

16.13

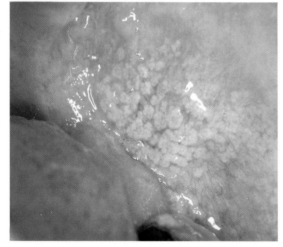

16.14

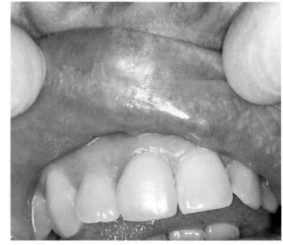

16.15

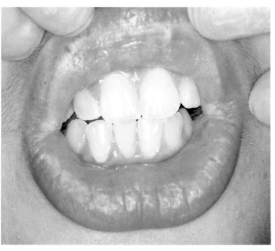

16.16

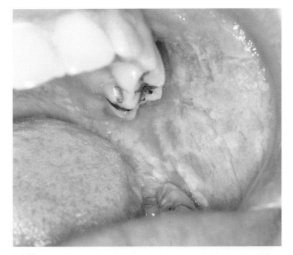

16.17

WHITE SPONGE NAEVUS
(Familial white folded gingivostomatosis)

White sponge naevus is a symptomless inconsequential autosomal dominant condition which manifests from infancy. The oral mucosa is thickened, folded, spongy and white or grey (**Figures 16.16** and **16.17**).

Lesions are bilateral in the oral mucosa and can affect oesophageal, nasal, vaginal or anal mucosa. Rare cases have iris coloboma.

ABNORMAL LABIAL FRAENUM

A labial maxillary fraenum may occasionally be associated with spacing between the central incisors — a maxillary median diastema (**Figure 16.18**).

Figure 16.19, the same patient as in **Figure 16.18**, shows the palatal attachment of the fraenum.

ABSENT UVULA

The uvula is rarely absent (**Figure 16.20**) and then usually as a result of trauma or surgery. The uvula may be hypoplastic in Cowden's syndrome (*see* page 289).

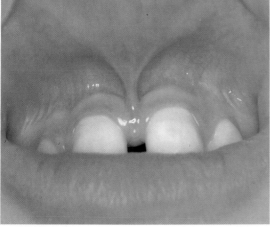

16.18

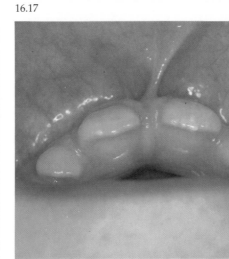

16.19

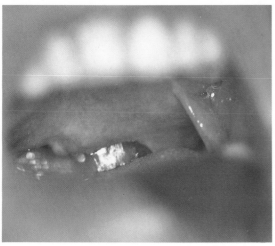

16.20

CLEIDOCRANIAL DYSPLASIA
(*Cleidocranial dysostosis*)

Cleidocranial dysplasia is an inherited defect of membrane bones, often an autosomal dominant trait. Defects involve mainly the skull and clavicles. Persistence of the metopic suture gives rise to a vertical midline furrow in the forehead with frontal bossing (**Figure 16.21**).

The sutures are still open and multiple wormian bones evident in the occipito-parietal region (**Figure 16.22**). The midface is hypoplastic.

The clavicles are hypoplastic or aplastic. In **Figure 16.23** the right clavicle is aplastic, the left hypoplastic. When the patient attempts to bring his shoulders forward and together, he can almost approximate them (**Figure 16.24**).

Radiography shows absence of the clavicles (**Figure 16.25**).

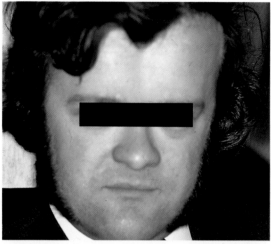

16.21

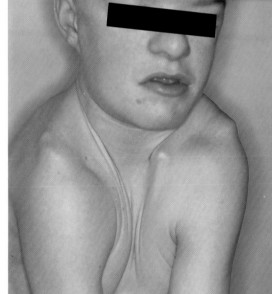

16.22

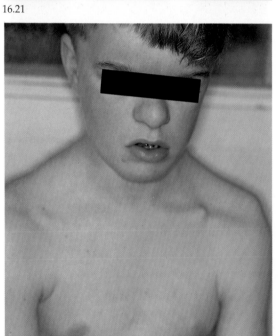

16.23

16.24

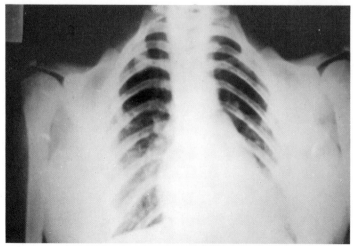

16.25

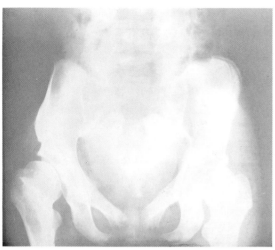

16.26

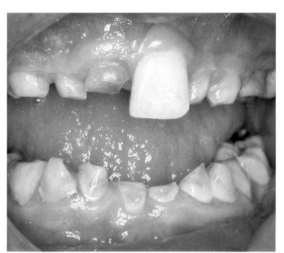

16.27

Pelvic anomalies may be seen in cleidocranial dysplasia (**Figure 16.26**) and kyphoscoliosis is common.

The dentition may be disrupted because of multiple supernumerary teeth and impactions (**Figure 16.27**).

Radiography shows multiple unerupted and impacted teeth (**Figure 16.28**) and dentigerous cysts (**Figure 16.29**).

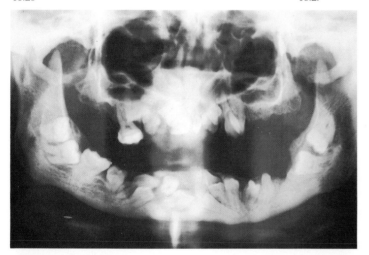

16.28

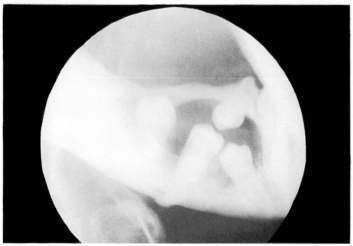

16.29

APERT'S SYNDROME (*Acrocephalo-syndactyly*)

Craniosynostosis, a high steep forehead, ocular hyperteleorism and antimongoloid slope to the eyes are characteristics of Apert's (**Figure 16.30**) and Crouzon's syndromes.

Apert's syndrome involves progressive synostosis of bones in the hands, feet (**Figure 16.31**) and vertebrae as well as ankylosis of joints.

Palatal anomalies are common (**Figure 16.32**), and one-third of patients have cleft palate. Maxillary hypoplasia is seen.

CROUZON'S SYNDROME (*Craniofacial dysostosis*)

Craniosynostosis, ocular hyperteleorism and proptosis are characteristics of Crouzon's syndrome (**Figure 16.33**). Teeth may be missing, peg-shaped or enlarged.

Radiography shows craniosynostosis and abnormal skull morphology and pronounced digital impressions ('copper-beaten skull') (**Figure 16.34**).

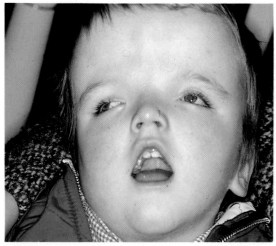

16.30

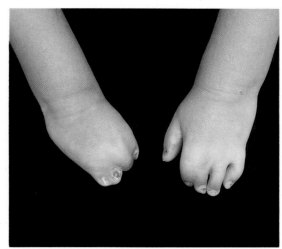

16.31

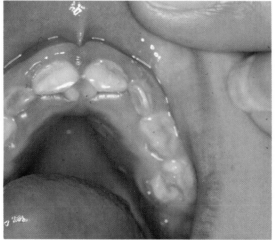

16.32

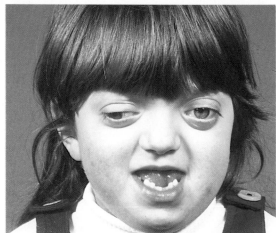

16.33

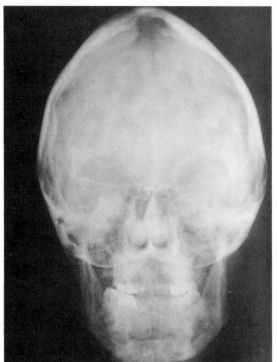

16.34

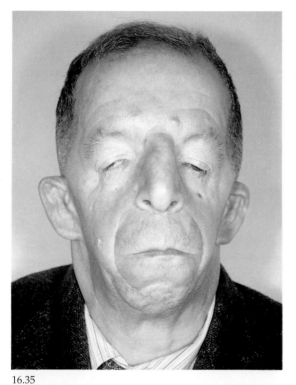

16.35

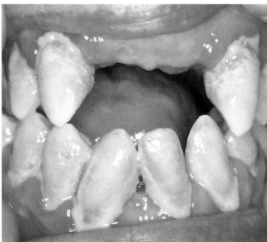

16.36

16.37

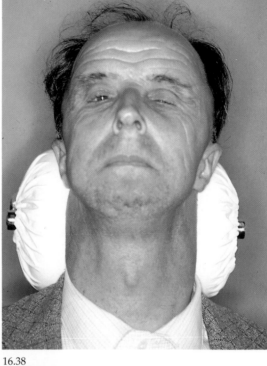

16.38

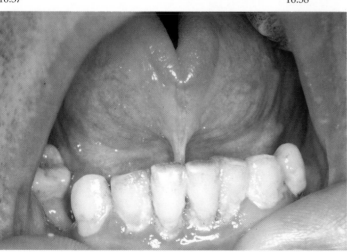

16.39

TREACHER COLLINS' SYNDROME (*Mandibulofacial dysostosis*)

The face in Treacher Collins' syndrome is characteristic, with pronounced anti-mongoloid slanting of the eyes, zygomatic and mandibular hypoplasia and low-set malformed ears (**Figure 16.35**). It is an autosomal dominant condition, often with deafness, caused by a first branchial arch anomaly.

Malocclusion is common (**Figure 16.36**). Cleft palate is seen in about one-third of patients.

PIERRE ROBIN SEQUENCE (SYNDROME)

In severe congenital micrognathia with a cleft palate there may be glossoptosis and respiratory embarrassment (**Figure 16.37**). Periodic dyspnoea is often evident from birth. There may also be congenital cardiac anomalies and mental handicap.

HALLERMANN–STREIFF SYNDROME (*Oculomandibulo dyscephaly*)

The Hallermann–Streiff syndrome is characterized by dyscephaly, hypotrichosis, microphthalmia, cataracts, beaked nose, micrognathia (**Figure 16.38**), and proportionate short stature. Radiological findings can include a large, poorly ossified skull with decreased ossification in the sutural areas, an increase in the number of wormian bones, severe mid-facial hypoplasia, a prominent nasal bone, and obtuse or nearly straight gonial angles. Potential complications are related to the narrow upper airway.

Teeth may be supernumerary (**Figure 16.39**) or malformed or absent. Natal teeth may sometimes be seen in affected infants.

CHONDRO-ECTODERMAL DYSPLASIA (*Ellis–van Creveld syndrome*)

Dwarfism, polydactyly, ectodermal dysplasia affecting nails and teeth (**Figure 16.40**; lateral incisors are missing), multiple fraenae, hypoplastic teeth and polydactyly (**Figure 16.41**) characterize this syndrome.

OSTEOGENESIS IMPERFECTA (*Fragilitas ossium*)

Osteogenesis imperfecta is a group of rare disorders in which a defect in type I collagen leads to fragile bones that fracture with minimal trauma. Autosomal dominant and recessive types have been described. There are several subtypes varying in severity and in features such as otosclerosis, blue sclerae (**Figure 16.42**; *see also* **Figure 10.54**), hypermobile joints, cardiac valve defects (mitral valve prolapse or aortic incompetence) and dentinogenesis imperfecta.

The primary dentition may be affected by dentinogenesis imperfecta in some types of osteogenesis imperfecta (**Figure 16.43**). The permanent dentition may be unaffected.

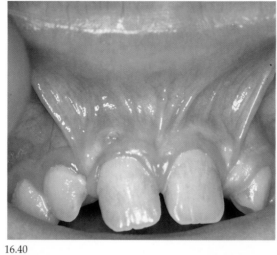

16.40

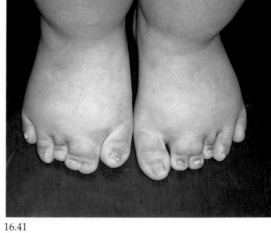

16.41

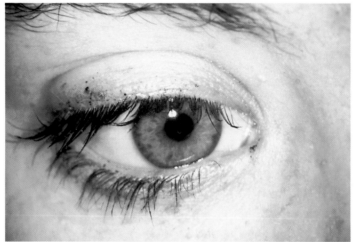

16.42

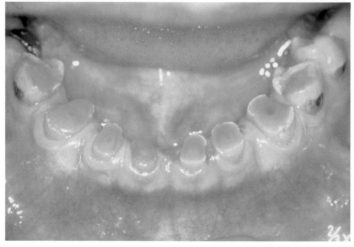

16.43

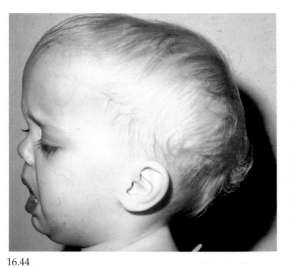

16.44

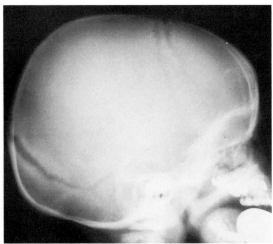

16.45

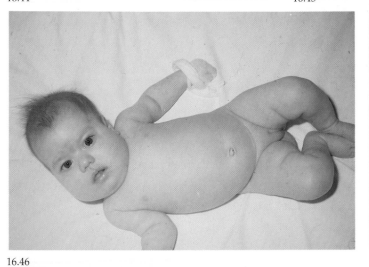

16.46

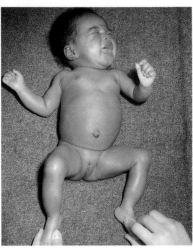

16.47

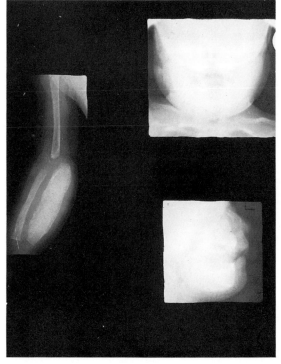

16.48

OSTEOPETROSIS (*Albers-Schoenberg syndrome*)

Osteopetrosis is a rare inherited disorder of bone. The autosomal recessive malignant type is lethal in early life but the autosomal dominant type is compatible with life. The maxilla is hypoplastic (**Figure 16.44**) and sinuses obliterated.

The bones are extremely dense (**Figure 16.45**); teeth often have short roots and may erupt late or not at all. The dense bone causes a predisposition to osteomyelitis. Bone marrow transplantation as therapy can lead to graft-versus-host disease.

VAN BUCHEM'S DISEASE

Generalized osteosclerosis with hyperostosis of calvaria, mandible and clavicles, syndactyly and facial palsy are seen in van Buchem's disease (sclerosteosis).

CAFFEY'S DISEASE (*Infantile cortical hyperostosis*)

This is a rare, possibly autosomal dominant condition, that presents often with swellings around the eyes or over the mandible (**Figure 16.46**). The condition resembles cherubism but appears at 2–4 months of age. The teeth are neither hypoplastic nor delayed in eruption.

There are tender, soft tissue swellings over the tibiae (**Figure 16.47**), with fever, anaemia and irritability. These features are extremely similar to those seen in child abuse, or osteomyelitis.

Radiographs show periosteal new bone formation (**Figure 16.48**).

ICHTHYOSIS

The disorders of cornification (ichthyoses) comprise acquired and inherited disorders characterized clinically by generalized scaling and histologically by hyperkeratosis. They may arise through defects in the production or maintenance of a normal cornified cell compartment.

Perioral involvement is not uncommon (**Figure 16.49**) and there may be enamel hypoplasia, delayed tooth eruption, periodontal disease and caries. Hyperkeratotic plaques have been described on the tongue.

Scales may involve many sites (**Figure 16.50**), depending on the type of ichthyosis. The most common is ichthyosis vulgaris, which is an autosomal dominant condition affecting the extremities in particular, including the nails (**Figure 16.51**) but rarely the mouth.

HEREDITARY PALMOPLANTAR KERATOSES

This heterogeneous group of disorders may occasionally be associated with oral disease. In particular, this is so in the Papillon–Lefèvre syndrome (*see* page 186). Oral mucosal hyperkeratosis is seen in the focal palmoplantar and oral mucosa hyperkeratosis syndrome. Dental dysplasia has been seen in other variants.

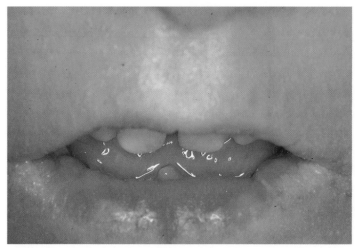

16.49

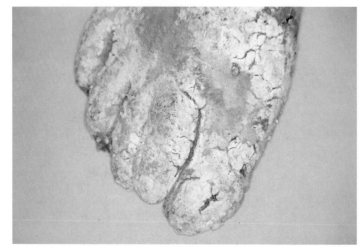

16.50

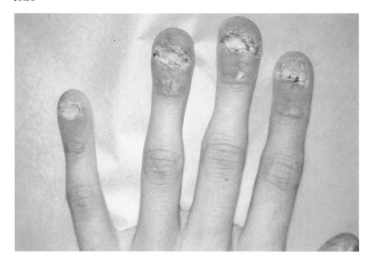

16.51

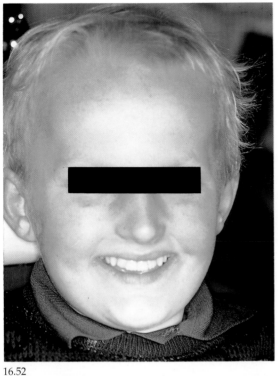

16.52

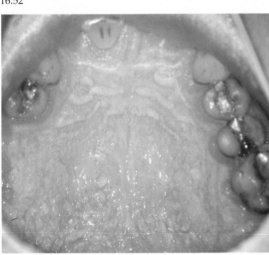

16.54

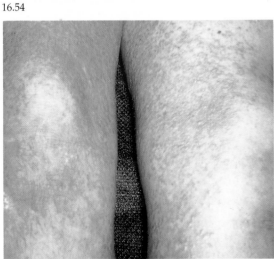

16.56

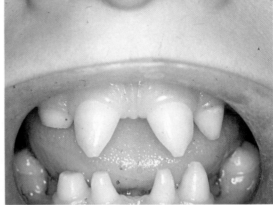

16.53

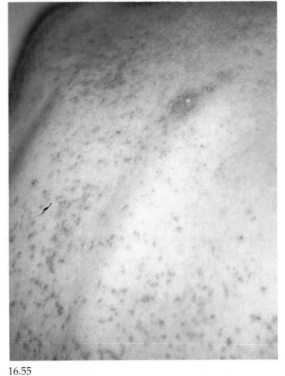

16.55

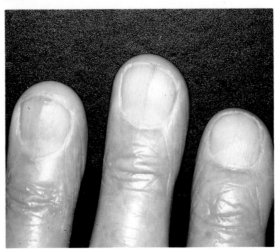

16.57

ECTODERMAL DYSPLASIA

Hypohidrotic ectodermal dysplasia is a genetic disorder, usually sex-linked, characterized by sparse hair (hypotrichosis) (**Figure 16.52**), absent sweat glands (hypohidrosis) and consequent fever, respiratory infections, missing teeth (hypodontia) and sometimes frontal bossing. Patients are otherwise well and mentally normal.

There is usually hypodontia (**Figure 16.53**; *see also* **Figure 10.5**) rather than anodontia (**Figure 16.52**; patient is wearing a denture), and the few teeth that are present often are of simple conical shape and erupt late. Dry mouth predisposes to caries.

Rare varieties include an autosomal dominant variety (the 'tooth and nail' type), characterized by hypodontia and hypoplastic nails, and a subtype in which teeth are normal (hypohidrotic ectodermal dysplasia with hypothyroidism).

DARIER'S DISEASE (*Dyskeratosis follicularis*)

Darier's disease is a rare autosomal dominant skin disorder characterized by multiple papules seen especially over the shoulders and upper arms. Oral lesions are seen in up to 40 per cent, starting as red papules that turn to white pebbly lesions seen especially in the palate, gingiva and dorsum of tongue (**Figure 16.54**).

Papules over shoulders and back (**Figure 16.55**), and knees (**Figure 16.56**) are seen with nail defects which include longitudinal splits and fragility such that nails tend to be wider than long (**Figure 16.57**).

WARTY DYSKERATOMA

This is a forme fruste of Darier's disease.

Oral lesions in the absence of skin lesions are termed warty dyskeratomas.

EHLERS–DANLOS SYNDROME

Ehlers–Danlos syndrome is a group of inherited disorders of collagen. Most types are inherited as autosomal dominant traits and involve abnormal collagen type III.

Hypermobility of joints is common, the skin is soft, extensible and fragile, purpura is common and there may be other defects, such as mitral valve prolapse. Patients may be able to touch the tip of their nose with their tongue. The teeth may be small with abnormally shaped roots and multiple pulp stones (**Figure 16.58**). Temporomandibular joint subluxation is common.

Type VIII or IX Ehlers–Danlos syndrome may be associated with early onset periodontal disease.

EPIDERMOLYSIS BULLOSA

Epidermolysis bullosa is a group of rare mainly inherited disorders of skin and mucosa, mostly characterized by vesiculation at the epithelial basement membrane zone in response to minor trauma, and often consequent scarring. Oral lesions are seen rarely in the non-scarring simplex type of epidermolysis bullosa, in which the vesiculation is intra-epithelial, but in most other forms, bullae may be seen in the mouth (**Figure 16.59**).

Bullae appear early in life, often precipitated by suckling, and break down to persistent ulcers that eventually heal with scarring. The tongue may become depapillated and scarred (**Figure 16.60**). Milia have been described intraorally in epidermolysis bullosa.

(Contd)

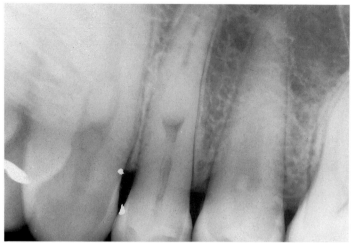

16.58

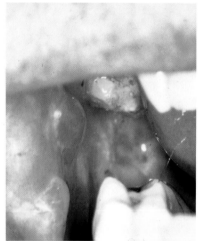

16.59

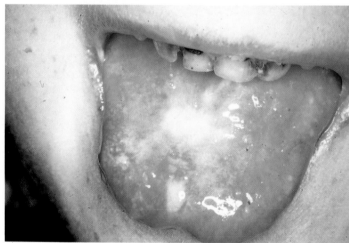

16.60

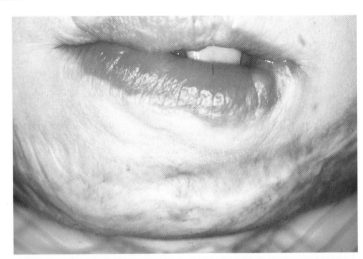

16.61

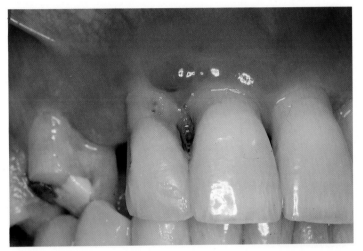

16.62

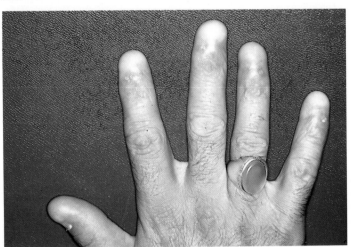

16.63

Scar formation may distort the lower lip (**Figure 16.61**). Enamel hypoplasia may be seen and, in view of the fragility of mucosa (**Figure 16.62**) oral hygiene tends to be neglected with subsequent caries and periodontal disease. Squamous cell carcinoma is a rare complication.

Scarring with the dystrophic form affects the extremities including the nails (**Figure 16.63**).

An acquired form of epidermolysis bullosa (epidermolysis bullosa acquisita) is a chronic blistering disease of skin and mucosa with autoantibodies to type VII procollagen of epithelial basement membrane.

INCONTINENTIA PIGMENTI
(*Bloch–Sulzberger disease*)

Incontinentia pigmenti is a type of ectodermal dysplasia. It is a rare dominant disorder that is either sex-linked or lethal to males. Virtually all surviving patients are female. Pigmented, vesicular or verrucous skin lesions are seen (**Figure 16.64**) often with mental handcap and visual defects.

Most patients have dental anomalies and both dentitions may exhibit anomalies. Hypodontia, conical teeth and delayed eruption are the usual features (**Figures 16.65** and **16.66**).

PACHYONYCHIA CONGENITA

In this autosomal dominant condition, the nails become thickened, hard and yellow, there is palmar and plantar hyperhidrosis and hyperkeratosis, and oral white lesions clinically resembling those of white sponge naevus. The dorsum of tongue is the common site, although other sites may be affected (**Figure 16.67**). Natal teeth may be seen in affected neonates.

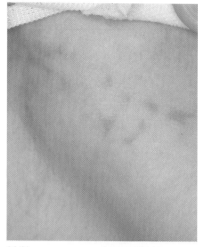

16.64

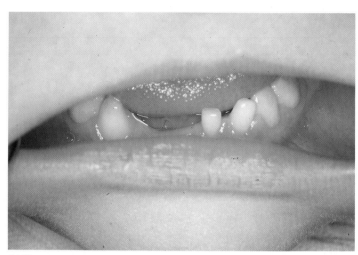

16.65

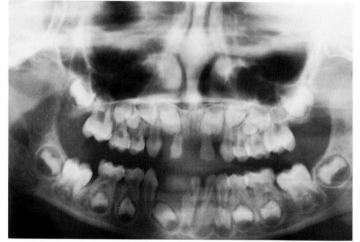

16.66

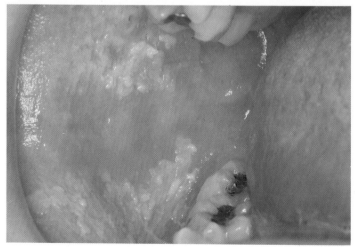

16.67

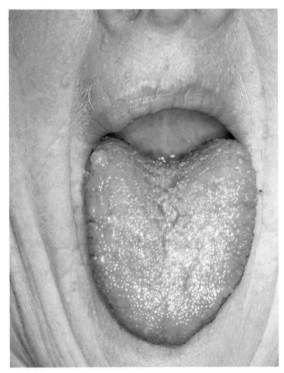

16.68

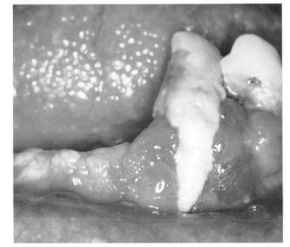

16.70

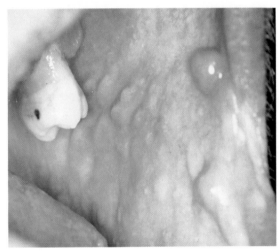

16.69

16.71

COWDEN'S SYNDROME (*Multiple hamartoma and neoplasia syndrome*)

This is an autosomal dominant condition of multiple hamartomas, with a predisposition to tumours, particularly carcinomas of breast, thyroid and colon. Papular oral lesions are common (**Figures 16.68** to **16.71**).

Other oral lesions may include fissured tongue, hypoplasia of the uvula, and maxillary and mandibular hypoplasia.

Large numbers of papillomatous lesions are seen on the skin especially over the neck, nose and ear (**Figure 16.72**).

Mucocutaneous lesions often precede the appearance of malignant disease elsewhere. Other manifestations of Cowden's syndrome may include small keratoses on the palms and soles; mental handicap and motor incoordination.

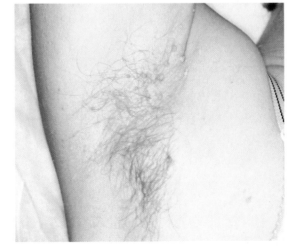

16.72

290

DOWN'S SYNDROME

Down's syndrome is a trisomic chromosome anomaly, in most instances affecting children of elderly mothers. There is a typical mongoloid appearance (**Figure 16.73**), with brachycephaly (**Figure 16.74**) and short stature. There are anomalies of many organs and virtually all patients have learning disabilities.

A fairly characteristic, though not pathognomonic feature is the presence of white spots (Brushfield spots) around the iris (**Figure 16.75**). Another feature is a single palmar crease (simian crease) and clinodactyly of the fifth finger (**Figure 16.76**).

Patients with Down's syndrome have multiple immune defects. Blepharitis and keratitis are common (**Figure 16.77**), as are hepatitis and upper respiratory infections (**Figure 16.78**). The dry mouth here is a consequence of mouth-breathing because of nasal obstruction.

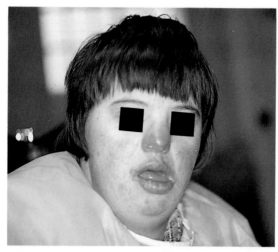

16.73

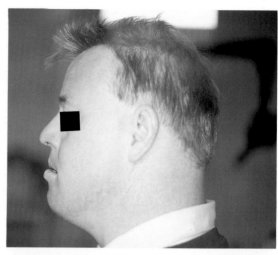

16.74

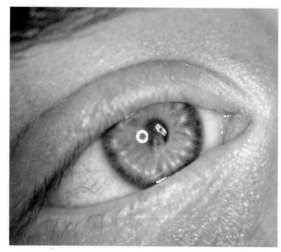

16.75

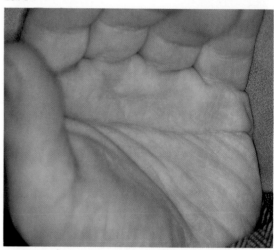

16.76

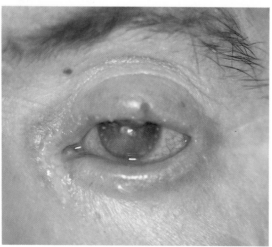

16.77

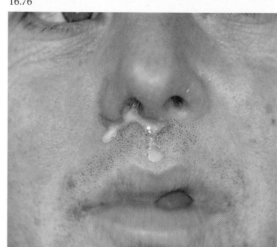

16.78

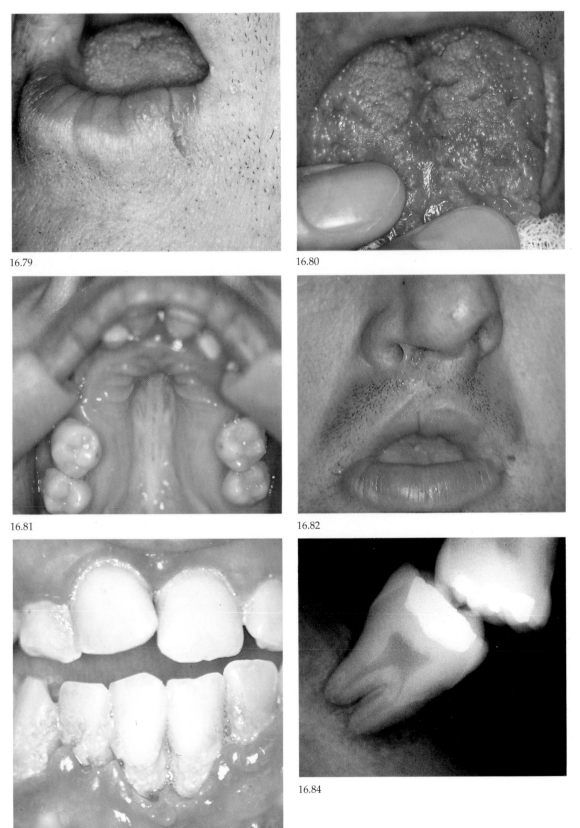

16.79

16.80

16.81

16.82

16.83

16.84

Cheilitis and cracking of the lips are common in Down's syndrome, possibly because of mouth-breathing (**Figure 16.79**). Macroglossia and fissured tongue are often seen (**Figure 16.80**).

The midface is hypoplastic and palatal anomalies common (**Figure 16.81**). Cleft lip and palate are more prevalent in Down's syndrome than in the general population (**Figure 16.82**).

Early loss of teeth is a feature, not only because of poor oral hygiene in many patients, but also because the teeth have short roots and there may be rapidly destructive periodontal disease (**Figures 16.83 and 16.84**).

EPILOIA
(*Tuberous sclerosis,
Bourneville–Pringle
disease*)

Tuberous sclerosis is an autosomal dominant condition of mental handicap, epilepsy, and skin lesions due to a defect on chromosome 9.

Adenoma sebaceum is the pathognomonic feature and is typically seen in the nasolabial fold (**Figures 16.85** and **16.86**). This is an angiofibroma that can be severely disfiguring and may involve other sites, such as the chin. Fibrous plaques on the forehead and shagreen patches elsewhere are other cutaneous features.

Most patients are both mentally handicapped and epileptic. Cerebral calcifications are seen (**Figure 16.87**). Ocular lesions (phakomas) and neurological complications (astrocytomas) may be seen.

Patients may also have cardiac rhabdomyoma or renal hamartomas (cysts or angiomyolipomas).

Subungual fibromas (Koenen's tumours) are another pathognomonic feature (**Figure 16.88**) and may be seen with longitudinal ridging of the nails.

Papilliferous oral mucosa lesions may be seen (**Figure 16.89**) in 10% (angiofibromas).

Pit-shaped enamel defects are a feature and there may be phenytoin-induced gingival hyperplasia.

Finally, depigmented 'ash leaf' naevi may be seen on the trunk (**Figure 16.90**).

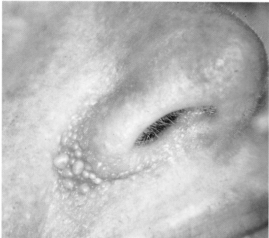

16.85

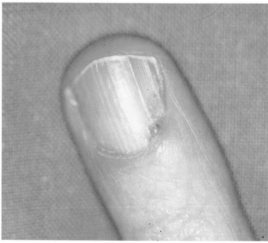

16.86

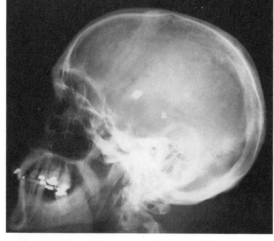

16.87

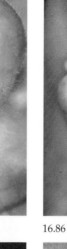

16.88

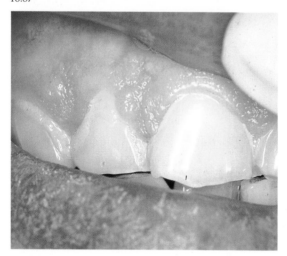

16.89

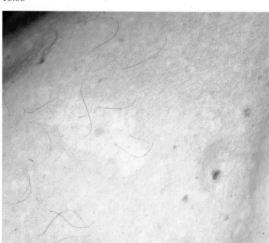

16.90

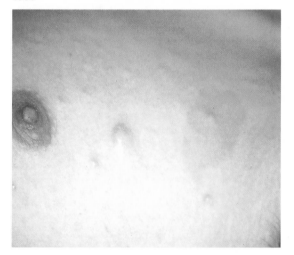

16.91

VON RECKLINGHAUSEN'S DISEASE (*Generalized neurofibromatosis*)

The disease known as neurofibromatosis is now recognized to consist of distinct variants that differ from each other genetically, microscopically, and clinically. Neurofibromatosis type I (NF-I) is often referred to as Von Recklinghausen's disease of skin. Neurofibromatosis type II (NF-II) is a much more uncommon manifestation that probably results from a structural defect in chromosome 22, as opposed to NF-I, which is related to chromosome 17. Although neurofibromas occur in NF-II, neurilemmomas and acoustic neuromas are the predominant neural tumours; bilateral acoustic neuromas are the hallmark of the disease. NF-II largely afflicts the central nervous system and has a more gradual onset than and different clinical features from NF-I. One of the most feared complications of NF-I is development of cancer, which is estimated to occur in about 5% of cases. The most common associated malignancy is the neurofibrosarcoma but this is rare in the mouth.

Cutaneous and subcutaneous neurofibromas (**Figure 16.91**), with skin hyperpigmentation are the features of Von Recklinghausen's disease (NF-I). This is an autosomal dominant condition but many cases are new mutations.

Café-au-lait hyperpigmented patches are seen, especially in the axillary region (**Figure 16.92**; this illustration also shows an adjacent neurofibroma).

Dystrophic kyphoscoliosis is common (**Figure 16.93**) and there may sometimes be mental handicap and epilepsy, or rarely renal artery stenosis or phaeochromocytoma. Acoustic neuromas are not common — many earlier reports were of a distinct condition of bilateral acoustic neurofibromatosis (NF-II). However, optic nerve or optic chiasmal gliomas may be present.

Neurofibromas may affect any part of the body, including the oral cavity, typically the tongue or palate (**Figure 16.94**).

Most patients also have small dome-shaped brown hamartomas (Lisch nodules) on the front of the iris, on slit-lamp examination.

16.92

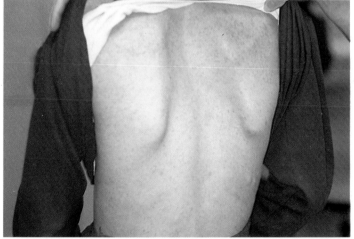

16.93

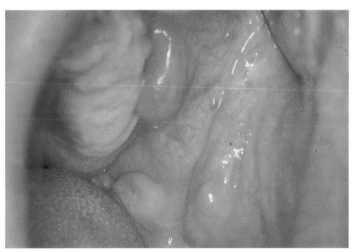

16.94

STURGE–WEBER SYNDROME (*Encephalofacial angiomatosis*)

An angioma affects the upper face (**Figure 16.95**) and usually extends into the occipital lobe of the brain, producing epilepsy and often glaucoma, hemiplegia and mental handicap.

The haemangioma often appears to be limited to the area of distribution of one or more of the divisions of the trigeminal nerve (**Figure 16.96**). There may be neuralgia. The affected area is somewhat swollen and hypertrophic.

Radiography shows calcification intracranially in the angioma (**Figure 16.97**).

The haemangioma may extend intraorally and be associated with hypertrophy of the affected jaw, macrodontia, and accelerated tooth eruption (**Figure 16.98**). Since the patients are often treated with phenytoin there is frequently also gingival hyperplasia.

GORLIN'S SYNDROME (*Gorlin–Goltz syndrome, multiple basal cell naevi syndrome*)

Gorlin's syndrome is an autosomal dominant condition of multiple basal cell naevi (**Figure 16.99**), with odontogenic keratocysts, especially in the mandible, and other features. Frontal and parietal bossing and a broad nasal root give the typical facial appearance.

Multiple basal cell naevi, often with milia, appear in childhood or adolescence, mainly over the nose, eyelids and cheeks (**Figure 16.100**). Rarely are the abdomen or extremities affected.

(Contd)

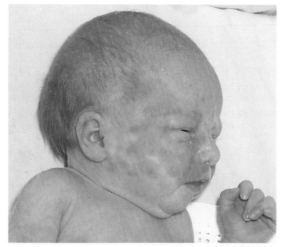

16.95

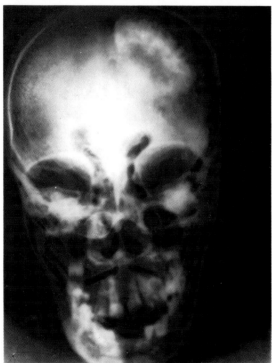

16.97

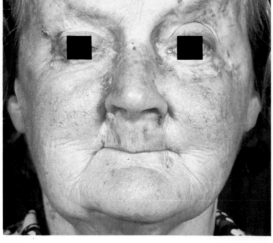

16.99

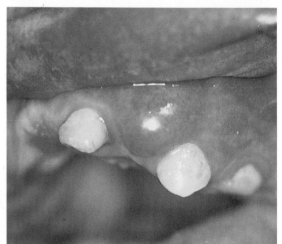

16.96

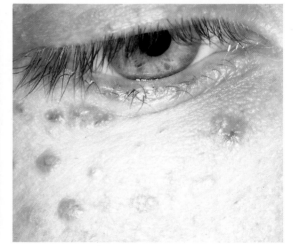

16.98

16.100

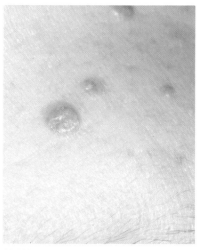

16.101

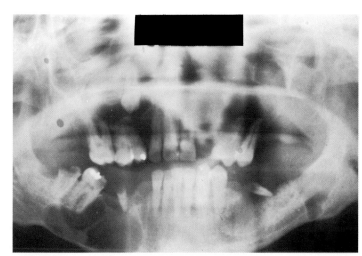

16.102

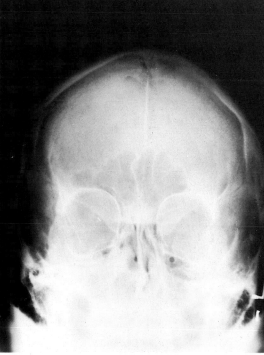

16.103

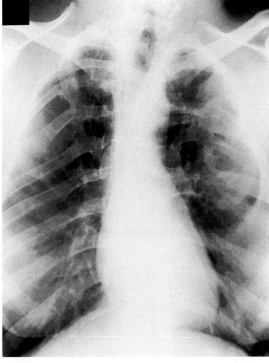

16.104

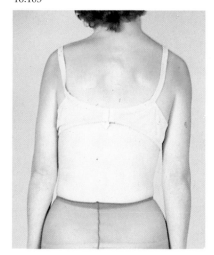

16.105

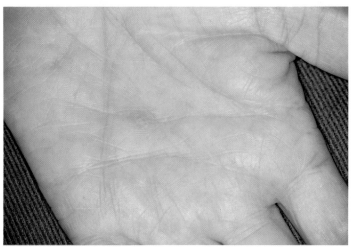

16.106

Figure 16.101 shows a close up of a naevus that is developing into a basal cell carcinoma. Only about 50 per cent of adult patients have significant numbers of naevoid basal cell carcinomas and only rarely are the lesions aggressive.

Keratocysts develop mainly in the mandible as shown by radiography (**Figure 16.102**). These develop during the first 30 years of life.

Cleft lip and/or palate are seen in about 5 per cent of cases.

Calcification of the falx cerebri (**Figure 16.103**) is a common feature, seen in over 80 per cent of patients.

Medulloblastomas and other brain tumours have been reported in up to 5 per cent of patients, as have a range of neoplasms of other tissues, especially cardiac fibromas.

There are many skeletal anomalies but bifid ribs are a common feature (**Figure 16.104**).

Kyphoscoliosis is often seen (**Figure 16.105**) and vertebral defects are common.

Other occasional associations include pseudo-hypoparathyroidism and diabetes mellitus.

Pits may be seen in the soles or palms (**Figure 16.106**). Occasionally, basal cell carcinomas arise in these pits.

PEUTZ–JEGHER'S SYNDROME (*Lentigo polyposis*)

Peutz–Jegher's syndrome is an autosomal dominant disorder, consisting of circumoral melanosis with intestinal polyposis. Polyps are mainly in the small intestine. Brown or black small macules are seen around the mouth (**Figure 16.107**), nose and sometimes eyes, and intraorally at any site, although rarely on the tongue or floor of the mouth. The pigmentation is typically spray-like and brown and precedes detection of the polyps.

Peutz–Jegher's syndrome may occasionally be associated with malignant neoplasms of the gastrointestinal tract, ovary, cervix, testis and breast.

MELANOTIC NAEVUS

Most intraoral melanotic naevi are seen on the hard palate (**Figure 16.108**) or in the buccal mucosa (**Figure 16.109**). Most are circumscribed, small, greyish or brownish macules and are benign.

The most common are intramucosal naevi (**Figure 16.109**), seen typically in the palate or buccal mucosa as brown macules or papules. Less common are oral melanotic macules and compound, junctional and blue naevi.

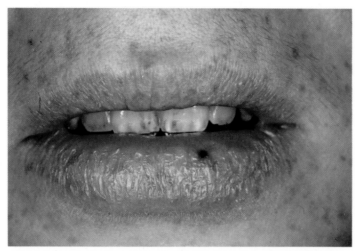

16.107

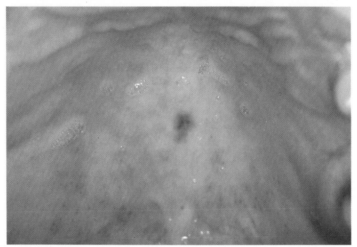

16.108

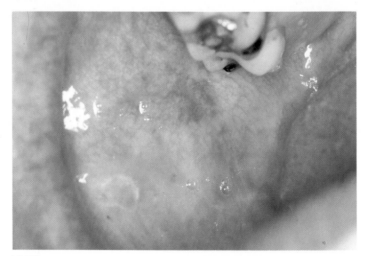

16.109

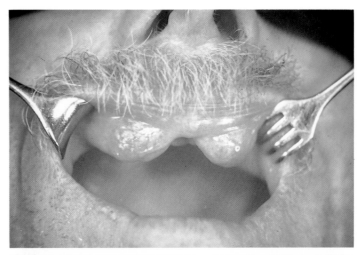

16.110

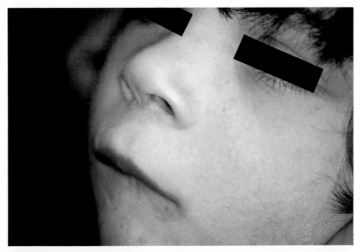

16.111

ASCHER'S SYNDROME

The combination of double lip (**Figure 16.110**) with sagging eyelids (blepharochalasis) and non-toxic thyroid enlargement is termed Ascher's syndrome.

DE LANGE SYNDROME (*Amsterdam dwarf*)

De Lange syndrome is a rare congenital disorder of 'fish mouth' with a long philtrum (**Figure 16.111**), eyebrows that meet (synophrys), dwarfism and mental handicap.

The mandible is hypoplastic and the palate is small and may be cleft (**Figure 16.112**). Teeth are often small and delayed in eruption.

Hands and feet are small and there is often syndactyly or oligodactyly (**Figure 16.113**).

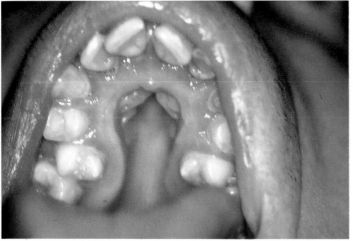

16.112

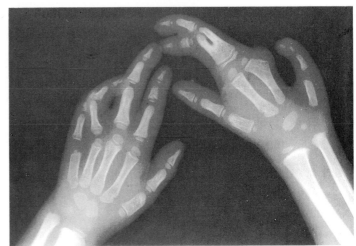

16.113

CRI-DU-CHAT SYNDROME

Deletion of the short arm of chromosome 5 is a rare disorder characterized by a cry like a cat in infancy, and facial dysmorphogenesis (**Figure 16.114**). Most patients are of short stature, mentally handicapped, and often have cardiac and skeletal anomalies.

Micrognathia, high-arched palate, enamel hypoplasia and a poorly defined mandibular angle are the main features. Microcephaly (**Figure 16.115**), small pituitary fossa and large frontal sinuses may be seen on radiography.

PATAU'S SYNDROME

Cleft lip (often bilateral) and cleft palate with micrognathia are orofacial features of trisomy 13 (**Figure 16.116**).

OROFACIAL–DIGITAL SYNDROME (OFD)

Multiple fibrous bands may be associated with cleft or lobulated tongue, polydactyly and often a midline cleft of the upper lip in Mohr's syndrome (OFD type II; **Figure 16.117**).

In OFD type I, the tongue may be bifid or lobed, with cleft lip or palate and hypodontia or supernumerary teeth, fraenae and fraenulae are short and there is hypertelorism, mental changes, and brachy-, syn-, or clino-dactyly.

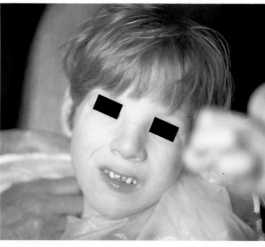

16.114

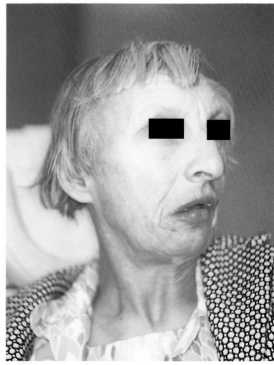

16.115

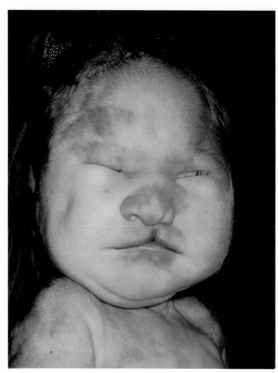

16.116

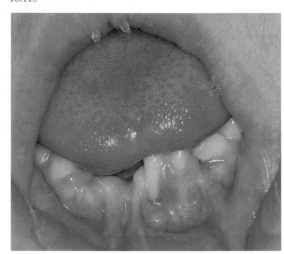

16.117

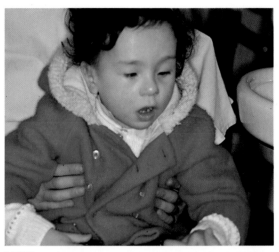

16.118

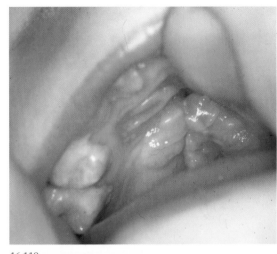

16.119

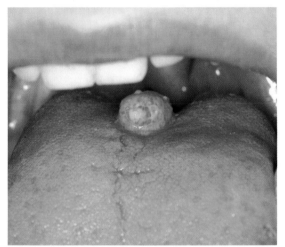

16.120

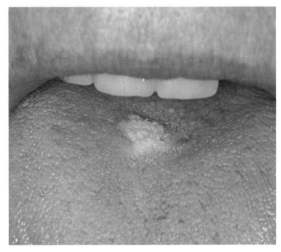

16.121

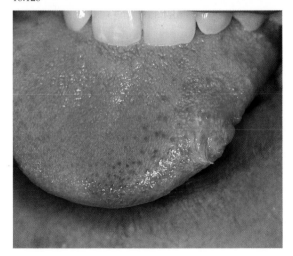

16.122

SMITH–LEMLI–OPITZ SYNDROME

This is a rare autosomal recessive syndrome consisting of ptosis, broad nose and anteverted nostrils, low-set ears and micrognathia (**Figure 16.118**). Most have some syndactyly, growth retardation, and learning disability.

The maxillary alveolar ridges are broad and the palate high-arched or cleft (**Figure 16.119**).

THYROID (LINGUAL)

The thyroid arises from an invagination of lingual mucosa. Occasionally, thyroid tissue remains in the tongue (**Figure 16.120**). Complications may include hypothyroidism in up to 20%, dysplasia, dysarthria or dyspnoea. A radionuclide scan will define exactly what thyroid tissue is present, and where, since in about two-thirds of cases no thyroid tissue is present in the neck.

VERRUCOUS NAEVUS

Naevus unius lateris is a warty proliferation of unknown aetiology (**Figure 16.121**).

ABNORMAL LINGUAL PAPILLAE

Figure 16.122 shows an isolated congenital anomaly of the tongue.

300

LABAND SYNDROME

Hereditary gingival fibromatosis is frequently an isolated condition of little consequence apart from a cosmetic problem and occasional associations with hypertrichosis and/or epilepsy. There are, however, several uncommon or rare eponymous syndromes described in which gingival fibromatosis can be a feature: these include the Zimmermann–Laband, Murray–Puretic–Drescher, Rutherfurd, Cowden and Cross syndromes (*see* **Table 16**).

The Laband syndrome consists of gingival hyperplasia (**Figure 16.123**) together with hypoplastic terminal phalanges (**Figure 16.124**) and other defects.

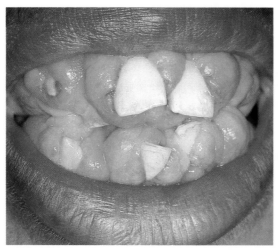

16.123

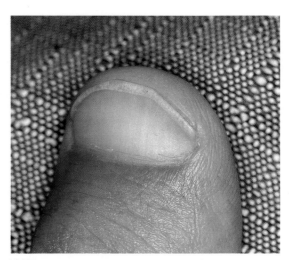

16.124

Table 16 SYNDROMES ASSOCIATED WITH GINGIVAL FIBROMATOSIS

Syndrome	Inheritance	Main features apart from gingival fibromatosis
Zimmermann–Laband	AD	Ears and nose thickened and enlarged Nail dysplasia Terminal phalanges hypoplastic Joint hyper-extensibility Hepatosplenomegaly
Murray–Puretic–Drescher	AR	Hyaline fibrous tumours over scalp, neck and limbs Osteolysis of terminal phalanges Recurrent infections
Rutherfurd	AD	Retarded tooth eruption Corneal opacities
Cowden	AD	Giant fibroadenoma of breast Hypertrichosis Multiple hamartomas
Cross	AR	Hypopigmentation Microphthalmia with cloudy corneas Learning disability Athetoid cerebral palsy
Gingival fibromatosis	AD	± Hypertrichosis ± Epilepsy ± Learning disability
Gingival fibromatosis with progressive deafness	AD	Progressive sensorineural deafness

AD = autosomal dominant.
AR = autosomal recessive.

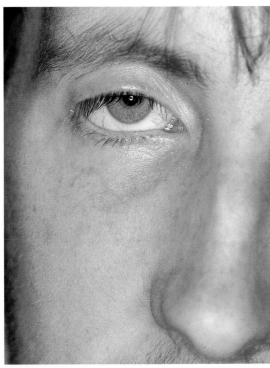

16.125

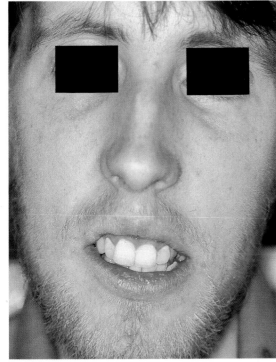

16.127

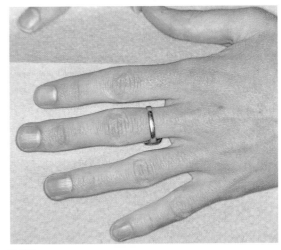

16.126

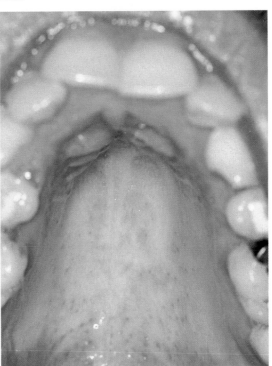

16.128

MYOTONIC DYSTROPHY (*Steinert syndrome*)

Myotonic dystrophy (dystrophia myotonica) is the most disabling form of myotonia and can lead to ptosis (**Figure 16.125**), facial weakness, cataracts, testicular atrophy and frontal baldness. Other complications include cardiac conduction defects, respiratory impairment, mild endocrinopathies, intellectual deterioration and personality changes.

There is atrophy of the temporalis, masseter and sternomastoid muscles, and distal limb weakness and wasting (**Figure 16.126**).

Atrophy of the masticatory muscles leads to an open mouth posture (myopathic facies; **Figure 16.127**). Myotonia in the tongue causes difficulty in speaking (dysarthria). There may also be dysphagia and increased caries.

There are pronounced changes in dental arch form with open occlusal relationships, expanded arches and labially or buccally displaced teeth often with diastemas, and a high arched palate (**Figure 16.128**).

17 INJURY, POISONING AND IATROGENIC DISEASE

For further details *see* Section 1.5, page 56.

304

BURNS

Burns are most common after the ingestion of hot foods and are seen especially on the palate or tongue, for example, 'pizza-palate' (**Figures 17.1** and **17.2**).

Cold injury is uncommon, but follows cryosurgery. Electrical burns are also uncommon, seen usually in pre-school children who bite electric flex. Very rarely, burns are caused by irradiation or natural products such as the houseplant *Dieffenbachia*, or the enzyme bromelin in pineapple.

Some patients attempt to relieve oral pain by holding an analgesic tablet at the site of pain (**Figure 17.3**).

Aqueous chlorhexidine is an excellent oral antiseptic but often produces superficial tooth discoloration, as shown in **Figure 17.4**. Over-enthusiastic or undiluted use of concentrated solutions may rarely produce burns as shown. Taste disturbances and salivary gland swelling are other rare sequelae.

EROSIONS

Chemicals such as acids (chromic, trichloracetic, phosphoric) may be used during dental procedures and can cause ulcers. Self-curing resins, especially epoxy resins for oral use may also produce erosions (**Figure 17.5**), as may various mouthwashes.

Rubber-based or silicone-based impression materials occasionally produce an erosive reaction (**Figure 17.6**).

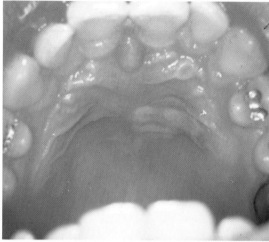
17.1

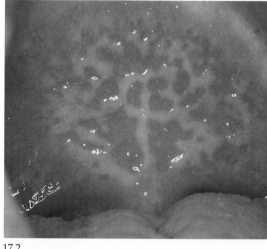
17.2

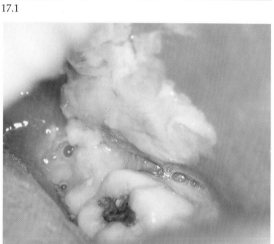
17.3

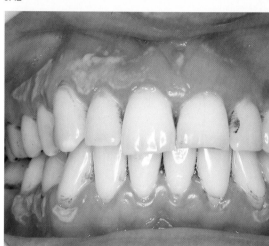
17.4

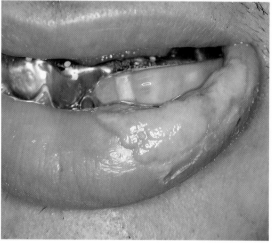
17.5

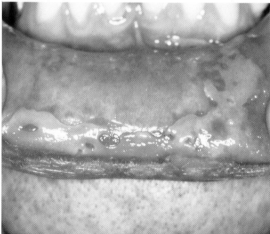
17.6

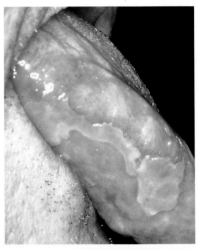

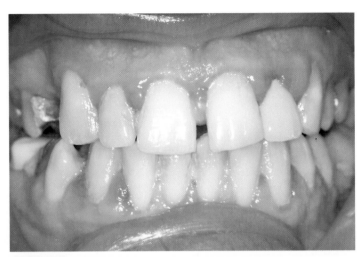

17.7   17.8

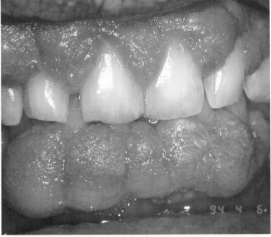

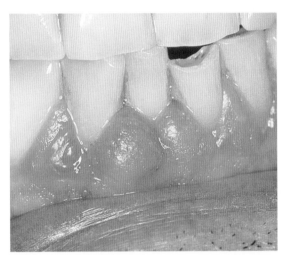

17.9   17.10

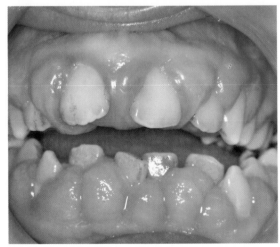

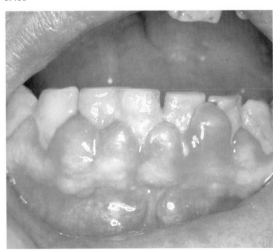

17.11   17.12

LICHENOID LESIONS

Lesions resembling lichen planus, lupus erythematosus, pemphigoid or pemphigus may be drug-induced. Non-steroidal anti-inflammatory agents, antidiabetic, antihypertensive and antimalarial drugs are causes of lichenoid lesions (**Figure 17.7** was a reaction to methyldopa; *see also* Section 1.5, page 56), as are some restorative materials and graft-versus-host disease.

DRUG-INDUCED GINGIVAL HYPERPLASIA

Gingival enlargement may occur in patients receiving phenytoin, cyclosporin and calcium-channel blocker therapy, particularly nifedipine (**Figures 17.8** and **17.9**; *see also* Section 1.5, page 56), diltiazem, felodipine and amlodipine (**Figure 17.10**). It is suggested that the gingival overgrowth is due to impaired collagen resorption secondary to defective fibroblast function.

The anticonvulsant phenytoin is the drug which classically can produce gingival hyperplasia (**Figure 17.11**). Poor oral hygiene exacerbates the hyperplasia, which appears interdentally 2–3 months after treatment is started. The papillae enlarge to a variable extent, with relatively little tendency to bleed.

Cyclosporin is a commonly-used immunosuppressive drug that can cause gingival hyperplasia closely resembling that induced by phenytoin. It is seen mainly anteriorly (**Figure 17.12**) and labially and is exacerbated by poor oral hygiene and concurrent administration of nifedipine.

(Contd)

DRUG-INDUCED GINGIVAL HYPERPLASIA (*Contd*)

Drugs that produce gingival hyperplasia may also induce hirsutism (**Figure 17.13**).

DRUG-INDUCED ULCERATION

A range of drugs may produce oral ulceration (*see* Section 1.5, page 56). The most consistent association is with cytotoxic agents, but the example in **Figure 17.14** was caused by tranexamic acid.

COCAINE-INDUCED GINGIVAL LESIONS

Cocaine is sometimes deliberately rubbed into the gingivae or vestibule. Gingival/ulceration and necrosis, accompanied by a brief 'high', can accompany local use of cocaine. The powerful vasoconstrictive effects of the cocaine are probably responsible for some of the local destruction. Tissue damage can develop within a few days of regular application of cocaine causing both soft- and hard-tissue destruction, although lesions usually heal when there is a cessation of the cocaine abuse.

Oral neglect with caries and gingivitis are seen in **Figure 17.15** in a juvenile who applied cocaine and amphetamine (mixed with sugar) to his maxillary gingiva, consequently with a gingival reaction and caries. Cocaine can also produce a vestibular burn (**Figure 17.16**).

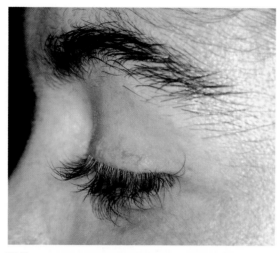

17.13

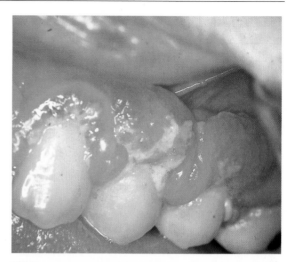

17.14

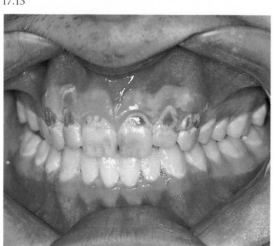

17.15

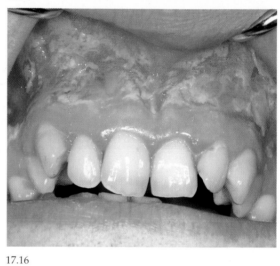

17.16

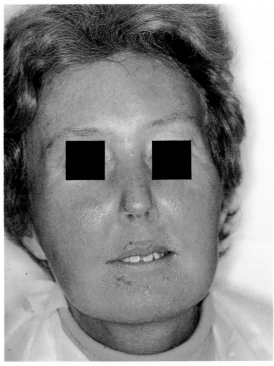

17.17

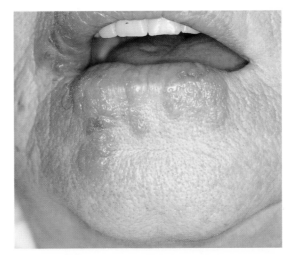

17.18

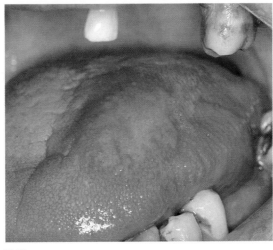

17.20

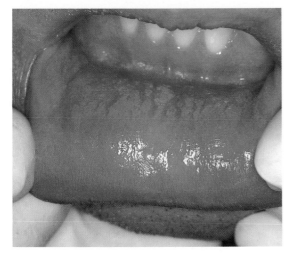

17.19

ALLERGIC REACTIONS

Rubber products, such as dental dam (**Figure 17.17**), eugenol and other essential oils (**Figure 17.18**) and various dentifrices (**Figure 17.19**) can occasionally induce allergic reactions (*see also* **Figure 10.324**).

Drugs rarely may induce a fixed drug eruption (**Figure 17.20**).

CANDIDOSIS

Median rhomboid glossitis (**Figure 17.21**) is predisposed by smoking.

Oral thrush can be induced by use of a corticosteroid inhaler (**Figure 17.22**; *see also* **Figure 2.156**). Lesions typically are seen in the fauces.

Mucosal staining from the use of gentian violet to treat candidosis (**Figure 17.23**) is now uncommon.

EPILEPSY

Epileptics often suffer repeated orofacial trauma causing soft tissue lacerations and scarring (**Figure 17.24**), and damage to teeth and/or jaws.

Anti-epileptic drugs given to pregnant mothers may cause fetal orofacial defects. These have been recorded both with phenytoin and sodium valproate.

Phenytoin can induce gingival hyperplasia (*see* page 305).

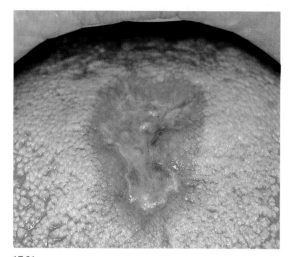

17.21

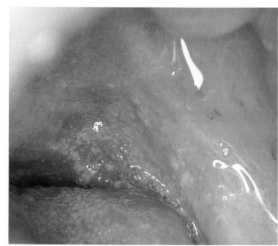

17.22

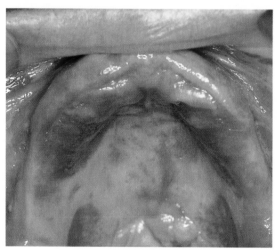

17.23

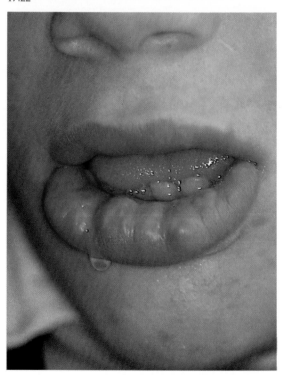

17.24

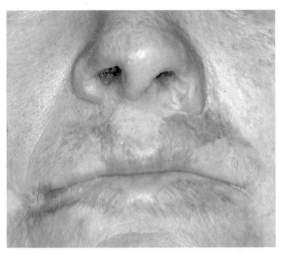

17.25

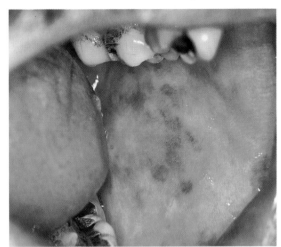

17.26

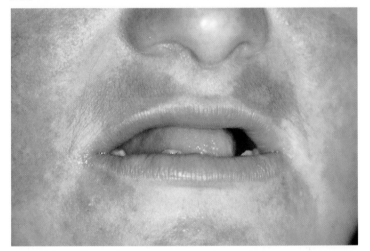

17.27

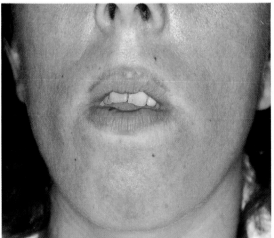

17.28

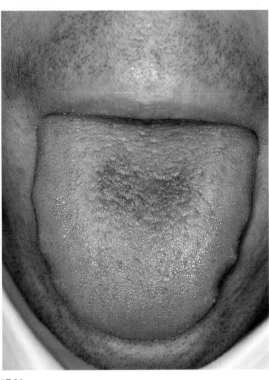

17.29

DRUG-INDUCED HYPER-PIGMENTATION

Long-term use of phenytoin can have wide-reaching adverse effects including hyperpigmentation (**Figure 17.25**). Hyperpigmentation also may be caused by antimalarials (**Figure 17.26**), ACTH, clofazimine, zidovudine, ketoconazole, busulphan and phenothiazines (*see* Section 1.5, page 56).

Long-term use of tranquillizers, such as chlorpromazine, may produce orofacial hyperpigmentation (**Figure 17.27**), xerostomia and facial dyskinesias.

Various chemicals that may produce a photosensitive dermatitis and pigmentation include furocumarine, bergamot oil and eugenol which may be found in perfumes, sprays, creams, mouthwashes and breath fresheners.

Chloasma (perioral hyperpigmentation) may arise during pregnancy or in patients using the oral contraceptive (**Figure 17.28**) or various other products (*see* Section 1.5, page 56).

Chlorhexidine and tobacco use may cause superficial staining (**Figure 17.29**), as may iron, bismuth subsalicylate and various other substances.

310

BETEL NUT STAINING

Betel use, typically in a quid with tobacco, not only causes discoloration of the mucosa (**Figure 17.30**) but can predispose to carcinoma.

TOOTH STAINING

Betel can also stain the teeth (**Figure 17.31**).

Other causes are discussed in Chapter 10 (*see* **Figures 10.27–10.72**).

POISONING

Heavy metal poisoning is now fortunately rare. Bismuth (**Figure 17.32**) and lead cause a line at the gingival margin where sulphides are deposited in areas of poor oral hygiene.

Arsenic poisoning is now rare and usually follows the ingestion of pesticides containing arsenates. Arsenic binds to keratins and chronic intoxication leads to mucositis, pigmentation (**Figure 17.33**), and facial oedema.

Arsenic poisoning causes 'rain-drop' hyper-pigmentation of the skin with hyperkeratosis of the palms (**Figure 17.34**) and soles and white transverse striae on the nails (Mees' lines).

A wide range of other poisons can cause oral problems. These may include burning mouth, ulceration, oedema, changes in salivation, changes in taste, hyperpigmentation or changes in sensation (*see* Section 1.5, page 56).

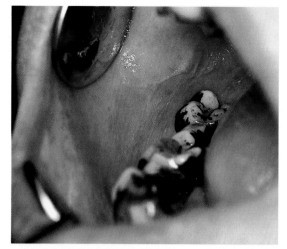

17.30

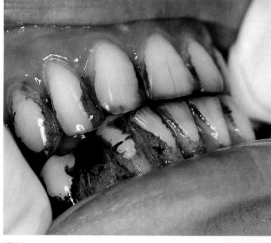

17.31

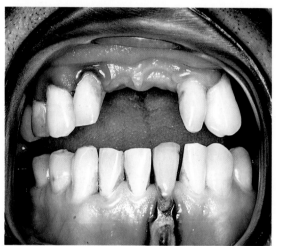

17.32

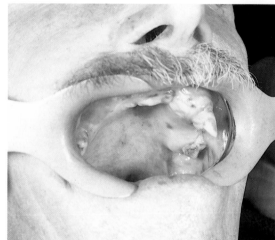

17.33

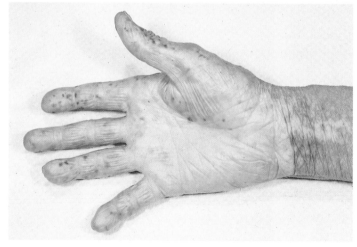

17.34

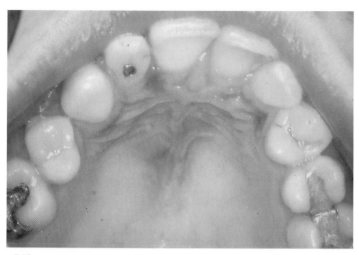

17.35

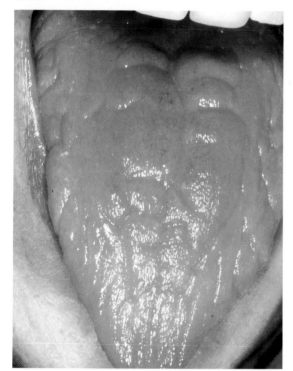

17.36

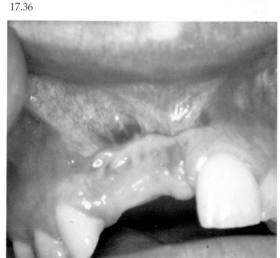

17.38

FOREIGN BODIES

Foreign bodies may result from facial trauma and may even enter the maxillary antrum. Palatal pigmentation from a foreign body (a pencil lead) is shown in **Figure 17.35**.

XEROSTOMIA

Various drugs may produce xerostomia (**Figure 17.36**). Atropinics or sympathomimetics may be responsible — especially some tranquillizers, antihypertensives and antidepressants (*see* Section 1.5, page 56).

PARAFUNCTION

The lingual indentations caused by the teeth can readily be seen in **Figure 17.37**). Parafunction can also contribute to attrition (*see* page 176), cheek-biting (*see* page 217), and facial arthromyalgia (*see* page 266).

AMALGAM TATTOO

Dental amalgam is a common cause of oral hyperpigmentation (**Figure 17.38**). Here amalgam had been used as a retrograde root-filling material, causing discoloration high towards the vestibule (*see also* **Figure 15.16**).

Amalgam can also be incorporated into the tissues during conservative dentistry. A bluish-black macule is usually seen in the gingiva or vestibule, especially in the mandible in the premolar–molar region (**Figure 17.39**).

17.37

17.39

ACRODYNIA

Chronic mercury exposure, from mercuric oxide (calomel) in teething powders, was a common cause of acrodynia up until the early 1950s. Now rare, acrodynia may be caused by mercury from paints, ointments, broken fluorescent light bulbs, or metallic mercury. Most cases are in children up to the age of 8 years, and present with profuse sweating, rashes, photophobia, alopecia, and puffiness and pink colour of the face (**Figure 17.40**), hands and feet (Pink disease).

Oral ulcers, disturbed tooth development and tooth exfoliation may be seen in severe acrodynia (**Figure 17.41**).

In many ways acrodynia resembles Kawasaki's disease (mucocutaneous lymph node syndrome).

TRAUMATIC HYPERPLASIA

Suction discs formerly used to help denture retention may produce hyperplasia in the palatal vault, as seen in **Figure 17.42**. Such a suction disc is shown in **Figure 17.43**.

TRAUMATIC ULCERS

See page 209.

DENTURE-INDUCED HYPERPLASIA

See page 191.

TRAUMA TO DENTITION

See page 176.

TOOTH EROSION

See page 176.

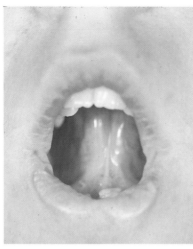

17.40

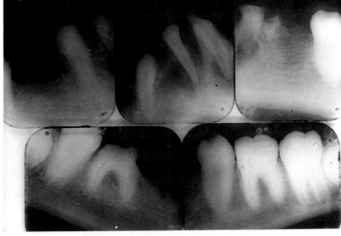

17.41

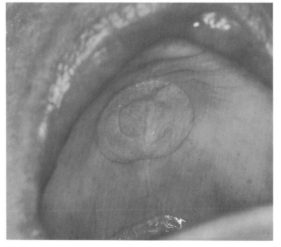

17.42

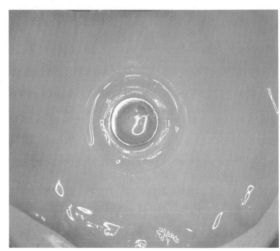

17.43

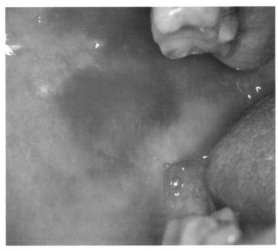

17.44

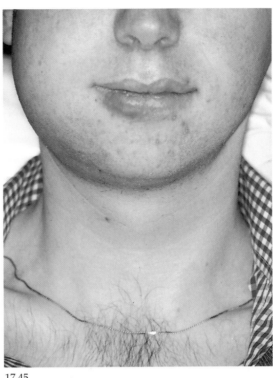

17.45

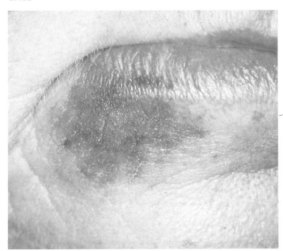

17.46

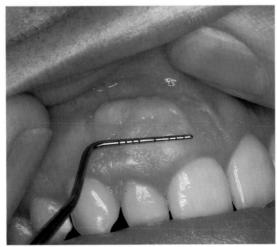

17.47

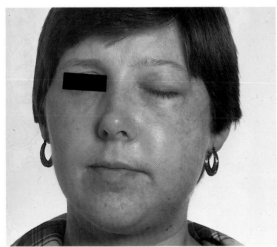

17.48

IATROGENIC INJURY

Dental local analgesic injections, especially regional blocks, commonly produce a small haematoma (**Figure 17.44**) which is usually inconsequential unless intramuscular, when it can cause trismus, or unless infected.

Extraoral swelling may be produced by a haematoma (**Figure 17.45**). Blood may track through fascial planes of the neck to cause extensive bruising, even down to the chest wall.

Post-operative oedema is particularly common after oral surgical procedures. **Figure 17.46** shows bruising from careless handling of the tissues.

Damage to nerves during surgery may produce paraesthesiae or permanent neurological deficit. Lingual nerve damage causes loss of sensation and taste sensation; inferior alveolar nerve damage can produce mental nerve sensory changes; and facial nerve damage can lead to facial palsy (*see* page 151) or Frey's syndrome (*see* page 317).

CICATRIZATION

Intraoral scarring is usually minimal except in severe tissue loss or some types of epidermolysis bullosa and mucous membrane pemphigoid. Keloids (**Figure 17.47**) are rare intraorally.

SURGICAL EMPHYSEMA

Dental instrumentation using air-turbine handpieces or air syringes occasionally introduces air into the tissues, producing surgical emphysema (**Figure 17.48**), recognized by acute swelling, crackling on palpation. Early recognition is essential to prevent such life-threatening complications as airway obstruction, deep neck infection or mediastinitis.

314

ANGIOEDEMA

Allergic angioedema is a type 1 response mediated by leukotrienes and vasoactive amines released from mast cells and basophils in an IgE-mediated response to an allergen. Labial swelling is a common presentation (**Figure 17.49**).

Allergens can be as varied as systemically administered drugs (such as penicillin) or topically contacted allergens in foodstuffs (such as benzoic and sorbic acids) (*see* Section 1.5, page 56).

Non-allergic angioedema can arise in patients receiving angiotensin-converting enzyme (ACE) inhibitors.

Hereditary angioedema (HANE) is a familial condition transmitted as an autosomal dominant trait, manifesting with angioedema often precipitated by mild trauma, such as that associated with dental treatment.

Hereditary angioedema is due to a decreased or defective inhibitor of the activated first component of complement (C1). Diseases occasionally associated with HANE are a lupus-like syndrome, coronary arteritis and autoimmune conditions, including Sjögren's syndrome, rheumatoid arthritis and thyroiditis: possibly because of disturbed immunoregulation.

C1 esterase deficiency is occasionally acquired, especially in lymphoproliferative disorders.

Swelling of the face, mouth and neck (**Figure 17.50**) in either type of angioedema may embarrass the airway. There may also be swelling of abdominal viscera and the extremities.

Figure 17.51 is the patient shown in **Figure 17.50**, seen between episodes.

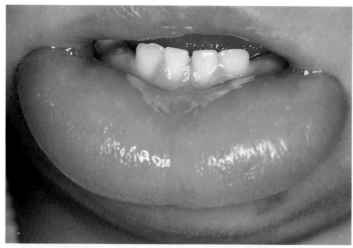

17.49

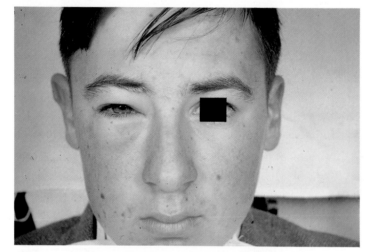

17.50

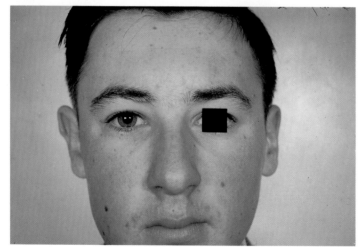

17.51

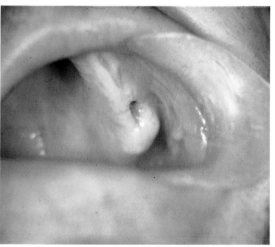

17.52

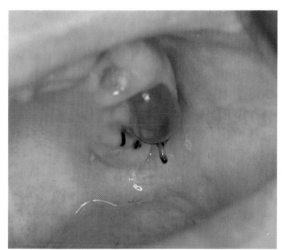

17.53

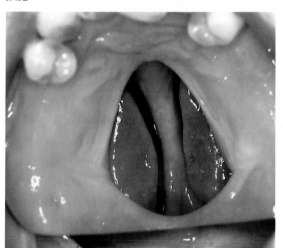

17.54

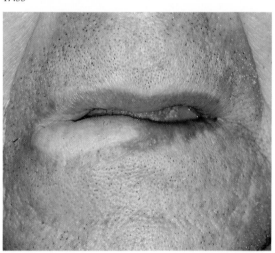

17.55

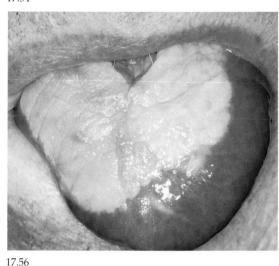

17.56

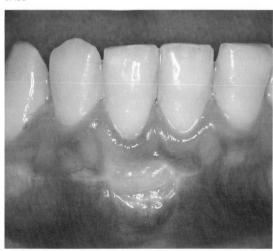

17.57

OROANTRAL FISTULA

Oroantral fistula (OAF) is almost invariably traumatic in aetiology, usually following extraction of an upper molar or premolar tooth (**Figure 17.52**). Fluid passes from the mouth into the sinus, which may become infected.

Occasionally, the antral lining prolapses through an OAF (**Figure 17.53**).

ORONASAL FISTULA

Surgery, such as the removal of a palatal neoplasm, may produce this defect (**Figure 17.54**).

GRAFTS

Skin graft of the defect following excision of a carcinoma remains paler (**Figure 17.55**) than the vermilion of the lip.

Intraorally, a skin graft becomes wrinkled and white (**Figure 17.56**). The ungrafted (red) part of the dorsum of tongue shown here is abnormal because of 'field-change' dysplasia.

Mucosal grafts from the palate for periodontal treatment are less white than skin grafts (**Figure 17.57**).

RADIATION INJURY

Radiotherapy involving the mouth and salivary glands invariably produces mucositis and often xerostomia (**Figure 17.58**). These, and other orofacial complications, are dose-dependent. Xerostomia predisposes to dental caries.

Pseudomembranous (**Figure 17.59**) and erythematous candidosis are common, especially where xerostomia is pronounced.

Endarteritis obliterans produces mucosal scarring (**Figure 17.60**), decreases the vascular supply to bone, predisposing to osteoradionecrosis (*see* page 198) and, if involving muscle, produces trismus. Irradiation of the tongue often produces taste loss.

Scarring is later followed by the appearance of telangiectasia (**Figure 17.61**).

Irradiation of developing teeth can cause hypoplasia, stunted root formation, and retarded eruption (**Figure 17.62**). Irradiation of the mandibular condyle, or other growth areas, can result in facial deformity.

The skin in the path of teletherapy tends to lose pigment, scar, and develop telangiectasia (**Figure 17.63**).

Previous irradiation predisposes to subsequent neoplasia: for example, radiotherapy to oropharyngeal neoplasms predisposes to subsequent salivary neoplasms.

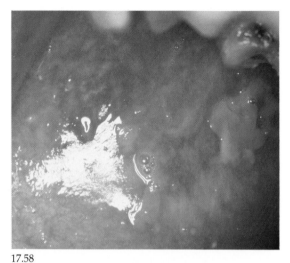

17.58

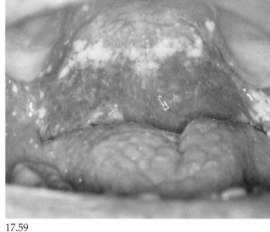

17.59

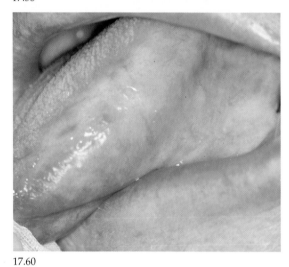

17.60

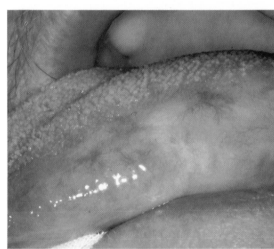

17.61

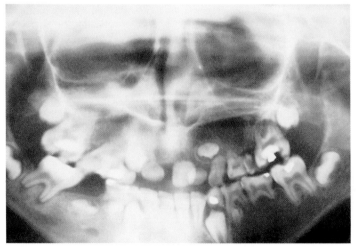

17.62

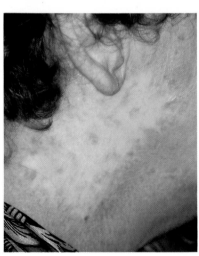

17.63

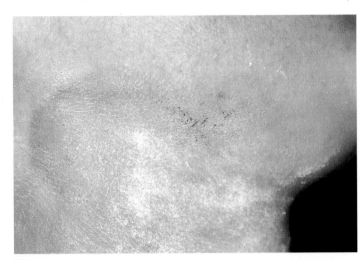

17.64

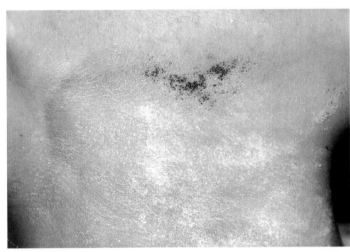

17.65

FREY'S SYNDROME
(*Gustatory sweating*)

Gustatory sweating is a rare clinical problem characterized by sweating, flushing, a sense of warmth, and occasional mild pain over an area of skin of the face while eating foods that produce a strong salivary stimulus. The disorder usually involves the area of skin innervated by the auriculotemporal nerve (Frey's syndrome) and is often termed the auriculotemporal syndrome.

Sweating of the skin over the area of innervation can easily be induced by the patient sucking on a piece of orange (**Figure 17.64**). A starch–iodine test confirms the precise areas of sweating (**Figure 17.65**).

Gustatory sweating is usually a consequence of interruption and alteration in the neural supply to sweat glands and blood vessels in an area of skin of the face and is usually a result of surgery. The syndrome follows between 6% and 60% of parotidectomies but has also been recorded after submandibular salivary gland surgery (**Figures 17.64 and 17.65**) and orthognathic surgery. Less commonly, gustatory sweating follows facial injury or infection. Diabetes mellitus is a rare cause. During subsequent regeneration, parasympathetic fibres are misdirected down previously sympathetic pathways such that normal parasympathetic stimulation results in a sympathetic-driven vasomotor effect of sweating and flushing of the skin. The typical lag time of months to years between neural damage and onset of clinical signs suggests that altered regeneration is the likely pathogenesis of most instances of gustatory sweating, but other theories of the cause of gustatory sweating have been postulated. Gustatory lacrimation, rhinorrhoea, and otorrhoea have also been described.

FACIAL PALSY

Inferior dental (alveolar) regional nerve local analgesic injections, if misplaced, may track through the parotid gland to reach the facial nerve and cause transient facial palsy (**Figure 17.66**). Any iatrogenic damage to the facial nerve (especially parotid surgery) can cause facial palsy.

BODY ART

Oral piercing is an unusual practice, may involve a variety of objects and may be seen in persons with other forms of body art (*see also* **Figure 10.287**). The placing of so-called jewellery, usually stainless-steel studs, rings or barbells, apparently has sexual connotations and in the oral region is typically seen in the lower lip. The so-called labrette piercing is usually a central piercing of the lip below the vermilion carrying a stud or ring (**Figure 17.67**).

The practice of tongue-piercing is a cause of some concern since oedema could be pronounced, widespread and a hazard to the airway. Thereafter, the permanent jewellery is placed and worn constantly, to avoid the perforation closing over spontaneously (**Figure 17.68**). Speech can be impaired and the teeth may be damaged by the jewellery.

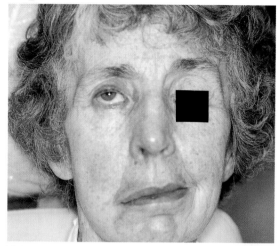

17.66

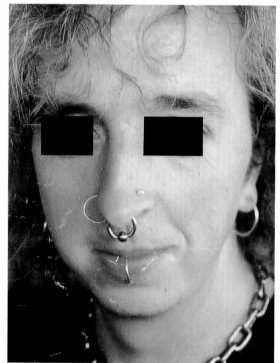

17.67

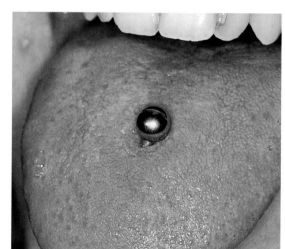

17.68

FURTHER READING

Figures in italic refer to page number in text.

Chapter 2

62   Boyd BW, Oral infection with associated lymphadenopathy due to *Mycobacterium chelonei*, *Ala Med* (1984) **54**:9–10.

Dimitrakopoulos I, Zouloumis L, Lazaridis N et al, Primary tuberculosis of the oral cavity, *Oral Surg Oral Med Oral Pathol* (1991) **72**:712–15.

Michaud M, Blanchette G, Tomich CF, Chronic ulceration of the hard palate: first clinical sign of undiagnosed pulmonary tuberculosis, *Oral Surg Oral Med Oral Pathol* (1984) **57**:63–7.

Volpe F, Schwimmer A, Barr C, Oral manifestations of disseminated *Mycobacterium avium–intracellulare* in a patient with AIDS, *Oral Surg Oral Med Oral Pathol* (1985) **60**:567–70.

Waldman RH, Tuberculosis and the atypical mycobacteria, *Otolaryngol Clin North Am* (1982) **15**:581–96.

63   Brazin SA, Leprosy (Hansen's disease), *Otolaryngol Clin North Am* (1982) **15**:597–611.

Helm FR, Gongloff RK, Wescott WB, Bilateral mixed density lesions in the body of the mandible, *J Am Dent Assoc* (1987) **115**:315–17.

64   Li KI, Kiernan S, Wald ER et al, Isolated uvulitis due to *Haemophilus influenzae* type b, *Pediatrics* (1984) **74**:1054–7.

Scully C, Vaccinia of the lip, *Br Dent J* (1977) **143**:57-9.

Wynder SG, Lampe RM, Shoemaker ME, Uvulitis and *Hemophilus influenzae* b bacteraemia, *Pediatr Emerg Care* (1986) **2**:23-5.

65   Badger GR, Oral signs of chickenpox (varicella): report of two cases, *ASDC J Dent Child* (1980) **47**:349–51.

Porter SR, Malamos D, Scully C, Mouth–skin interface: 3: Infections affecting skin and mouth, *Update* (1986) **33**:399–404.

66   Pallett AP, Nicholls MWN, Varicella-zoster: reactivation or reinfection, *Lancet* (1986) **i**:160.

Reichart PA, Oral manifestations of recently described viral infections, including AIDS, *Curr Opin Dent* (1991) **1**:377–83.

Schubert MM, Oral manifestations of viral infections in immunocompromised patients, *Curr Opin Dent* (1991) **1**:384–97.

Scully C, Bagg J, Viral infections in dentistry, *Curr Opin Dent* (1992) **2**:102–15.

Wright WE, Davis ML, Geffen DB et al, Alveolar bone necrosis and tooth loss: a rare complication associated with herpes zoster infection of the fifth cranial nerve, *Oral Surg Oral Med Oral Pathol* (1983) **56**:39–46.

67   Kalman CM, Laskin OL, Herpes zoster and zosteriform herpes simplex virus infections in immunocompetent adults, *Am J Med* (1986) **81**:775–80.

Mandal BK, Herpes zoster and the immunocompromised, *J Infect* (1987) **14**:1–5.

McKenzie CD, Gobetti JP, Diagnosis and treatment of orofacial herpes zoster: report of cases, *J Am Dent Assoc* (1990) **120**:679–81.

Scully C, Epstein J, Porter S et al, Viruses and chronic disorders involving the human oral mucosa, *Oral Surg Oral Med Oral Pathol* (1991) **72**:537–44.

68   Smith S, Ross JR, Scully C, An unusual oral complication of herpes zoster infection, *Oral Surg Oral Med Oral Pathol* (1984) **57**:388–9.

69 Corey L, Spear PG, Infections with herpes simplex viruses, *N Engl J Med* (1986) **314:**686–91, 749–57.

Epstein J, Scully C, Cytomegalovirus: a virus of increasing relevance to oral medicine and pathology, *J Oral Pathol Med* (1993) **22:**348–53.

Grossman ME, Stevens AW, Cohen PR, Brief report: herpetic geometric glossitis, *N Engl J Med* (1993) **329:**1859–60.

Jones AC, Freedman PD, Phelan JA et al, Cytomegalovirus infections of the oral cavity. A report of six cases and review of the literature, *Oral Surg Oral Med Oral Pathol* (1993) **75:**76–85.

Miller CS, Redding SW, Diagnosis and management of orofacial herpes simplex virus infections, *Dent Clin North Am* (1992) **36:**879–95.

Scully C, Infectious diseases. In: Mason DK, Millard D, eds, *2nd World Workshop on Oral Medicine* (University of Michigan Press: Ann Arbor, 1995) 3–104.

Scully C, Ulcerative stomatitis gingivitis and rash: a diagnostic dilemma, *Oral Surg Oral Med Oral Pathol* (1985) **59:**261–3.

Scully C, Orofacial herpes simplex virus infections: current concepts on the epidemiology, pathogenesis and treatment and disorders in which the virus may be implicated, *Oral Surg Oral Med Oral Pathol* (1989) **68:**701–10.

Spruance SL, The natural history of recurrent oral-facial herpes simplex virus infection, *Semin Dermatol* (1992) **11:**200–6.

70 Gill MJ, Arlette J, Buchan KA, Herpes simplex virus infection of the hand, *J Am Acad Dermatol* (1990) **22:**111–16.

Higgins CR, Schofield JK, Tatnall FM et al, Natural history, management and complications of herpes labialis, *J Med Virol* (1993) **Suppl 1:**22–6.

Spruance SL, Prophylactic chemotherapy with acyclovir for recurrent herpes simplex labialis, *J Med Virol* (1993) **Suppl 1:**27–32.

Stanberry LR, Herpes virus latency and recurrence, *Progr Med Virol* (1986) **33:**61–77.

Straus SE, Herpes simplex virus infection: biology, treatment and prevention, *Ann Intern Med* (1985) **103:**404–19.

71 Greenberg MS, Cohen SG, Boosz B et al, Oral herpes simplex infections in patients with leukaemia, *J Am Dent Assoc* (1987) **114:**483–6.

Jarrett M, Herpes simplex infections, *Arch Dermatol* (1983) **119:**99–103.

Scully C, Oral infections in the immunocompromised patient, *Br Dent J* (1992) **172:**401–7.

Wingard JR, Oral complications of cancer therapies. Infectious and non-infectious systemic consequences, *NCI Monographs* (1990) **9:**21–6.

72 Amler RW, Measles in young adults: the case for vigorous pursuit of immunisation, *Postgrad Med* (1985) **77:**251–8.

Glick M, Goldman HS, Viral infections in the dental setting: potential effects on pregnant HCWs, *J Am Dent Assoc* (1993) **124:**79–86.

Hoeprich PD, ed. *Infectious Disease: A Modern Treatise of Infectious Process,* 3rd edn (Harper and Row Publications: New York, 1983) 815–23.

Levy D, Measles: past, present and future, *NY State J Med* (1984) **84:**483–4.

Mitchell CD, Balfour HH Jr, Measles control: so near yet so far, *Prog Med Virol* (1985) **31:**1–42.

73   Gray ES, Human parvovirus infection, *J Pathol* (1987) **153**:310–12.

Whitley RJ, Parvovirus infection, *N Engl J Med* (1985) **313**:111–12.

74   Greenspan JS, Greenspan D, Oral aspects of the acquired immunodeficiency syndrome (AIDS). In: MacKenzie IC, Squier CA, Dabelsteen E, eds, *Oral Mucosal Diseases: Biology, Etiology and Therapy* (Laegeforeningens Forlag: Copenhagen, 1987) 65–9.

McCarthy GM, Host factors associated with HIV-related oral candidiasis. A review, *Oral Surg, Oral Med, Oral Pathol* (1992) **73**:181–6.

Scully C, Epstein JB, Porter SR et al, Recognition of oral lesions of HIV infection. 1. Candidosis, *Br Dent J* (1990) **169**:295–6.

Scully C, Laskaris G, Pindborg J et al, Oral manifestations of HIV infection and their management. I. More common lesions, *Oral Surg Oral Med Oral Pathol* (1991) **71**:158–66.

Scully C, Laskaris G, Pindborg J et al, Oral manifestations of HIV infection and their management. II. Less common lesions, *Oral Surg Oral Med Oral Pathol* (1991) **71**:167–71.

75   Axell T, Baert AE, Brocheriou C et al, An update of the classification and diagnostic criteria of oral lesions in HIV infection, *J Oral Pathol Med* (1991) **20**:97–100.

Axell T, Baert AE, Brocheriou C et al, Revised classification of HIV-associated oral lesions, *Br Dent J* (1991) **170**:305–6.

Leggott PJ, Oral manifestations of HIV infection in children, *Oral Surg Oral Med Oral Pathol* (1992) **73**:187–92.

Pindborg JJ, Scully C, Orofacial manifestations of HIV infection, *Medicine International* (1990) **76**:3172–4.

Porter SR, Scully C, Luker J et al, Oral manifestations of HIV infection, *Update* (1990) **40**:1173–80.

Porter SR, Scully C, HIV: the surgeon's perspective. Part 2. Diagnosis and management of non-malignant oral manifestations, *Br J Oral Maxillofac Surg* (1994) **32**:231–40.

Porter SR, Scully C, HIV: the surgeon's perspective. Part 3. Diagnosis and management of malignant neoplasms, *Br J Oral Maxillofac Surg* (1994) **32**:241–7.

Scully C, McCarthy G, Management of oral health in persons with HIV infection, *Oral Surg Oral Med Oral Pathol* (1992) **73**:215–25.

Scully C, Porter SR, Orofacial manifestations in infection with human immunodeficiency viruses, *Lancet* (1988) **1**:976–7.

Scully C, Porter SR, An ABC of oral health care in patients with HIV infection, *Br Dent J* (1991) **170**:149–50.

Scully C, Cawson RA, Porter SR, AIDS review, *Br Dent J* (1986) **161**:53–60.

Scully C, Epstein JB, Porter S et al, Recognition of oral lesions of HIV infection. 2. Hairy leukoplakia and Kaposi's sarcoma, *Br Dent J* (1990) **169**:332–3.

76   Greenspan D, Greenspan JS, Significance of oral hairy leukoplakia, *Oral Surg Oral Med Oral Pathol* (1992) **73**:151–4.

Schiodt M, Greenspan D, Daniels TE et al, Clinical and histologic spectrum of oral hairy leukoplakia, *Oral Surg Oral Med Oral Pathol* (1987) **64**:716–20.

Scully C, Epstein JB, Porter S et al, Recognition of oral lesions of HIV infection. 2. Hairy leukoplakia and Kaposi's sarcoma, *Br Dent J* (1990) **169**:332–3.

322

77 Eversole LR, Viral infections of the head and neck among HIV-seropositive patients, *Oral Surg Oral Med Oral Pathol* (1992) **73**:155–63.

78 Holmstrup P, Westergaard J, HIV-associated periodontal diseases. In: Lang NP, Karring T, eds, *Proceedings of the 1st European Workshop on Periodontology* (Quintessence Books: London, 1994) 439–61.

Scully C, Epstein JB, Porter S et al, Recognition of oral lesions of HIV infection. 3. Gingival and periodontal disease and less common lesions, *Br Dent J* (1990) **169**:370–2.

79 Heinic GS, Greenspan D, Greenspan JS, Oral CMV lesions and the HIV infected. Early recognition can help prevent morbidity, *J Am Dent Assoc* (1993) **124**:99–105.

MacPhail LA, Greenspan D, Feigal DW et al, Recurrent aphthous ulcers in association with HIV infection. Description of ulcer types and analysis of T-lymphocyte subsets, *Oral Surg Oral Med Oral Pathol* (1991) **71**:678–83.

80 Epstein J, Scully C, Neoplastic disease in the head and neck of patients with AIDS, *Int J Oral Maxillofac Surg* (1992) **2**:219–26.

Epstein JB, Silverman S Jr, Head and neck malignancies associated with HIV infection, *Oral Surg Oral Med Oral Pathol* (1992) **73**:193–200.

81 Porter SR, Glover S, Scully C, Oral hyperpigmentation and adrenocortical hypofunction in a patient with acquired immunodeficiency syndrome, *Oral Surg Oral Med Oral Pathol* (1990) **70**: 59–60

82 Bell EJ, Williams GR, Grist NR et al, Enterovirus infections, *Update* (1983) **26**:967–78.

Myer C, Cotton RT, Salivary gland disease in children: a review, *Clin Pediatr* (1986) **25**:314–22.

Scully C, Viruses and salivary gland disease, *Oral Surg Oral Med Oral Pathol* (1988) **66**:179–83.

Scully C, Non-neoplastic diseases of the major and minor salivary glands: a summary update, *Br J Oral Maxillofac Surg* (1992) **30**:244–7.

83 Grist NR, Bell EJ, Assaad F, Enteroviruses in human disease, *Prog Med Virol* (1978) **24**:114–57.

Kucera LS, Myrvik QN, *Fundamentals of Medical Virology,* 2nd edn (Lea and Febiger: Philadelphia, 1985) 216–28.

84 Conway SP, Coxsackie B2 virus causing simultaneous hand, foot and mouth disease and encephalitis, *J Infect* (1987) **15**:191.

Goh KT, Doraisingham S, Tan JC et al, An outbreak of hand, foot and mouth disease in Singapore, *Bull WHO* (1982) **60**:965–9.

Ishimaru Y, Nakano S, Yamaoka K et al, Outbreaks of hand, foot and mouth disease by Enterovirus 71, *Arch Dis Child* (1980) **55**:583–8.

Thomas I, Janniger CK, Hand, foot and mouth disease, *Cutis* (1993) **52**:265–6.

85 Johnson PA, Avery C, Infectious mononucleosis presenting as a parotid mass with associated facial nerve palsy, *Int J Oral Maxillofac Surg* (1991) **20**:193–5.

Leading article, New clinical manifestations of Epstein–Barr virus infection, *Lancet* (1982) **ii**:1253–5.

Leading article, EBV and persistent malaise, *Lancet* (1985) **i**:1017–18.

Wolf H, Seibl R, Benign and malignant disease caused by EBV, *J Invest Dermatol* (1984) **83** (Suppl):88–95.

86 Ablashi DV, Levine PH, Papas T, First international symposium on Epstein–Barr virus and associated malignant disease, *Cancer Res* (1985) **45**:3981–4.

Adler-Storthz K, Ficarra G, Woods KV et al, Prevalence of Epstein–Barr virus and human papillomavirus in oral mucosa of HIV-infected patients, *J Oral Pathol Med* (1992) **21**:164–70.

Epstein MA, Historical background: Burkitt's lymphoma and Epstein–Barr virus, *IARC Sci Publ* (1985) **60**:17–27.

Maddern BR, Werkhaven J, Wessel HB et al, Infectious mononucleosis with airway obstruction and multiple cranial nerve paresis, *Otolaryngol Head Neck Surg* (1991) **104**:529–32.

Purtilo DT, Tatsumi E, Manolov G, Epstein–Barr virus as an etiologic agent in the pathogenesis of lymphoproliferative and aproliferative diseases in immune deficient patients, *Int Rev Exp Pathol* (1985) **27**:113–83.

Sullivan JL, Epstein–Barr virus and the X-linked lymphoproliferative syndrome, *Adv Pediatr* (1983) **30**:365–99.

87 Garlick JA, Taichman LB, Human papillomavirus infection of the oral mucosa, *Am J Dermatopathol* (1991) **13**:386–95.

Green TL, Eversole LP, Leider AS, Oral and labial verruca vulgaris: clinical, histologic and immunohistochemical evaluation, *Oral Surg Oral Med Oral Pathol* (1986) **62**:410–16.

Scully C, Prime S, Maitland N, Papillomaviruses: their possible role in oral disease, *Oral Surg Oral Med Oral Pathol* (1985) **60**:166–74.

Scully C, Cox M, Maitland N et al, Papillomaviruses: their current status in relation to oral disease, *Oral Surg Oral Med Oral Pathol* (1988) **65**:526–32.

Whitaker SB, Wiegand SE, Budnick SD, Intraoral molluscum contagiosum, *Oral Surg Oral Med Oral Pathol* (1991) **72**:334–6.

88 Samaranayake LP, Scully C, Oral disease and sexual medicine, *Br J Sexual Med* (1988) **15**:138–43, 174–80.

Terezhalmy GT, Oral manifestations of sexually-related diseases, *Ear Nose Throat J* (1983) **62**:287–96.

89 Cousteau C, Leyder P, Laufer J, Syphilis primaire buccale: un diagnostic parfois difficile, *Rev Stomatol Chir Maxillofac* (1984) **85**:391–8.

Manton SL, Eggleston SI, Alexander I et al, Oral presentation of secondary syphilis, *Br Dent J* (1986) **160**:237–8.

90 Asvesti C, Anastassiadis G, Kolokotronis A et al, Oriental sore: a case report, *Oral Surg Oral Med Oral Pathol* (1992) **73**:56–8.

Castling B, Layton SA, Pratt RJ, Cutaneous leishmaniasis, *Oral Surg Oral Med Oral Pathol* (1994) **78**:91–2.

Crissey JT, Denenholz DA, Syphilis, *Clin Dermatol* (1984) **2**:1–166.

Kerdel-Vegas F, American leishmaniasis, *Int J Dermatol* (1982) **21**:291–303.

Marsden PD, Sampaio RN, Rocha R, Mucocutaneous leishmaniasis: an unsolved clinical problem, *Trop Doct* (1977) **7**:7–11.

Schuppli R, Leishmaniasis: a review, *Dermatologica* (1982) **165**:1–6.

324

Sitheeque MA, Qazi AA, Ahmed GA, A study of cutaneous leishmaniasis involvement of the lips and perioral tissues, *Br J Oral Maxillofac Surg* (1990) **28**:43–6.

Yusuf H, Battacharya MH, Syphilitic osteomyelitis of the mandible, *Br J Oral Surg* (1982) **20**:122–8.

91   Gonzalez T, Galvan E, Hernandez-Beriain JA et al, Destructive arthritis of the temporomandibular joint in a patient with Reiter's syndrome and human immunodeficiency virus infection, *J Rheumatol* (1991) **18**:1771–2.

International symposium on yaws and other endemic treponematoses (Washington DC, April 1984), *Rev Inf Dis* (1985) **7** (Suppl 2):217–351.

Keat A, Rowe I, Reiter's syndrome and associated arthritides, *Rheum Dis Clin North Am* (1991) **17**:25–42.

92   Enwonwu CO, Infectious oral necrosis (cancrum oris) in Nigerian children, *Community Dent Oral Epidemiol* (1985) **13**:190–4.

Holbrook WP, Bacterial infections of oral soft tissues, *Curr Opin Dent* (1991) **1**:404–10.

Johnson BD, Engel D, Acute necrotising ulcerative gingivitis: a review of diagnosis, etiology and treatment, *J Periodontol* (1986) **57**:141–50.

Lin JY, Wang DW, Peng CT et al, Noma neonatorum: an unusual case of noma involving a full-term neonate, *Acta Paediatrica* **81**:720–2.

Osuji OO, Necrotizing ulcerative gingivitis and cancrum oris (noma) in Ibadan, Nigeria, *J Periodontol* (1990) **61**:769–72.

Sabiston CB, A review and proposal for the etiology of acute necrotising gingivitis, *J Clin Periodontol* (1986) **13**:727–34.

Sawyer D, Nwoku AJ, Cancrum oris (noma): past and present, *J Dent Child* (1981) **48**:138–41.

93   Horowitz BJ, Edelstein SW, Lippman L, Sexual transmission of candida, *Obstet Gynecol* (1987) **69**:883–6.

Oelz O, Schaffner A, Frick P et al, *Trichosporon capitatum*: thrush-like oral infection, local invasion, fungaemia and metastatic abscess formation in a leukaemic patient, *J Infect* (1983) **6**:183–5.

Schnell JD, Epidemiology and prevention of peripartal mycoses, *Chemotherapy* (1982) **28** (Suppl 1):68–72.

94   Odds FC, Candida infections: an overview, *CRC Critical Rev Microbiol* (1987) **15**:1–5.

Scully C, Chronic atrophic candidosis, *Lancet* (1986) **ii**:437–8.

95   Holmstrup P, Bessermann M, Clinical, therapeutic and pathogenic aspects of chronic oral multifocal candidiasis, *Oral Surg Oral Med Oral Pathol* (1984) **56**:388–95.

Ohman SC, Dahlen G, Moller A et al, Angular cheilitis: a clinical and microbial study, *J Oral Pathol* (1986) **15**:213–17.

Warnakulasuriya KA, Samaranayake LP, Peiris JS, Angular cheilitis in a group of Sri Lankan adults: a clinical and microbiologic study, *J Oral Pathol Med* (1991) **20**:172–5.

Wright BA, Fenwick F, Candidiasis and atrophic tongue lesions, *Oral Surg Oral Med Oral Pathol* (1981) **51**:55–61.

96   Heimdahl A, Nord CE, Oral yeast infections in immunocompromised and seriously diseased patients, *Acta Odontol Scand* (1990) **48**:77–84.

Nielson H, Dangaard K, Schiodt M, Chronic mucocutaneous candidosis: a review, *Tandlaegkbladet* (1985) **89:**667–73.

Porter SR, Scully C, Candidosis endocrinopathy syndrome, *Oral Surg Oral Med Oral Pathol* (1986) **61:**573–8.

Porter S, Haria S, Scully C et al, Chronic candidiasis, enamel hypoplasia and pigmentary anomalies, *Oral Surg Oral Med Oral Pathol* (1992) **73:**312–14.

97   Smith CB, Candidiasis: pathogenesis, host resistance and predisposing factors. In: Bodey GP, Feinstein V, eds, *Candidiasis* (Raven Press: New York, 1985) 53.

98   Almeida O, Scully C, Oral lesions in the systemic mycoses, *Curr Opin Dent* (1991) **1:**423–8.

Almeida O de P, Jacks J, Scully C et al, Orofacial manifestations of paracoccidioidomycosis (South American blastomycosis), *Oral Surg Oral Med Oral Pathol* (1991) **72:**430–5.

Goodwin RA, Shapiro JL, Thurman GH et al, Disseminated histoplasmosis: clinical and pathologic correlations, *Medicine* (1980) **59:**1–33.

Jones AC, Bentsen YT, Freedman PD, Mucormycosis of the oral cavity, *Oral Surg Oral Med Oral Pathol* (1993) **75:**455–60.

Lehrer RI, Howard DH, Sypherd PS et al, Mucormycosis, *Ann Intern Med* (1980) **93:**93–100.

Oda D, MacDougall L, Fritsche T et al, Oral histoplasmosis as a presenting disease in acquired immunodeficiency syndrome, *Oral Surg Oral Med Oral Pathol* (1990) **70:**631–6 (published erratum appears in *Oral Surg Oral Med Oral Pathol* (1991) **71:**76).

Scully C, Almeida O, Orofacial manifestations of the systemic mycoses, *J Oral Pathol Med* (1992) **21:**289–94.

99   Beck-Mannagetta J, Necek D, Grasserbauer M, Solitary aspergillosis of maxillary sinus: complication of dental treatment, *Lancet* (1983) **i:**1280.

Schubert MM, Head and neck aspergillosis in patients undergoing bone-marrow transplantation, *Cancer* (1986) **57:**1092–6.

100   Bozzo L, Lima IA, Almeida O et al, Oral myiasis caused by sarcophagidae in an extraction wound, *Oral Surg Oral Med Oral Pathol* (1992) **74:**733–5.

Lopes MA, Zaia AA, Almeida OPD et al, Larva migrans affecting the mouth, *Oral Surg Oral Med Oral Pathol* (1994) **77:**362–7.

101   Douglas JG, Gillon J, Logan RFA et al, Sarcoidosis and coeliac disease: an association? *Lancet* (1984) **ii:**13–15.

James DG, Sharma OP, Overlap syndromes with sarcoidosis, *Postgrad Med J* (1985) **61:**769–71.

Macleod RI, Snow MH, Hawkesford JE, Sarcoidosis of the tongue, *Br J Oral Maxillofac Surg* (1985) **23:**243–6.

Mendelsohn SS, Field EA, Woolgar J, Sarcoidosis of the tongue, *Clin Exp Dermatol* (1992) **17:**47–8.

Van Maarsseveen ACMT, van der Waal I, Stam J et al, Oral involvement in sarcoidosis, *Int J Oral Surg* (1982) **11:**21–9.

102   Bowman KF, Barbery RT, Swango LJ et al, Cutaneous forms of bovine popular stomatitis in man, *JAMA* (1981) **246:**2813–18.

Chapter 3

104   Boyle P, MacFarlane GJ, Zheng T et al, Recent advances in the epidemiology of head and neck cancer, *Curr Opin Oncol* (1992) **4:**471–7.

326

Kleinman DV, Swango PA, Pindborg JJ et al, Toward assessing trends in oral mucosal lesions: lessons learned from oral cancer, *Adv Dental Res* (1993) **7**:32–41.

Morton RP, Missotten FEM, Pharoah POD, Classifying cancer of the lip: an epidemiologic perspective, *Eur J Cancer Clin Oncol* (1983) **19**:875–9.

Peterson DE, *Head and Neck Management of the Cancer Patient: Developments in Oncology* (Kluwer: The Hague, 1986).

Pindborg JJ, *Oral Cancer and Precancer* (John Wright & Sons Ltd: Bristol, 1980).

Scully C, Oral cancer: new insights into pathogenesis, *Dental Update* (1993) **20**:95–100.

Scully C, Boyle P, Tedesco B, The recognition and diagnosis of cancer arising in the mouth, *Postgrad Doc* (1992) **15**:134-41.

Ward-Booth P, Scully C, The management of mouth cancer, *Postgrad Doc* (1992) **15**:166–75.

Woods KV, Shillitoe EJ, Spitz MR et al, Analysis of human papillomavirus DNA in oral squamous cell carcinomas, *J Oral Pathol Med* (1993) **22**:101–8.

105 Davis S, Severson RK, Increasing incidence of cancer of the tongue in the United States among young adults, *Lancet* (1987) **ii**:910–11.

Macfarlane GJ, Boyle P, Scully C, Rising mortality from cancer of the tongue in young Scottish males, *Lancet* (1987) **ii**:912.

106 Craig RM Jr, Vickers VA, Correll RW, Erythroplastic lesion on the mandibular marginal gingiva, *J Am Dent Assoc* (1989) **119**:543–4.

Fitzpatrick PJ, Tepperman BS, Carcinoma of the floor of the mouth, *J Can Assoc Radiol* (1982) **33**:148–53.

Henk J, Langdon J, *Malignant Tumours of the Oral Cavity* (Edward Arnold: London, 1985).

107 Awange DO, Onyango JF, Oral verrucous carcinoma: report of two cases and review of literature, *East Afr Med J* (1993) **70**:316–18.

Gupta PC, Pindborg JJ, Mehta FS, Comparison of carcinogenicity of betal quid with and without tobacco: an epidemiological review, *Ecol Dis* (1982) **1**:213–19.

McDonald JS, Crissman JD, Gluckman JL, Verrucous carcinoma of the oral cavity, *Head Neck Surg* (1982) **5**:22–8.

108 Baden E, Prevention of cancer of the oral cavity and pharynx, *Cancer* (1987) **37**:49–62.

Scully C, Malamos D, Levers BGH et al, Sources and patterns of referrals of oral cancer: the role of general practitioners, *Br Med J* (1986) **293**:599–601.

Tandon DA, Bahadur S, Rath GK, Carcinoma of the soft palate, *J Laryngol Otol* (1992) **106**:130–2.

109 Antoniadis K, Karakasis D, Tzarou V et al, Benign cysts of the parotid gland, *Int J Oral Maxillofac Surg* (1990) **19**:139–40.

Illes RW, Brian MB, A review of tumours of the salivary gland, *Surg Gynecol Obstet* (1986) **163**:399–404.

Isaacson G, Shear M, Intraoral salivary gland tumours: a retrospective study of 201 cases, *J Oral Pathol* (1983) **12**:57–62.

110 Austin JR, Crockett DM, Pleomorphic adenoma of the palate in a child, *Head Neck* (1992) **14**:58–61.

Chan MNY, Radden BG, Intraoral salivary gland neoplasms: a retrospective study of 98 cases, *J Oral Pathol* (1986) **15:**339–42.

Hunter RM, Davis BW, Gray GF et al, Primary malignant tumours of salivary origin: a 52-year review, *Ann Surg* (1983) **49:**82–9.

Rasp G, Permanetter W, Malignant salivary gland tumours: squamous cell carcinoma of the submandibular gland in a child, *Am J Otolaryngol* (1992) **13:**109–12.

111 Keszler A, Dominguez FU, Ameloblastoma in childhood, *J Oral Maxillofac Surg* (1986) **44:**609–13.

Redman RS, Keegan BP, Spector CJ et al, Peripheral ameloblastoma with unusual mitotic activity and conflicting evidence regarding histogenesis, *J Oral Maxillofac Surg* (1994) **52:**192–7.

Reichart PA, Ries P, Considerations on the classification of odontogenic tumours, *Int J Oral Surg* (1983) **12:**323–33.

Slootweg PJ, Muller H, Malignant ameloblastoma or ameloblastic carcinoma, *Oral Surg Oral Med Oral Pathol* (1984) **57:**168–76.

Stuart DJ, Unicystic ameloblastoma of the mandible, *Br J Oral Maxillofac Surg* (1984) **22:**307–10.

112 Bahar M, Anavi Y, Abraham A et al, Primary malignant melanoma in the parotid gland, *Oral Surg Oral Med Oral Pathol* (1990) **70:**627–30.

Eisen D, Voorhees JJ, Oral melanoma and other pigmented lesions of the oral cavity, *J Am Acad Dermatol* (1991) **24:**527–37.

Hirshberg A, Leibovich P, Buchner A, Metastases to the oral mucosa: analysis of 157 cases, *J Oral Pathol Med* (1993) **22:**385–90.

Hoyt DJ, Jordan T, Fisher SR, Mucosal melanoma of the head and neck, *Arch Otolaryngol Head Neck Surg* (1989) **115:**1096–9.

Keller EE, Gunderson LL, Bone disease metastatic to the jaw, *J Am Dent Assoc* (1987) **115:**697–701.

MacIntyre DR, Briggs JC, Primary oral malignant melanoma, *Int J Oral Surg* (1984) **13:**160–5.

Marker P, Clausen PP, Metastases to the mouth and jaws from hepatocellular carcinomas, *Int J Oral Maxillofac Surg* (1991) **20:**371–4.

Nishimura Y, Yakata H, Kawasaki T et al, Metastatic tumours of the mouth and jaws: a review of the Japanese literature, *J Maxillofac Surg* (1982) **10:**253–8.

Patton LL, Brahim JS, Baker AR, Metastatic malignant melanoma of the oral cavity, *Oral Surg Oral Med Oral Pathol* (1994) **78:**51–6.

Peckitt NS, Wood GA, Malignant melanoma of the oral cavity. A case report, *Oral Surg Oral Med Oral Pathol* (1990) **70:**161–4.

Rapini RP, Golitz LE, Greer RO et al, Primary malignant melanoma of the oral cavity, *Cancer* (1985) **55:**1543–51.

Sooknundun M, Kacker SK, Kapila K et al, Oral malignant melanoma (a case report and review of the literature), *J Laryngol Otol* (1986) **100:**371–5.

van der Waal RI, Snow GB, Karim AB et al, Primary malignant melanoma of the oral cavity: a review of eight cases, *Br Dent J* (1994) **176:**185–8.

Woodwards RT, Shepherd NA, Hensher R, Malignant melanoma of the parotid gland: a case report and literature review, *Br J Oral Maxillofac Surg* (1993) **31:**313–15.

328

113 Baden E, Al Saati T, Caverivière P et al, Hodgkin's lymphoma of the oropharyngeal region, *Oral Surg Oral Med Oral Pathol* (1987) **64**:88–94.

Eisenbud L, Sciubba J, Mir R et al, Oral presentations in non-Hodgkin's lymphoma: a review of 31 cases, *Oral Surg Med Oral Pathol* (1983) **56**:151–6.

Maxymiw WG, Patterson BJ, Wood RE et al, B-cell lymphoma presenting as a midfacial necrotizing lesion, *Oral Surg Oral Med Oral Pathol* (1992) **74**:343–7.

114 Baden E, Carter R, Intraoral presentation of American Burkitt's lymphoma after extraction of a mandibular left third molar *J Oral Maxillofac Surg* (1987) **45**:689–93.

Kasha EE Jr, Parker CM, Oral manifestations of cutaneous T cell lymphoma, *Int J Dermatol* (1990) **29**:275–80.

Perez-Reyes N, Farhi DC, Squamous cell carcinoma of head and neck in patients with well-differentiated lymphocytic lymphoma, *Cancer* (1987) **59**:540–4.

115 Broadbent V, Pritchard J, Histiocytosis X: current controversies, *Arch Dis Child* (1985) **60**:605–8.

Cronin AJ, Stevenson ARL, Austin BW, Eosinophilic granuloma of the oral region: a potential diagnostic problem, *Aust Dent J* (1991) **36**:113–19.

Favera BE, McCarthy RC, Mieran GW, Histiocytosis X, *Hum Pathol* (1983) **14**:663–76.

116 Barnett ML, Cole RJ, Mycosis fungoides with multiple oral mucosal lesions, *J Periodontol* (1985) **56**:690–3.

Brousset P, Pages M, Chittal SM et al, Tumour phase of mycosis fungoides in the tongue, *Histopathology* (1992) **20**:87–9.

Evans GE, Dalziel KL, Mycosis fungoides with oral involvement, *Int J Oral Maxillofac Surg* (1987) **16**:634–7.

Osserman EF, Melini G, Butler VP, Multiple myeloma and related plasma cell dyscrasias, *JAMA* (1987) **258**:2930–7.

Patel SP, Hotterman OA, Mycosis fungoides: an overview, *J Surg Oncol* (1983) **22**:221–6.

Raubenheimer EJ, Danth J, Van Wilpe E, Multiple myeloma: a study of 10 cases, *J Oral Pathol* (1987) **16**:383–8.

Sirois DA, Miller AS, Harwick RD et al, Oral manifestations of cutaneous T-cell lymphoma. A report of eight cases, *Oral Surg Oral Med Oral Pathol* (1993) **75**:700–5.

Vicente A, Marti RM, Martin E et al, Mycosis fungoides with oral involvement, *Int J Dermatol* (1991) **30**:864–6.

Yaegaki K, Kameyama T, Takenaka M et al, Myelomatosis (IgD) discovered by oral manifestations, *Int J Oral Surg* (1985) **14**:381–4.

117 Cooley RO, Sanders BJ, The pediatrician's involvement in prevention and treatment of oral disease in medically compromised children, *Pediatr Clin North Am* (1991) **38**:1265–88.

Dreizen S, McCredie KB, Keating MJ, Chemotherapy-associated oral haemorrhages in adults with acute leukaemia, *Oral Surg Oral Med Oral Pathol* (1983) **55**:572–8.

Dreizen S, McCredie KB, Keating MJ et al, Malignant gingival and skin infiltrates in adult leukemia, *Oral Surg Oral Med Oral Pathol* (1983) **55**:572–8.

Schubert MM, Sullivan KM, Recognition, incidence, and management of oral graft-versus-host disease, *NCI Monographs* (1990) **9**:135–43.

118   Barrett AP, A long-term prospective clinical study of oral complications during conventional chemotherapy for acute leukemia, *Oral Surg Oral Med Oral Pathol* (1987) **63**:313-16.

Dreizen S, McCredie KB, Bodey GP et al, Quantitative analysis of the oral complications of anti-leukemia chemotherapy, *Oral Surg Oral Med Oral Pathol* (1986) **62**:650–3.

Sherr CJ, Leukemia and lymphoma, *Cell* (1987) **48**:727–9.

119   Dreizen S, McCredie KB, Bodey GP et al, Microbial mucocutaneous infections in acute adult leukaemia, *Postgrad Med* (1986) **79**:107–18.

Mintz SM, Anavi Y, Maxillary osteomyelitis and spontaneous tooth exfoliation after herpes zoster, *Oral Surg Oral Med Oral Pathol* (1992) **73**:664–6.

Scully C, MacFarlane TW, Orofacial manifestations in childhood malignancy: clinical and microbiological findings during remission, *ASDC J Dent Child* (1983) **50**:121–5.

120   Cigliano B, De Fazio P, Esposito P, Neonatal congenital epulis, *Int J Oral Maxillofac Surg* (1985) **14**:456–7.

Lack EE, Gingival granular cell tumours of the newborn (congenital epulis): a clinical and pathologic study of 21 patients, *Am J Surg Pathol* (1981) **5**:37–46.

Zuker RM, Buenechea R, Congenital epulis: review of the literature and case report, *J Oral Maxillofac Surg* (1993) **51**:1040–3.

121   Kaban LB, Mulliken JB, Vascular anomalies of the maxillofacial region, *J Oral Maxillofac Surg* (1986) **44**:203–13.

Stal S, Hamilton S, Spira M, Haemangioma, lymphangioma and vascular malformations of the head and neck, *Otolaryngol Clin North Am* (1986) **19**:769–96.

122   Laskaris G, Skouteris C, Maffucci's syndrome: report of a case with oral haemangiomas, *Oral Surg Med Oral Pathol* (1984) **57**:263–6.

Skouteris CA, More on hemangiomas in patients with Maffucci's syndrome, *J Oral Maxillofac Surg* (1994) **52**:205.

Wolf M, Engelberg S, Recurrent oral bleeding in Maffucci's syndrome: report of a case, *J Oral Maxillofac Surg* (1993) **51**:596–7.

Yavuzylimaz E, Yamalik N, Eratalay K et al, Oral-dental findings in a case of Maffucci's syndrome, *J Periodontol* (1993) **64**:673–7.

Zocchi D, Innao V, Calderoni P, Maffucci's syndrome: report of three cases and review of the literature, *Ital J Orthop Traumatol* (1983) **9**:263–6.

Chapter 4

124   Gilsen G, Nilsson KO, Matsson L, Gingival inflammation in diabetic children related to degree of metabolic control, *Acta Odont Scand* (1980) **38**:241–6.

Lamey PJ, Darwazeh AM, Frier BM, Oral disorders associated with diabetes mellitus, *Diabetic Medicine* (1992) **9**:410-16.

Murrah VA, Diabetes mellitus and associated oral manifestations: a review, *J Oral Pathol* (1985) **14**:271–81.

Porter SR, Haria S, Scully C et al, Chronic candidiasis, enamel hypoplasia and pigmentary anomalies, *Oral Surg Oral Med Oral Pathol* (1992) **74**:312-14.

Walls AW, Soames JV, Dental manifestations of autoimmune hypoparathyroidism, *Oral Surg Oral Med Oral Path* (1993) **75**:452–4 (published erratum appears in *Oral Surg Oral Med Oral Pathol* (1993) **75**:779).

125 Chuong R, Kaban LB, Kozakewich H, Central giant cell lesions on the jaw: a clinico-pathologic study, *J Oral Maxillofac Surg* (1986) **44**:708–13.

Kinirons MJ, Glasgow JFT, The chronology of dentinal defects related to medical findings in hypoparathyroidism, *J Dent* (1985) **13**:346–9.

Walls AWG, Soames JV, Dental manifestations of autoimmune hypoparathyroidism, *Oral Surg Oral Med Oral Pathol* (1993) **75**:452–4.

126 Karpf DB, Braunstein GD, Current concepts in acromegaly: aetiology, diagnosis and treatment, *Compr Ther* (1986) **12**:22–30.

Whelan J, Redpath T, Buckle R, The medical and anaesthetic management of acromegalic patients undergoing maxillofacial surgery, *Br J Oral Surg* (1982) **20**:77–83.

127 Brunt LM, Wells SA, The multiple endocrine neoplasia syndromes, *Invest Radiol* (1985) **20**:916–27.

Casino AJ, Sciubba JJ, Ohri G et al, Orofacial manifestations of the multiple endocrine neoplasia syndrome, *Oral Surg Oral Med Oral Pathol* (1981) **51**:516–20.

Lamey P-J, Carmichael F, Scully C, Oral pigmentation, Addison's disease and the results of screening for adreno-cortical insufficiency, *Br Dent J* (1985) **158**:297–8.

Moyer GN, Terezhalmy GT, O'Brian JT, Nelson's syndrome: another condition associated with mucocutaneous hyper-pigmentation, *J Oral Med* (1985) **1**:13–17.

128 Challacombe SJ, Scully C, Keevil B et al, Serum ferritin in recurrent oral ulceration, *J Oral Pathol* (1983) **12**:290–9.

Drummond JF, White DK, Damm DD, Megaloblastic anemia with oral lesions: a consequence of gastric by-pass surgery, *Oral Surg Oral Med Oral Pathol* (1985) **59**: 149–53.

Grattan CEH, Scully C, Oral ulceration: a diagnostic problem, *Br Med J* (1986) **292**: 1093–4.

Greenberg MS, Clinical and histologic changes of the oral mucosa in pernicious anaemia, *Oral Surg Oral Med Oral Pathol* (1981) **52**:38–42.

Loggi DG Jr, Regenye GR, Milles M, Pica and iron-deficiency anemia: a case report, *J Oral Maxillofac Surg* (1992) **50**:633–5.

McLoughlin IJ, Hassanyeh F, Pica in a patient with anorexia nervosa, *Br J Psychiatry* (1990) **156**:568–70.

Porter SR, Scully C, Aphthous stomatitis – an overview of aetiopathogenesis and management, *Clin Exp Dermatol* (1991) **16**:235–43.

Scully C, Porter SR, Recurrent aphthous stomatitis: current concepts of aetiology, pathogenesis and management, *J Oral Pathol Med* (1989) **18**:21–7.

129 Doppelt SH, Vitamin D, rickets and osteomalacia, *Orthop Clin North Am* (1984) **15**:671–86.

Ellis CN, Vanderveen EE, Rasmussen JE, Scurvy: a case caused by peculiar dietary habits, *Arch Dermatol* (1984) **120**:1212–14.

Solt DB, The pathogenesis, oral manifestations, and implications for dentistry of metabolic bone disease, *Curr Opin Dent* (1991) **1**:783–91.

130 Babejews A, Occult multiple myeloma associated with amyloid of the tongue, *Br J Oral Maxillofac Surg* (1985) **23**:298–303.

Franklin ED, The heavy chain diseases, *Harvey Lect* (1984) **78**:1–22.

Fuchs A, Jagirdar J, Schwartz IS, Beta 2 microglobulin amyloidosis (AB 2M) in patients undergoing long-term hemodialysis, *Am J Clin Pathol* (1987) **88**:302–7.

Geist JR, Geist SM, Wesley RK, Diagnostic procedures in oral amyloidosis, *Compendium* (1993) **14**:924, 926–8, 930.

Gertz MA, Kyle RA, Griffing WL et al, Jaw claudication in primary systemic amyloidosis, *Medicine (Baltimore)* (1986) **65**:173–9.

Glenner GG, Amyloid deposits and amyloidosis, *N Engl J Med* (1980) **302**:1283–92, 1333–43.

Myssiorek D, Alvi A, Bhuiya T, Primary salivary gland amyloidosis causing sicca syndrome, *Ann Otol Rhinol Laryngol* (1992) **101**:487–90.

Raymond AK, Sneige N, Batsakis JG, Pathology consultation: amyloidosis in the upper aerodigestive tracts, *Ann Otol Laryngol* (1992) **101**:794–6.

Reinish EI, Raviv M, Srolovitz H et al, Tongue, primary amyloidosis and multiple myeloma, *Oral Surg Oral Med Oral Pathol* (1994) **77**:121–5.

131 Bach G, Friedman R, Weissmann B et al, The defect in Hurler and Scheie syndromes: deficiency of α-1-iduronidase, *Proc Natl Acad Sci USA* (1972) **69**:2048–51.

Gardner DG, Oral manifestations of Hurler's syndrome, *Oral Surg Oral Med Oral Pathol* (1971) **32**:46–57.

Keith O, Scully C, Weidmann GM, Orofacial features of Scheie (Hurler–Scheie) syndrome (alpha-L-iduronidase deficiency) *Oral Surg Oral Med Oral Pathol* (1990) **70**:70–4.

Scully C, Orofacial manifestations of the Lesch–Nyhan syndrome, *Int J Oral Surg* (1981) **10**:380–3.

Sofaer JA, Single gene disorders. In: Jones JH, Mason DK, eds, *Oral manifestations of systemic disease* (Saunders: Eastbourne, 1980) 37.

132 Dahlen G, Bjorkander J, Gahnberg L et al, Periodontal disease and dental caries in relation to primary IgG subclass and other humoral immunodeficiencies, *J Clin Periodontol* (1993) **20**:7–13.

Engstrom GN, Engstrom PE, Hammarstrom L et al, Oral conditions in individuals with selective immunoglobulin A deficiency and common variable immunodeficiency, *J Periodontol* (1992) **63**:984–9.

Porter SR, Scully C, Orofacial manifestations in primary immunodeficiencies involving IgA deficiency, *J Oral Pathol Med* (1993) **22**:117–19.

Scully C, Porter SR, Immunodeficiency. In: Ivanyi L, ed. *Immunology of Oral Diseases* (MTP Press: Lancaster, 1986) 235–56.

Scully C, Porter SR, Primary immunodeficiencies. In: Jones JH, Mason DK, eds, *Oral Manifestations of Systemic Disease*, 2nd edn (Saunders: London, 1990).

Chapter 5

134 Ramasinghe AW, Warnakulasuriya KAAS, Tennekoon GE et al, Oral mucosal changes in iron deficiency anemia in a Sri Lankan female population, *Oral Surg Oral Med Oral Pathol* (1983) **55**:29–32.

Stockman JA, Iron deficiency anaemia: have we come far enough? *JAMA* (1987) **258**:1645–7.

Van Dis ML, Langlais RP, The thalassemias: oral manifestations and complications, *Oral Surg Oral Med Oral Pathol* (1986) **62**:229–33.

135 Hoffbrand AV, Pettit JE, Myeloproliferative disorders. In: *Essential Haematology*, 2nd edn (Blackwell Scientific Publications: Oxford, 1984) 182–93.

van Wingerden JJ, van Rensburg PG, Coetzee BP, Malignant fibrous histiocytoma of the parotid gland associated with polycythaemia, *Head Neck Surg* (1986) **8**:218–21.

136 Ficarra G, Miliani A, Adler-Storthz K et al, Recurrent oral condylomata acuminata and hairy leukoplakia: an early sign of myelodysplastic syndrome in an HIV-seronegative patient, *J Oral Pathol Med* (1991) **20**:398–402.

Flint SR, Sugerman P, Scully C et al, The myelodysplastic syndromes: case report and review, *Oral Surg Oral Med Oral Pathol* (1990) **70**:579–83.

Luker J, Scully C, Oakhill A, Gingival swelling as a manifestation of aplastic anaemia, *Oral Surg Oral Med Oral Pathol* (1991) **71**:55–6.

137 Hobson P, Dental care of children with haemophilia and related conditions, *Br Dent J* (1981) **151**:249–53.

Johnson RS, Diagnosis and treatment of von Willebrand's disease, *J Oral Maxillofac Surg* (1987) **45**:608–12.

Monsour PA, Kruger BJ, Harden RA, Prevalence and detection of patients with bleeding disorders, *Aust Dent J* (1986) **31**:104–10.

White GC, Lesesne HR, Hemophilia, hepatitis and acquired immunodeficiency, *Ann Intern Med* (1983) **98**:403–4.

Zakrzewska J, Gingival bleeding as a manifestation of von Willebrand's disease, *Br Dent J* (1983) **155**:157–60.

138 Barrett AP, Tvevsky J, Griffiths CJ, Thrombocytopenia induced by quinine, *Oral Surg Oral Med Oral Pathol* (1983) **55**:351–4.

Colvin BT, Thrombocytopenia, *Clin Haematol* (1985) **14**:661–81.

139 Baehni PC, Payot P, Tsai CC et al, Periodontal status associated with chronic neutropenia, *J Clin Periodontol* (1983) **10**:222–30.

Scully C, Gilmour C, Neutropenia and dental patients, *Br Dent J* (1986) **160**:43–6.

Scully C, Macfadyen E, Campbell A, Oral manifestations in cyclic neutropenia, *Br J Oral Surg* (1982) **20**:96–101.

140 Lubow RM, Cooley RL, Hartman KS et al, Plasma-cell gingivitis, *J Periodontol* (1984) **55**:235–41.

Macleod RI, Ellis JE, Plasma cell gingivitis related to the use of herbal toothpaste, *Br Dent J* (1989) **166**:375–6.

Scully C, Orofacial manifestations in chronic granulomatous disease of childhood, *Oral Surg Oral Med Oral Pathol* (1981) **51**:148–51.

Sollecito TP, Greenberg MS, Plasma cell gingivitis, *Oral Surg Oral Med Oral Pathol* (1992) **73**:690–3.

Timms MS, Sloan P, Association of supraglottic and gingival idiopathic plasmacytosis, *Oral Surg Oral Med Oral Pathol* (1991) **71**:451–3.

Timms MS, Sloan P, Pace Balzan A, Idiopathic plasmacytosis of the oral and supraglottic mucosa, *J Laryngol Otol* (1988) **102**:646–8.

White JW, Olsen KD, Banks PM, Plasma cell orofacial mucositis: report of a case and review of the literature, *Arch Dermatol* (1986) **122**:1321–4.

141 Barrett AP, Oral complications of bone marrow transplantation, *Aust NZ J Med* (1986) **16**:239–40.

Berkowitz RJ, Strandford S, Jones P et al, Stomatologic complications of bone marrow transplantation in a pediatric population, *Pediatr Dent* (1987) **9**:105–10.

Garfunkel AA, Tager N, Chausu S et al, Oral complications in bone marrow transplantation patients: recent advances, *Isr J Med Sci* (1994) **30**:120–4.

Locksley RM, Infection with varicella-zoster virus after marrow transplantation, *J Infect Dis* (1985) **152**:1172–81.

Seto BG, Oral mucositis in patients undergoing bone-marrow transplantation, *Oral Surg Oral Med Oral Pathol* (1985) **60**:493–7.

Chapter 6

144 Browning S, Hislop S, Scully C et al, The association between burning mouth syndrome and psychosocial disorders, *Oral Surg Oral Med Oral Pathol* (1987) **64**:171–4.

Feinmann C, Harris M, Psychogenic facial pain, *Br Dent J* (1984) **156**:165–9, 205–9.

Hunter S, The management of 'psychogenic' orofacial pain, *BMJ* (1992) **304**:329–30.

Maresky LS, van der Bijl P, Gird I, Burning mouth syndrome, *Oral Surg Oral Med Oral Pathol* (1993) **75**:303–7.

Remick RA, Blasberg B, Psychiatric aspects of atypical facial pain, *Can Dent Assoc J* (1985) **12**:913–16.

Rojo L, Silvestre J, Bagan JV et al, Psychiatric morbidity in burning mouth syndrome, *Oral Surg Oral Med Oral Pathol* (1993) **75**:308–11.

Scully C, La maladie du petit papier, *Br Dent J* (1993) **175**:289–92.

Scully C, Porter SR, Oral Medicine: 4. Orofacial pain, *Postgrad Dent* (1993) **3**:186–8.

Tourne LPM, Fricton JR, Burning mouth syndrome, *Oral Surg Oral Med Oral Pathol* (1992) **74**:158–67.

Wray D, Scully C, The sore mouth, *Medicine International* (1986) **2**:1134–8.

145 Cristobal MC, Aguilar A, Urbina F et al, Self-inflicted tongue ulcer: an unusual form of factitious disorder, *J Am Acad Dermatol* (1987) **17**:339–41.

Keith O, Flint S, Scully C, Lingual abscess in a patient with anorexia nervosa, *Br Dent J* (1989) **167**:71–2.

Lamey PL, McNab L, Lewis MAO et al, Orofacial artefactual disease, *Oral Surg Oral Med Oral Pathol* (1994) **77**:131–4.

Spigset O, Oral symptoms in bulimia nervosa, *Acta Odontol Scand* (1991) **49**:335–9.

Svirsky JA, Sawyer DR, Dermatitis artefacta of the paraoral region, *Oral Surg Oral Med Oral Pathol* (1987) **64**:259–63.

146 Fusco MA, Freedman PD, Black SM et al, Munchausen's syndrome: report of case, *J Am Dent Assoc* (1986) **112**:210–14.

Goss AN, Poly dental addiction, *Aust Dent J* (1986) **31**:421–3.

Michalowski R, Munchausen's syndrome: a new variety of bleeding type: self-inflicted cheilorrhagia glandularis, *Dermatologica* (1985) **170**:93–7.

Scully C, Eveson JW, Porter SR, Munchausen's syndrome: oral presentations, *Br Dent J* (1995) **178**:65–7.

Chapter 7

148   Barrett AP, Schifter M, Trigeminal neuralgia, *Aust Dent J* (1993) **38**:198–203.

Lazar ML, Greenlee RG, Naarden AL, Facial pain of neurologic origin mimicking oral pathologic conditions: some current concepts and treatment, *J Am Dent Assoc* (1980) **100**:884–8.

Loesser JD, Tic douloureux and atypical facial pain, *Can Dent Assoc J* (1985) **12**: 917–23.

Schnurr RF, Brooke RI, Atypical odontalgia, *Oral Surg Oral Med Oral Pathol* (1992) **73**:445–8.

Scully C, The mouth in general practice: 3: Oral and facial pain, *Dermatology in Practice* (1982) **1**:16–18.

Sweet WH, The treatment of trigeminal neuralgia (tic douloureux), *N Engl J Med* (1986) **315**:174–7.

Zakrzewska JM, Nally FF, Flint SR, Cryotherapy in the management of paroxysmal trigeminal neuralgia: four-year follow-up of 39 patients, *J Maxillofac Surg* (1986) **14**: 5–7.

149   Burt RK, Sharfman WH, Karp BI et al, Mental neuropathy (numb chin syndrome), *Cancer* (1992) **70**:877–81.

Flint S, Scully C, Isolated trigeminal sensory neuropathy: a heterogeneous group of disorders, *Oral Surg Oral Med Oral Pathol* (1990) **69**:153–6.

Lecky BRF, Hughes RAC, Murray NMF, Trigeminal sensory neuropathy, *Brain* (1987) **110**:1463–85.

Scully C, Orofacial manifestations of disease: 6: Neurological, psychiatric and muscular disorders, *Hospital Update* (1986) **6**:135–9.

Westerhof W, Bos JD, Trigeminal trophic syndrome: a successful treatment with transcutaneous electrical stimulation, *Br J Dermatol* (1983) **108**:601–4.

150   Cartwright RA, Boddy J, Barnard D et al, Association between Bell's palsy and lymphoid malignancies, *Leuk Res* (1985) **9**:31–3.

Glanvill P, Pether JVC, Lyme disease, *Br Med J* (1987) **294**:1226.

Hanner P, Badr G, Rosenhall U et al, Trigeminal dysfunction in patients with Bell's palsy, *Acta Otolaryngol (Stockh)* (1986) **101**:224–30.

Hattori T, Tokugawa K, Fukushige J et al, Facial palsy in Kawasaki disease, *Pediatrics* (1987) **146**:601–2.

Leading article, Bell's palsy, *Lancet* (1982) **i**:663.

Neiuwmeyer PA, Koch PAM, Visser SL et al, Bell's palsy: a polyneuropathy, *Clin Otolaryngol* (1982) **7**:293–8.

151   Ficarra G, Oral lesions of iatrogenic and undefined etiology and neurologic disorders associated with HIV infection, *Oral Surg Oral Med Oral Pathol* (1992) **73**:201–11.

Meienberg O, Muri R, Nuclear and infranuclear disorders, *Baillieres Clin Neurol* (1992) **1**:417–34.

Scully C, Cawson RA, Neurological disease. In: Scully C, Cawson RA, eds, *Medical Problems in Dentistry*, 3rd edn (Wright: Bristol, 1992)

Wortham E, Blumenthal H, Diplopia: a review of 48 cases of isolated ocular cranial neuropathy, *J Okla Stat Med Assoc* (1985) **78**:99–103.

152 Dhamoon SK, Iqbal S, Collins GH, Ipsilateral hemiplegia and the Wallenberg syndrome, *Arch Neurol* (1984) **41**:179–80.

Luker J, Scully C, The lateral medullary syndrome, *Oral Surg Oral Med Oral Pathol* (1990) **69**:322–4.

Marentette JL, Goding GS Jr, Levine SC, Rehabilitation of the lower cranial nerves, *Neurosurg Clin N Am* (1993) **4**:573–80.

Persson M, Osterberg T, Granerus AK et al, Influence of Parkinson's disease on oral health, *Acta Odontol Scand* (1992) **50**:37–42.

Chapter 8

154 Abraham-Inpijn L, Oral and otal manifestations as the primary symptoms in Wegener's granulomatosis, *J Head Neck Pathol* (1983) **2**:20–2.

Allen CM, Camisa C, Salewski C et al, Wegener's granulomatosis: report of three cases with oral lesions, *J Oral Maxillofac Surg* (1991) **49**:294–8.

Eufinger H, Machtens E, Akuamoa-Boateng E, Oral manifestations of Wegener's granulomatosis. Review of the literature and report of a case, *Int J Oral Maxillofac Surg* (1992) **21**:50–3.

Fauci AS, Haynes BF, Katz P et al, Wegener's granulomatosis: prospective clinical and therapeutic experience with 85 patients for 21 years, *Ann Intern Med* (1983) **98**:76–85.

Hansen LS, Silverman S, Pons VG et al, Limited Wegener's granulomatosis, *Oral Surg Oral Med Oral Pathol* (1985) **60**:524–31.

Israelson H, Binnie WH, Hurt WC, The hyperplastic gingivitis of Wegener's granulomatosis, *J Periodontol* (1981) **52**:81–7.

Lustmann J, Segal N, Markitziu A, Salivary gland involvement in Wegener's granulomatosis, *Oral Surg Oral Med Oral Pathol* (1994) **77**:254–9.

Lutcavage GJ, Schaberg SJ, Arendt DA et al, Gingival mass with massive soft tissue necrosis, *J Oral Maxillofac Surg* (1991) **49**:1332–8.

Parion E, Seymour RA, Macleod RK et al, Wegener's granulomatosis: a distinct gingival lesion, *J Clin Periodontol* (1992) **19**:64–6.

Patten SF, Tomecki KJ, Wegener's granulomatosis: cutaneous and oral mucosal disease, *J Am Acad Derm* (1993) **28**:710–18.

155 Flint SR, Keith O, Scully C, Hereditary haemorrhagic telangiectasia, *Oral Surg Oral Med Oral Pathol* (1988) **66**:440–4.

Peery WH, Clinical spectrum of hereditary haemorrhagic telangiectasia, *Am J Med* (1987) **82**:989–97.

156 Patterson A, Barnard N, Scully C et al, Necrosis of the tongue in a patient with intestinal infarction, *Oral Surg Oral Med Oral Pathol* (1992) **74**:582–6.

Scully C, Eveson JW, Barrett AW et al, Necrosis of the lip in giant cell arteritis, *J Oral Maxillofac Surg* (1993) **51**:581–3.

Chapter 9

158 Brook I, The clinical microbiology of Waldeyer's ring, *Otolaryngol Clin North Am* (1987) **20**:259–72.

Brook I, Walker RI, Possible role of anaerobic bacteria in the persistence of streptococcal tonsillar infection, *US Navy Med* (1981) **72**:26–9.

159 Gleeson M, Diagnosing maxillary sinusitis, *BMJ* (1992) **305**:662–3.

Umetsu DT, Ambrosino DM, Quinti I, Recurrent sinopulmonary infection and impaired antibody response to bacterial capsular polysaccharide antigen in children with selective IgG subclass deficiency, *N Engl L Med* (1985) **313**:1247–51.

Chapter 10

162   Alexander SA, Serino R, Ceen RF, Deciduous tooth anomalies and partial anodontia, *Oral Surg Oral Med Oral Pathol* (1985) **60**:230.

O'Dowling IB, McNamara TG, Congenital absence of permanent teeth among Irish school-children, *J Ir Dent Assoc* (1990) **36**:136–8.

Porter SR, Scully C, Diseases affecting the teeth, *Medicine International* (1990) **76**:3145–9.

Ruprecht A, Batniji S, el-Neweihi E, Incidence of oligodontia (hypodontia), *J Oral Med* (1986) **41**:43–6.

Tso MS, Crawford PJ, Miller J, Hypodontia, ectodermal dysplasia and sweat pore count, *Br Dent J* (1985) **158**:56–60.

163   Brook AH, A unifying aetiological explanation for anomalies of human tooth number and size, *Arch Oral Biol* (1984) **29**:373–8.

Guzman R, Elliott MA, Rossie KM, Odontodysplasia in a pediatric patient: literature review and case report, *Pediatric Dent* (1990) **12**:45–8.

Ruprecht A, Batniji S, el-Neweihi E, Incidence of supernumerary teeth, *Ann Dent* (1984) **43**:18–21.

Sabah E, Eden E, Unal T, Odontodysplasia: report of a case, *J Clin Pediatr Dent* (1992) **16**:115–18.

Scully C, Defects affecting the teeth, *Update* (1983) **26**:2203–8.

Scully C, Cawson RA, Common dental disorders, *Medicine International* (1986) **2**:1129–34.

Scully C, Porter SR, Oral Medicine: 1. Teeth and periodontium, *Postgrad Dent* (1992) **2**:93–100.

164   Amler NH, Gemination – anomalous tooth development, *Ann Dent* (1983) **42**:33–4.

Caliskan MK, Traumatic gemination – triple tooth. Survey of the literature and report of a case, *Endodontics & Dental Traumatology* (1992) **8**:130–3.

Chen RJ, Wang CC, Gemination of a maxillary premolar, *Oral Surg Oral Med Oral Pathol* (1990) **69**:656.

Gazit E, Lieberman MA, Macrodontia of maxillary central incisors: case reports, *Quintessence International* (1991) **22**:883–7.

Grover PS, Lorton L, Gemination and twinning in the permanent dentition, *Oral Surg Oral Med Oral Pathol* (1985) **59**:313–18.

Kohavi D, Shapira J, Tissue regeneration principles applied to separation of fused teeth, *J Clin Periodontol* (1990) **17**:623–9.

Smith GA, Double teeth, *Br Dent J* (1980) **148**:163–4.

165   Consolo U, Massignan C, Salgarelli A et al, Dens invaginatus. Review of the literature and presentation of two clinical cases, *Stomatologia Mediterranea* (1990) **10**:269–76.

Davis PJ, Brook AH, Presentation of talon cusp, diagnosis, clinical features, associations and possible aetiology, *Br Dent J* (1986) **160**:84–8.

Hill FJ, Dens evaginatus and its management, *Br Dent J* (1984) **156**:400–2.

Ju Y, Dens evaginatus – a difficult diagnostic problem?, *J Clin Pediatr Dent* (1991) **15**:247–8.

Kieser JA, van der Merwe CA, Classificatory reliability of the Carabelli trait in man, *Arch Oral Biol* (1984) **29**:795–801.

Loh HS, Lim SS, Facial infection arising from dens evaginatus, *Br Dent J* (1985) **158**:367–8.

Ruprecht A, Batniji S, Sastry KA, el-Neweihi E, The incidence of dental invagination, *J Pedodont* (1986) **10**:265–72.

Su HL, Dens evaginatus: report of case of continued root development after Ca(OH)$_2$ apexification, *ASDC J Dent Child* (1992) **59**:285–8.

Wong MT, Augsburger RA, Management of dens evaginatus, *General Dentistry* (1992) **40**:300–3.

166 Crawford PJM, Evans RD, Aldred MJ, Amelogenesis imperfecta: autosomal dominant hypomaturation–hypoplasia type with taurodontism, *Br Dent J* (1988) **164**:71–3.

Elzay RP, Chamberlain DH, Differential diagnosis of enlarged dental pulp chambers: a case report of amelogenesis imperfecta with taurodontism, *ASDC J Dent Child* (1986) **53**:388–90.

Jaspers MT, Witkop CJ, Taurodontism: an isolated trait associated with syndromes and X-chromosomal aneuploidy, *Am J Hum Genet* (1980) **32**:396–413.

167 American Dental Association Council on Dental Therapeutics, *Fluoride Compounds: Accepted Dental Therapeutics*, 39th edn (1982) 344–68.

Moller IJ, Fluorides and dental fluorosis, *Int Dent J* (1982) **32**:135–7.

Murray JJ, Rugg-Gunn AJ, *Fluorides in Caries Prevention*, 2nd edn (Wright: Bristol, 1982), 207–17.

Pindborg JJ, Aetiology of development of enamel defects not related to fluorosis *Int Dent J* (1982) **32**:122–34.

168 Davies PH, Lewis DH, Dilaceration: a surgical/orthodontic solution, *Br Dent J* (1984) **156**:16–18.

Goodman AH, Armelagos GJ, The chronological distribution of enamel hypoplasia in human permanent incisor and canine teeth, *Arch Oral Biol* (1985) **30**:503–7.

Lowe PL, Dilaceration caused by a direct penetrating injury, *Br Dent J* (1985) **159**:373–4.

Sarnat H, Moss SJ, Diagnosis of enamel defects, *NY State Dent J* (1985) **51**:103–4.

Seow WK, Enamel hypoplasia in the primary dentition: a review, *ASDC J Dent Child* (1991) **58**:441–52.

169 Aldred MJ, Crawford PJM, Rowe W et al, Scanning electron microscopic study of primary teeth in X-linked amelogenesis imperfecta, *J Oral Pathol Med* (1992) **21**:186–92.

Crawford PJM, Aldred MJ, X-linked amelogenesis imperfecta, *Oral Surg* (1992) **73**:449–55.

De Sort KD, Amelogenesis imperfecta: the genetics, classification and treatment, *J Prosthet Dent* (1983) **49**:786–92.

Sundell S, Valentin J, Hereditary aspects and classification of hereditary amelogenesis imperfecta, *Community Dent Oral Epidemiol* (1986) **14**:211–16.

338

170 Escobar VH, Goldblatt LI, Bixler D, A clinical, genetic and ultrastructural study of 'snow-capped teeth': amelogenesis imperfecta hypomaturation type, *Oral Surg Oral Med Oral Pathol* (1981) **52**:607–12.

Kerebel B, Daculsi G, Ultrastructural study of amelogenesis imperfecta, *Calcif Tissue Res* (1977) **24**:191–7.

Wright JT, Analysis of kindred with amelogenesis imperfecta, *J Oral Pathol* (1985) **14**:366–74.

171 Gage JP, Dentinogenesis imperfecta: a new perspective, *Aust Dent J* (1985) **30**:285–90.

Lukinmaa PL, Ranta H, Ranta K et al, Dental findings in osteogenesis imperfecta, *J Craniofac Genet Dev Biol* (1987) **7**:115–25.

Nicholls AC, Pope FM, Heterogeneity of osteogenesis imperfecta congenita, *Lancet* (1980) **i**:820–1.

Smith R, Francis MJO, Houghton GR, *The Brittle Bone Syndrome: Osteogenesis Imperfecta* (Butterworths: London, 1983) 41–68.

Sunderland EP, Smith CJ, The teeth in osteogenesis and dentinogenesis imperfecta, *Br Dent J* (1980) **149**:287–9.

172 Alvarez MP, Crespi PV, Shanske AL, Natal molars in Pfeiffer syndrome type 3: a case report, *J Clin Pediatr Dent* (1993) **18**:21–4.

Chow MH, Natal and neonatal teeth, *J Am Dent Assoc* (1980) **100**:215–16.

Dick HM, Honore LH, Dental structures in benign ovarian cystic teratomas (dermoid cysts), *Oral Surg Oral Med Oral Pathol* (1985) **60**:299–307.

Leung AKC, Natal teeth, *Am J Dis Child* (1986) **140**:249–51.

Sciubba JJ, Younai F, Epipalatus: a rare intraoral teratoma, *Oral Surg Oral Med Oral Pathol* (1991) **71**:476–81.

173 Kurol J, Infraocclusion of primary molars: an epidemiological and familial study, *Community Dent Oral Epidem* (1981) **9**:94–102.

Peterson LJ, Rationale for removing impacted teeth: when to extract or not to extract, *J Am Dent Assoc* (1992) **123**:198–204.

Rosenthal P, Ramos A, Mungo R, Management of children with hyper-bilirubinemia and green teeth, *J Pediatr* (1986) **108**:103–5.

174 Davies AK, Cundall RB, Dandiker Y et al, Photo-oxidation of tetracycline absorbed on hydroxyapatite in relation to the light-induced staining of teeth, *J Dent Res* (1985) **64**:936–9.

Peterson CK, Tetracycline effects on teeth preclude use in children and pregnant or lactating women, *Postgrad Med* (1984) **76**:24–34.

Scopp IW, Kazandjian G, Tetracycline-induced staining of teeth, *Postgrad Med* (1986) **79**:202–3.

175 Arends J, Christoffersen J, The nature of the early caries lesion in enamel, *J Dent Res* (1986) **65**:2–11.

Holloway PJ, The role of sugar in the aetiology of dental caries, *J Dent* (1983) **11**:189–213.

Scully C, Dental caries: progress in microbiology and immunology, *J Infect* (1981) **3**:107–33.

Winter GB, Problems involved with the use of comforters, *Int Dent J* (1980) **30**:28.

176 Asher C, Read MJF, Early enamel erosion in children associated with excessive consumption of citric acid, *Br Dent J* (1987) **162**:384–7.

Dahl BL, Carlsson GE, Ekfeldt A, Occlusal wear of teeth and restorative materials. A review of classification, etiology, mechanisms of wear, and some aspects of restorative procedures, *Acta Odontol Scand* (1993) **51**:299–311.

'In the News': Swimming pool tooth erosion – hazard detected in US, *Can Dent Assoc J* (1983) **49**:744–5.

Konig KG, Root lesions, *Int Dent J* (1990) **40**:283–8.

Milosevic A, Tooth wear: an aetiological and diagnostic problem, *Eur J Prosthodont Res Dent* (1993) **1**:173–8.

Nunn JH, Durning P, Fragile X (Martin Bell) syndrome and dental care, *Br Dent J* (1990) **168**:160–2.

Peak J, Eveson J, Scully C, Oral manifestations of Rett's syndrome, *Br Dent J* (1992) **172**:248–9.

Russell MD, The relationship of occlusal wear to occlusal contact area, *J Oral Rehabil* (1983) **10**:383–91.

Smith BG, Knight JK, A comparison of patterns of toothwear and aetiological factors, *Br Dent J* (1984) **157**:16–19.

Van Reenen JF, Briedenhahn SJ, Tooth-mutilating practices amongst the Damara of SW Africa (Namibia), *Tydskr Tandheelkd Ver S Afr* (1985) **40**:537–9.

Whittaker DK, Mutilated teeth, *Dental Update* (1984) **11**:555–62.

177 Fairburn CG, Cooper PJ, The clinical features of bulimia nervosa, *Br J Psychiatry* (1984) **144**:238–46.

Feiglin B, Root resorption, *Aust Dent J* (1986) **31**:12–22.

Spigset O, Oral symptoms in bulimia nervosa. A survey of 34 cases, *Acta Odontol Scand* (1991) **49**:335–9.

Taylor VE, Sneddon J, Bilateral facial swelling in bulimia, *Br Dent J* (1987) **163**:115–17.

178 Andersson L, Blomlof L, Lindskog S, Tooth ankylosis: clinical, radiographic and histological assessment, *Int J Oral Surg* (1984) **13**:423–31.

Leider AS, Garbarino VE, Generalized hypercementosis, *Oral Surg Oral Med Oral Pathol* (1987) **63**:375–80.

179 Gill Y, Scully C, Orofacial odontogenic infections: review of microbiology and current treatment, *Oral Surg Oral Med Oral Pathol* (1990) **70**:155–8.

Kannangara DW, Thadepalli H, McQuirter JL, Bacteriology and treatment of dental infections, *Oral Surg Oral Med Oral Pathol* (1980) **50**:103–9.

Newman MG, Anaerobic oral and dental infection, *Rev Infect Dis* (1984) **1** (Suppl): 5107–14.

Williams BL, McCann GF, Schoenknecht FD, Bacteriology of dental abscesses of endodontic origin, *J Clin Microbiol* (1983) **18**:770–4.

180 Garulnick W, Odontogenic infections, *Br Dent J* (1984) **156**:440–7.

Haidar Z, Facial sinuses: cases of mistaken identity, *Ann Dent* (1985) **44**:9–11.

Lewis MAO, MacFarlane TW, McGowan DA, A microbiological and clinical review of the acute dentoalveolar abscess, *Br J Oral Maxillofac Surg* (1990) **28**:359–66.

181 Shear M, *Cysts of the Oral Regions*, 2nd edn (Wright: Bristol, 1983) 114–41.

340

Wood NK, Periapical lesions, *Dent Clin North Am* (1984) **28**:725–66.

182 Lindhe JH, *Textbook of Clinical Periodontology* (Munksgaard: Copenhagen, 1985) Chapters 3 and 4.

Page RC, Gingivitis, *J Clin Periodontol* (1986) **13**:345–59.

Scully C, Porter SR, Disorders of the gums and periodontium, *Medicine International* (1990) **76**:3150–3.

183 Nisengard RJ, Nieders M, Desquamative lesions of the gingiva, *J Periodontol* (1981) **52**:500–10.

Steelman R, Self-injurious behaviour: report of a case and follow-up, *J Oral Med* (1986) **41**:108–11.

Watson PJ, Gingival recession, *J Dent* (1984) **12**:29–35.

184 Ahl DR, Hilgeman JL, Periodontal emergencies, *Dent Clin North Am* (1986) **30**:459–72.

Nitzan DW, Tal O, Sela MN et al, Pericoronitis: a reappraisal of its clinical and microbiological aspects, *J Oral Maxillofac Surg* (1985) **43**:510–16.

Smith RG, Davies RM, Acute lateral periodontal abscesses, *Br Dent J* (1986) **161**:176–8.

185 Davies RM, Smith RG, Porter SR, Destructive forms of periodontal disease in adolescents and young adults, *Br Dent J* (1985) **158**:429–35.

Gillet R, Johnson NW, Bacterial invasion of the periodontium in a case of juvenile periodontitis, *J Clin Periodontol* (1982) **9**:93–100.

Page RC, Altman LC, Ebersole JL et al, Rapidly progressive periodontitis: a distinct clinical condition, *J Periodontol* (1983) **54**:197–209.

Socransky SS, Haffajee AD, Goodson JM et al, New concepts of destructive periodontal disease, *J Clin Periodontol* (1984) **11**:21–32.

Tonetti MS, Etiology and pathogenesis. In: Lang NP, Karring T, eds, *Proceedings of the 1st European Workshop on Periodontology* (Quintessence Books: London, 1994) 54–89.

Watanabe K, Prepubertal periodontitis: a review of diagnostic criteria, pathogenesis, and differential diagnosis, *J Periodontal Res* (1990) **25**:31–48.

186 Efeoglu J, Porter SR, Mutlu S et al, Papillon–Lefèvre syndrome affecting two siblings, *Br J Paediatric Dent* (1990) **6**:115–20.

Puliyel JM, Iyer KSS, A syndrome of keratosis palmo-plantaris congenita, pes planus, onychogryphosis, periodontosis, arachnodactyly and a peculiar acro-osteolysis, *Br J Dermatol* (1986) **115**:243–8.

Sloan P, Soames JV, Murray JJ et al, Histopathological and ultrastructural findings in a case of Papillon–Lefèvre syndrome, *J Periodontol* (1984) **55**:482–5.

Tinanoff N, Tanzer JM, Kornman KS et al, Treatment of the periodontal component of the Papillon–Lefèvre syndrome, *J Clin Periodontol* (1986) **13**:6–10.

187 Addy M, Moran J, Griffiths A et al, Extrinsic tooth discoloration by metals and chlorhexidine: I. Surface protein denaturation of dietary precipitation, *Br Dent J* (1985) **159**:281–5.

Eriksen HM, Kantanen H, Nordbo H et al, Characterisation of salivary proteins from stainers and non-stainers adsorbed to hydroxyapatite, *Acta Odontol Scand* (1985) **43**:115–20.

188 Addy M, Moran J, Extrinsic tooth discoloration by metals and chlorhexidine: II. Clinical staining produced by chlorhexidine, iron and tea, *Br Dent J* (1985) **159**:331–4.

Driessens FC, Borggreven JM, Verbeeck R et al, On the physiochemistry of plaque calcification and the phase composition of dental calculus, *J Periodont Res* (1985) **20**:329–36.

Lockhart PB, Gingival pigmentation as the sole presenting sign of chronic lead poisoning in a mentally-retarded adult, *Oral Surg Oral Med Oral Pathol* (1981) **52**:143–9.

Mandel ID, Calculus revisited: a review, *J Clin Periodontol* (1986) **13**:249–57.

189 Bakaeen G, Scully C, Hereditary gingival fibromatosis in a family with Zimmermann–Laband syndrome, *J Oral Pathol Med* (1991) **20**:457–9.

'Emphasis', Plaque: current approaches to prevention and control, *J Am Dent Assoc* (1984) **109**:690–702.

Gould AR, Escobar VH, Symmetrical gingival fibromatosis, *Oral Surg Oral Med Oral Pathol* (1981) **51**:62–7.

Newman MG, Current concepts on the pathogenesis of periodontal disease: microbiology emphasis, *J Periodontol* (1985) **56**:734–9.

Porter SR, Scully C, Periodontal aspects of systemic disease: classification. In: Lang NP, Karring T, eds, *Proceedings of the 1st European Workshop on Periodontology* (Quintessence Books: London, 1994) 375–414.

Takagi M, Yamamoto H, Mega H et al, Heterogeneity in the gingival fibromatoses, *Cancer* (1991) **68**:2202–12.

190 Moskow BS, Bloom A, Embryogenesis of the gingival cyst, *J Clin Periodontol* (1983) **10**:119–39.

Wysocki GP, Brannon RB, Gardner DG et al, Histogenesis of the lateral periodontal cyst and the gingival cyst of the adult, *Oral Surg Oral Med Oral Pathol* (1980) **48**:327–9.

191 Lee KW, The fibrous epulis and related lesions, *Periodontics* (1986) **6**:277–99.

Macleod RI, Soames JW, Epulides: a clinicopathological study of a series of 200 consecutive lesions, *Br Dent J* (1987) **163**:51–3.

Needleman IG, Salah MW, Metastatic breast carcinoma presenting with multiple gingival epulides, *Br Dent J* (1992) **172**:448–50.

Porter SR, Scully C, Periodontal aspects of systemic disease: classification. In: Lang NP, Karring T, eds, *Proceedings of the 1st European Workshop on Periodontology* (Quintessence Books, London 1994) 375–414.

192 Henderson D, Poswillo D, *A Colour Atlas and Textbook of Orthognathic Surgery: the Surgery of Facial Skeletal Deformity* (Wolfe Medical Publications Ltd: London, 1985).

Profitt WR, On the aetiology of malocclusion: the North Croft Lecture 1985, *Br J Orthod* (1986) **13**:1–12.

193 Kribbs PJ, Chesnut CH 3d, Osteoporosis and dental osteopenia in the elderly, *Gerodontology* (1984) **3**:101–6.

Larsson E, The prevalence and aetiology of prolonged dummy- and finger-sucking habits, *Eur J Orthod* (1985) **7**:172–6.

342

Luke LS, The effects of thumb-sucking on oro-facial structures and speech: a review, *Compend Contin Educ Dent* (1983) **4**:575–9.

194 Shear M, *Cysts of the Oral Regions*, 2nd edn (J Wright: Bristol, 1983).

Shear M, The odontogenic keratocyst: recent advances, *Dtsch Zahnartztl Z* (1985) **40**:510–13.

195 Angelopoulou E, Angelopoulos AP, Lateral periodontal cyst: review of the literature and report of a case, *J Periodontol* (1990) **61**:126–31.

Lindh C, Larsson A, Unusual joint–bone cysts, *J Oral Maxillofac Surg* (1990) **48**:258–63.

Shear M, Cysts of the jaws: recent advances, *J Oral Pathol* (1985) **14**:43–59.

Wysocki GP, The differential diagnosis of globulomaxillary radiolucencies, *Oral Surg Oral Med Oral Pathol* (1981) **51**:281–6.

196 Greval RS, Sofat JR, Nasopalatine cyst: a case report, *J Indian Dent Assoc* (1985) **57**:143–6.

197 Adekeye EO, Cornah J, Osteomyelitis of the jaws: a review of 141 cases, *Br J Maxillofac Surg* (1985) **23**:24–35.

Jacobsson S, Diffuse sclerosing osteomyelitis of the mandible, *Int J Oral Surg* (1984) **13**:363–85.

Shroyer JV, Lew D, Abreo F et al, Osteomyelitis of the mandible as a result of sickle cell disease: report and literature review, *Oral Surg Oral Med Oral Pathol* (1991) **72**:25–8.

198 Carlson ER, The radiobiology, treatment and prevention of osteoradionecrosis of the mandible, *Recent Results Cancer Res* (1994) **134**:191–9.

Coffin F, The incidence and management of osteoradionecrosis of the jaws following head and neck radiotherapy, *Br J Radiol* (1983) **56**:851–7.

Daramola JO, Ajagbe HA, Chronic osteomyelitis of the mandible in adults, *Br J Oral Surg* (1982) **20**:58–62.

Epstein J, Osteoradionecrosis: clinical experience and proposal for classification, *J Oral Maxillofac Surg* (1987) **45**:104–10.

Marciani RO, Ownby HE, Osteoradionecrosis of the jaws, *J Oral Maxillofac Surg* (1986) **44**:218–23.

Murray CG, Daley TE, Zimmerman SO, The relationship between dental disease and radiation necrosis of the mandible, *Oral Surg Oral Med Oral Pathol* (1980) **49**:99–104.

Pyykonen H, Malmstrom M, Oikarinen VS et al, The effects of radiation treatment of tongue and floor of mouth cancer on the dentition, saliva secretion, mucous membranes and lower jaw, *Int J Oral Maxillofac Surg* (1986) **15**:401–9.

Sanger JR, Matloub HS, Yousif NJ et al, Management of osteoradionecrosis of the mandible, *Clin Plast Surg* (1993) **20**:517–30.

199 Field EA, Speechley JA, Rotter E et al, Dry socket incidence compared after 12-year interval, *Br J Oral Maxillofac Surg* (1985) **23**:419–27.

Turner PS, A clinical study of 'dry socket', *Int J Oral Surg* (1982) **11**:226–31.

200 Eggen S, Natvig B, Relationship between torus mandibularis and number of present teeth, *Scand J Dent Res* (1986) **94**:233–40.

Jones K, Korzcak P, The diagnostic significance and management of Gardner's syndrome, *Br J Oral Maxillofac Surg* (1990) **28**:80–4.

Lello GE, Makek M, Stafne's mandibular lingual cortical defect: discussion of aetiology, *J Maxillofac Surg* (1985) **13**:172–6.

Rezai RF, Torus palatinus, an exostosis of unknown aetiology: review of the literature, *Compend Contin Educ Dent* (1985) **6**:149–52.

Sondergaard JO, Bulow S, Jarvinen H et al, Dental anomalies in familial adenomatous polyposis coli, *Acta Odont Scand* (1987) **45**:61–3.

Sondergaard J O, Rasmussen MS, Videbaek H et al, Mandibular osteomas in sporadic colorectal carcinoma, *Scand J Gastroenterol* (1993) **28**:23–4.

Traboulsi EI, Krush AJ, Gardner EJ et al, Prevalence and importance of pigmented ocular fundus lesions in Gardner's syndrome, *N Eng J Med* (1987) **316**:661–7.

Wolf J, Jarvinen HJ, Hietanen J, Gardner's dento-maxillary stigmas in patients with familial adenomatosis coli, *Br J Oral Maxillofac Surg* (1986) **24**:410–16.

201 Avery BS, A sialocoele and unusual parotid fistula: case report, *Br J Oral Surg* (1980) **18**:40–4.

Brook I, Diagnosis and management of parotitis, *Arch Otolaryngol Head Neck Surg* (1992) **118**:469–71.

Galili B, Marmary Y, Juvenile recurrent parotitis: clinicoradiologic follow-up study and the beneficial effect of sialography, *Oral Surg Oral Med Oral Pathol* (1986) **61**:550–6.

Pfaltz CR, Chilla R, Sialadenosis and sialadenitis: pathophysiological and diagnostic aspects, *Adv Otorhinolaryngol* (1981) **26**:1–249.

Pruett TL, Simmons RL, Nosocomial Gram-negative bacillary parotitis, *JAMA* (1984) **251**:252–3.

Seifert G, Miehlke A, Haubrich J et al, *Diseases of the Salivary Glands: Pathology, Diagnosis, Treatment, Facial Nerve Surgery* (Thieme: Stuttgart, New York, 1986) 78-84.

Zhao-ju Z, Song-ling W, Jia-rui Z et al, Chronic obstructive parotitis, *Oral Surg Oral Med Oral Pathol* (1992) **73**:434-40.

202 Blair SW, Wood GD, Obstructive sialadenitis, *Int J Oral Surg* (1980) **9**:63–7.

Isacsson G, Persson NE, The gigantiform salivary calculus, *Int J Oral Surg* (1982) **11**:135–9.

Kabakkaya Y, Dogan M, Yigitoglu MR et al, Bilateral parotid duct fistula, *Ann Otol Rhinol Laryngol* (1993) **102**:375–7.

Seifert G, Miehlke A, Haubrich J et al, *Diseases of the Salivary Glands: Pathology, Diagnosis, Treatment, Facial Nerve Surgery* (Thieme: Stuttgart, New York, 1986) 85–90.

Yamane GM, Scharlock SE, Jain R et al, Intra-oral minor salivary gland sialolithiasis, *J Oral Med* (1984) **39**:85–90.

Zachariades N, Bilateral recurrent submandibular obstructive sialadenitis, *J Oral Med* (1985) **40**:86–103.

203 Epstein JB, Scully C, The role of saliva in oral health and the causes and effects of xerostomia, *J Can Dent Assoc* (1992) **58**:217–21.

Epstein JB, Stevenson-Moore P, Scully C, Management of xerostomia, *J Can Dent Assoc* (1992) **58**:140–3.

344

McClatchey KD, Appleblatt NH, Zarbo RJ et al, Plunging ranula, *Oral Surg Oral Med Oral Pathol* (1984) **57**:408–12.

Lamey PJ, Scully C, Diseases of the salivary glands, *Medicine International* (1990) **76**:3167–9.

Navazesh M, Ship II, Xerostomia: diagnosis and treatment, *Am J Otolaryngol* (1983) **4**:283–92.

Scully C, Porter SR, Oral Medicine: 3. Salivary disorders, *Postgrad Dent* (1993) **3**:150–3.

204 Brannon RB, Fowler CB, Hartman KS, Necrotizing sialometaplasia. A clinicopathologic study of sixty-nine cases and review of the literature, *Oral Surg Oral Med Oral Pathol* (1991) **72**:317–25.

Chilla R, Sialadenosis of the salivary glands of the head, *Adv Otorhinolaryngol* (1981) **26**:1–38.

Grillon GL, Lally ET, Necrotising sialometaplasia: literature review and presentation of five cases, *J Oral Surg* (1981) **39**:747–53.

Mesa ML, Gertler RS, Schneider LC, Necrotising sialometaplasia: frequency of histologic misdiagnosis, *Oral Surg Oral Med Oral Pathol* (1984) **57**:71–3.

Scully C, Eveson JW, Richards A, Adenomatoid hyperplasia in the palate: another sheep in wolf's clothing, *Br Dent J* (1992) **173**:141–2.

205 Hay KD, Reade PC, The use of an elimination diet in the treatment of recurrent aphthous ulceration of the oral cavity, *Oral Surg Oral Med Oral Pathol* (1984) **57**:504–7.

Porter SR, Scully C, Flint SR, Haematological status in recurrent aphthous stomatitis compared with other oral disease, *Oral Surg Oral Med Oral Pathol* (1988) **66**:41–4.

Scully C, Porter SR, Diseases of the oral mucosa, *Medicine International* (1990) **76**:3154–62.

Scully C, Porter SR, Oral Medicine: 2. Disorders affecting the oral mucosa (part 1), *Postgrad Dent* (1992) **2**:109–13.

Scully C, Porter SR, The mouth: 1. Skin diseases that can affect the mouth, *Dermatology in Practice* (1993) **1**:14–18.

Scully C, Porter SR, Oral medicine. 2. Disorders affecting the oral mucosa (part 2), *Postgrad Dent* (1993) **3**:142–7.

Scully C, Porter SR, The mouth 2: Signs and symptoms of oral disease, *Dermatology in Practice* (1994) **2**:14–17.

Vincent SD, Lilly GE, Clinical, historic, and therapeutic features of aphthous stomatitis. Literature review and open clinical trial employing steroids, *Oral Surg Oral Med Oral Pathol* (1992) **74**:79–86.

206 Grattan CEH, Scully C, Oral ulceration: a diagnostic problem, *Br Med J* (1986) **292**:1093–4.

Marshall GS, Edwards KM, Butler J et al, Syndrome of periodic fever, pharyngitis and aphthous stomatitis, *J Pediatr* (1987) **110**:43–6.

Rennie JS, Reade PC, Hay KD et al, Recurrent aphthous stomatitis, *Br Dent J* (1985) **159**:361–7.

Scully C, Matthews R, Mouth ulcers, *Update* (1983) **26**:693–780.

Scully C, Porter SR, Recurrent aphthous stomatitis: current concepts of etiology, pathogenesis and management, *J Oral Pathol Med* (1989) **18**:21–7.

207 Barnes CG, Behçet's syndrome, *J R Soc Med* (1984) **77**:816–18.

Cervera R, Navarro M, López-Soto A et al, Antibodies to endothelial cells in Behçet's disease: cell binding activity heterogeneity and association with clinical activity, *Ann Rheum Dis* (1994) **53**:265–7.

Hamza M, Orogenital ulcerations in mixed connective tissue disease, *J Rheumatol* (1985) **12**:643–4.

Masuda K, Urayama A, Kogure M et al, Double-masked trial of cyclosporin versus colchicine and long-term open study of cyclosporin in Behçet's disease, *Lancet* (1989) **1**:1093–6.

Wechsler B, Piette JC, Behçet's disease. Retains most of its mysteries, *BMJ* (1992) **304** (Edit):1199–200.

208 Firestein GS, Gruber HE, Weisman MH, Mouth and genital ulcers with inflamed cartilage: MAGIC syndrome, *Am J Med* (1985) **79**:65–72.

Jorizzo JL, Behçet's syndrome, *Arch Dermatol* (1986) **122**:556–8.

209 Symons AL, Rowe PV, Romanink K, Dental aspects of child abuse: review and case reports, *Aust Dent J* (1987) **32**:42–7.

Van Wyk CW, An oral lesion caused by fellatio, *Am J Forensic Med Pathol* (1981) **2**:217–19.

210 Behrman RE, Vaughan VC, *Nelson's Textbook of Paediatrics*, 12th edn (W B Saunders: Philadelphia, London, Toronto, 1983).

Chaudhry AP, Yamane GM, Sharlock SE et al, A clinicopathological study of intraoral lymphoepithelial cysts, *J Oral Med* (1984) **39**:79–84.

Harari MD, Clezy JKA, Sharp E, Glossal cysts in four infants, *Arch Dis Child* (1987) **62**:1173–4.

Jorgensen RJ, Shapira SD, Salinas CF et al, Intra-oral findings and anomalies in neonates, *Pediatrics* (1982) **69**:557–82.

211 Crotty CP, Factitious lip crusting, *Arch Dermatol* (1981) **117**:338–40.

Evans CD, Staphylococcal infection in median fissure of the lower lip, *Clin Exp Dermatol* (1986) **11**:289–91.

Reade PC, Sim R, Exfoliative cheilitis – a factitious disorder? *Int J Oral Maxillofac Surg* (1986) **15**:313–17.

Rosenquist B, Median lip fissure: etiology and suggested treatment, *Oral Surg Oral Med Oral Pathol* (1991) **72**:10–14.

Winchester L, Scully C, Prime SS et al, Cheilitis glandularis: a case affecting the upper lip, *Oral Surg Oral Med Oral Pathol* (1986) **62**:654–7.

212 Axell T, Holmstrup P, Kramer IRH et al, International seminar on oral leukoplakia and associated lesions related to tobacco habits, *Community Dent Oral Epidemiol* (1984) **12**:145–54.

Daley TD, Common acanthotic and keratotic lesions of the oral mucosa: a review, *J Can Dent Assoc* (1990) **56**:407–9.

Hansen LS, Olson JA, Silverman S, Proliferative verrucous leukoplakia, *Oral Surg Oral Med Oral Pathol* (1985) **60**:285–98.

McGuirt WF, Snuff-dippers carcinoma, *Arch Otolaryngol* (1983) **109**:757–60.

Shklar G, Oral leukoplakia, *N Engl J Med* (1986) **315**:1544–5.

213 Eveson JW, Oral premalignancy, *Cancer Surv* (1983) **2**:403–24.

Shibuya H, Amagasa T, Seto KI et al, Leukoplakia-associated multiple carcinomas in patients with tongue carcinoma, *Cancer* (1986) **57**:843–6.

Silverman S, Gorsky M, Lozado F, Oral leukoplakia and malignant transformation: a follow-up study of 257 patients, *Cancer* (1984) **53**:563–8.

214 Amagasa T, Yokoo E, Sato K et al, A study of the clinical characteristics and treatment of carcinoma in situ, *Oral Surg Oral Med Oral Pathol* (1985) **60**:50–5.

Lind PO, Malignant transformation in oral leukoplakia, *Scand J Dent Res* (1987) **95**:449–55.

215 Axell T, Henricsson V, Leukoedema – an epidemiologic study with special reference to the influence of tobacco habits, *Community Dent Oral Epidemiol* (1981) **9**:142–6.

Brooks JK, Balciunas BA, Geographic stomatitis: review of the literature and report of five cases, *J Am Dent Assoc* (1987) **115**:421–4.

Caniff JP, Mucosal diseases of uncertain etiology: III. Oral submucous fibrosis. In: Mackenzie IC, Squier CA, Dabelsteen E, eds, *Oral Mucosal Diseases: Biology, Etiology and Therapy* (Laegeforeningens Forlag: Copenhagen, 1987) 87–91.

Duncan SC, Su WPD, Leukoedema of the oral mucosa (possibly an acquired white sponge naevus), *Arch Dermatol* (1980) **116**:906–8.

Luker J, Scully C, Erythema migrans affecting the palate, *Br Dent J* (1983) **155**:385.

Pindborg JJ, Murti PR, Bhousle RB et al, Oral submucous fibrosis as a precancerous condition, *Scand J Dent Res* (1984) **92**:224–9.

Van Wyk CW, Ambrosio SC, Leukoedema: ultrastructural and histochemical observations, *J Oral Pathol* (1983) **12**:29–35.

216 Hudgins LJ, Inflammatory papillary hyperplasia: evaluation of two treatment modalities, *Ont Dent* (1986) **63**:11–16.

Westcott WB, Correll RW, Multiple papillary projections on the alveolar mucosa and palate, *J Am Dent Assoc* (1984) **108**:91–2.

217 Gilmour AG, Craven CM, Chustecki AM, Self-mutilation under combined inferior dental block and solvent intoxication, *Br Dent J* (1984) **156**:438–9.

La Blanc J, Epker BN, Lesch–Nyhan syndrome: surgical treatment of a case with lip-chewing, *J Maxillofac Surg* (1981) **9**:64–7.

218 El-Mofty SK, Swanson PE, Wick MR et al, Eosinophilic ulcer of the oral mucosa, *Oral Surg Oral Med Oral Pathol* (1993) **75**:716–22.

Renshaw AA, Rosai J, Benign atypical vascular lesions of the lip, *Am J Surg Pathol* (1993) **17**:557–65.

Sklavounou A, Laskaris G, Eosinophilic ulcer of the oral mucosa, *Oral Surg Oral Med Oral Pathol* (1984) **58**:431–6.

Wright JM, Rankin KV, Wilson JW, Traumatic granuloma of the tongue, *Head Neck Surg* (1983) **5**:363–6.

219 Dummett CO, Overview of normal oral pigmentation, *J Indiana Dent Assoc* (1980) **50**:13–18.

Dummett CO, Pertinent considerations in oral pigmentation, *Br Dent J* (1984) **158**:9–12.

Ho KKL, Dervan P, O'Loughlin S et al, Labial melanotic macule: a clinical histopathologic, and ultrastructural study, *J Am Acad Dermatol* (1993) **28**:33–9.

Kaugars GE, Heise AP, Riley WT et al, Oral melanotic macules. A review of 353 cases, *Oral Surg Oral Med Oral Pathol* (1993) **76**:59–61.

220 Axell T, Hedin A, Epidemiologic study of excessive oral melanin pigmentation with special reference to the influence of tobacco habits, *Scand J Dent Rev* (1982) **90**:434–42.

Brown FH, Houston GD, Smoker's melanosis. A case report, *J Periodontol* (1991) **62**:524–7.

Schawaf M, Gingival tattoo: an unusual gingival pigmentation – report of four cases, *J Oral Med* (1986) **41**:130–3.

221 Luker J, A case of lingual abscess, *Br Dent J* (1985) **159**:300.

Roberge RJ, Seizure-related oral lacerations: incidence and distribution, *J Am Dent Assoc* (1985) **111**:279–80.

Steelman R, Self-injurious behaviour: report of a case and follow-up, *J Oral Med* (1986) **41**:108–10.

222 Correll RW, Wescott WB, Jensen JL, Non-painful, erythematous circinate lesions of a protean nature on a fissured tongue, *J Am Dent Assoc* (1984) **109**:90–1.

Kullaa-Mikkonen A, Geographic tongue: a scanning electron microscopic study, *J Cutan Pathol* (1986) **13**:154–62.

Wysocki GP, Daley TD, Benign migratory glossitis in patients with juvenile diabetes, *Oral Surg Oral Med Oral Pathol* (1987) **63**:68–70.

223 Escobar V, Farman G, Arm RN, Oral gonococcal infection, *Int J Oral Surg* (1984) **13**:549–54.

Tikjob G, Petersen CS, Ousted M et al, Localisation of gonococci in the anterior oral cavity – a possible reservoir of the gonococcal infection? *Ann Clin Res* (1985) **17**:73–5.

Van der Wal N, Van der Waal I, Candida albicans in median rhomboid glossitis: a post-mortem study, *Int J Oral Maxillofac Surg* (1986) **15**:322–5.

Van der Wal N, Van der Kwast WA, Van der Waal I, Median rhomboid glossitis: a follow-up of 16 patients, *J Oral Med* (1986) **41**:117–20.

224 Paur RK, Paur HS, Lingual tonsillitis, *South Med J* (1986) **79**:1126–8.

Ribbon JW, Amon PM, Larson RA et al, 'Golden tongue' syndrome caused by *Ramichloridium schulzeri*, *Arch Dermatol* (1985) **121**:892–4.

225 Kullaa-Mikkonen A, Sorvari T, Lingua fissurata, *Int J Oral Maxillofac Surg* (1986) **15**:525–33.

Kullaa-Mikkonen A, Sorvari T, Kotilainen R, Morphological variations on the dorsal surface of the human tongue, *Proc Finn Dent Soc* (1985) **81**:104–10.

Murty GE, Fawcett S, The aetiology and management of glossodynia, *Br J Clin Pract* (1990) **44**:389–92.

226 Brook IM, King DJ, Miller ID, Chronic granulomatous cheilitis and its relationship to Crohn's disease, *Oral Surg Oral Med Oral Pathol* (1983) **56**:405–7.

Halme L, Meurman JH, Laine P et al, Oral findings in patients with active and inactive Crohn's disease, *Oral Surg Oral Med Oral Pathol* (1993) **76**:175–81.

Scully C, Cochran KM, Russell RI et al, Crohn's disease of the mouth: an indication of intestinal involvement, *Gut* (1982) **23**:198–201.

227 Kano Y, Shiohara T, Yagita A et al, Association between cheilitis granulomatosa and Crohn's disease, *J Am Acad Dermatol* (1993) **28**:801–2.

Lamey P-J, Lewis MAO, Rees TD et al, Sensitivity to cinnamonaldehyde component of toothpaste, *Br Dent J* (1990) **168**:115–18.

Meisel-Stosiek M, Hornstein OP, Stosiek N, Family study on Melkersson–Rosenthal syndrome. Some hereditary aspects of the disease and review of literature, *Acta Derm Venereol (Stockh)* (1990) **70**:221–6.

Patton DW, Ferguson MM, Forsyth A, Orofacial granulomatosis: a possible allergic basis, *Br J Oral Maxillofac Surg* (1985) **23**:235–42.

Shehade SA, Foulds IS, Granulomatous cheilitis and a positive Kveim test, *Br J Derm* (1986) **115**:619–22.

Wadlington WB, Riley HD Jr, Lowbeer L, The Melkersson–Rosenthal syndrome, *Pediatrics* (1984) **73**:502–6.

Wiesenfeld DW, Ferguson MM, Mitchell D et al, Orofacial granulomatosis: a clinical and pathological analysis, *Q J Med* (1985) **54**:101–13.

Williams PM, Greenberg MS, Management of cheilitis granulomatosa, *Oral Surg Oral Med Oral Pathol* (1991) **72**:436–9.

Winnie R, DeLuke DM, Melkersson–Rosenthal syndrome, *Int J Oral Maxillofac Surg* (1992) **21**:115-17.

Worsaae N, Christensen KO, Bondesen S et al, Melkersson–Rosenthal syndrome and Crohn's disease, *Br J Oral Surg* (1980) **18**:254–8.

Worsaae N, Pindborg JJ, Granulomatous gingival manifestations of Melkersson–Rosenthal syndrome, *Oral Surg Oral Med Oral Pathol* (1980) **49**:131–8.

Zimmer WM, Rogers RS, Reeve CM et al, Orofacial manifestations of Melkersson–Rosenthal syndrome, *Oral Surg Oral Med Oral Pathol* (1992) **74**:610–19.

228 Chan S, Scully C, Prime SS et al, Pyostomatitis vegetans: oral manifestation of ulcerative colitis, *Oral Surg Oral Med Oral Pathol* (1991) **72**:689–92.

Neville B, Laden SA, Smith SE et al, Pyostomatitis vegetans, *Am J Dermatopathol* (1985) **7**:69–77.

Maki M, Aine L, Lipsanen V et al, Dental enamel defects in first-degree relatives in coeliac disease patients, *Lancet* (1991) **337**:763.

Thornhill MH, Zakrewska JM, Gilkes JJH, Pyostomatitis vegetans: report of three cases and review of the literature, *J Oral Pathol Med* (1992) **21**:128–33.

Van Hale HM, Rogers RS, Zone JJ et al, Pyostomatitis vegetans: a reactive mucosal marker for inflammatory disease of the gut, *Arch Dermatol* (1985) **121**:94–8.

Wright KB, Holan G, Casamassimo PS et al, Alveolar bone loss in two children with short-bowel syndrome receiving total parenteral nutrition, *J Periodontol* (1991) **62**:272–5.

Chapter 11

230 Zaia AA, Graner E, Almeida OPD et al, Oral changes associated with biliary atresia and liver transplantation, *J Clin Paediatr Dent* (1993) **18**:39–42.

231 Richards A, Rooney J, Prime S et al, Primary biliary cirrhosis: sole presentation with rampant dental caries, *Oral Surg Oral Med Oral Pathol* (1994) **77**:16–18.

Chapter 12

234 Barnard N, Scully C, Epstein's syndrome: implications for the oral surgeon, *Oral Surg Oral Med Oral Pathol* (1993) **76**:32–4.

Bublitz A, Machat E, Scharer K et al, Changes in dental development in paediatric patients with chronic kidney disease, *Proc Eur Dial Transplant Assoc Eur Ren Assoc* (1981) **18**:517–23.

Liddington M, Richardson AJ, Higgins RM, Skin cancer in renal transplant recipients, *Br J Surg* (1989) **766**:1002–5.

Precious DS, Laba JP, Hinrichsen GJ, Dental considerations for patients on chronic dialysis and renal transplant recipients, *Can Dent Assoc J* (1981) **9**:595–9.

Richards A, Scully C, Eveson J et al, Epstein syndrome: oral lesions in a patient with nephropathy, deafness and thrombocytopenia, *J Oral Pathol Med* (1991) **20**:512–13.

Stoufi ED, Sonis ST, Shklar G, Significance of the head and neck in late infection in renal transplant recipients, *Oral Surg Oral Med Oral Pathol* (1986) **62**:524–8.

Ziccardi VB, Saini J, Demas PN et al, Management of the oral and maxillofacial surgery patient with end-stage renal disease, *J Oral Maxillofac Surg* (1992) **50**:1207–12.

235 Seow WK, Latham SC, The spectrum of dental manifestations in vitamin D-resistant rickets and implications for management, *Pediatr Dent* (1986) **8**:245–50.

Chapter 13

238 Chiodo GT, Rosenstein DI, Dental treatment during pregnancy: a preventive approach, *J Am Dent Assoc* (1985) **110**:365–8.

Levm RP, Pregnancy gingivitis, *J Md State Dent Assoc* (1987) **30**:27.

Pack ARC, Thomson ME, Effect of topical and systemic folic acid supplementation on gingivitis of pregnancy, *J Clin Periodontol* (1980) **7**:402–14.

Seymour RA, Heasman PA, Drugs and the periodontium, *J Clin Periodontol* (1988) **15**:1–16.

Wong RC, Ellis CN, Physiologic skin changes in pregnancy, *J Am Acad Dermatol* (1984) **10**:929–40.

239 Fechner RE, Fitz-Hugh GS, Pope TL Jr, Extraordinary growth of giant cell reparative granuloma during pregnancy, *Arch Otolaryngol* (1984) **110**:116–19.

Kirkham DB, Severe alveolar bone loss associated with pyogenic granuloma – a case report, *J Wis Dent Assoc* (1982) **58**:17–19.

Chapter 14

242 Barker FG, Lappard BJ, Seal DV, Streptococcal necrotizing fasciitis: comparison between histological and clinical features, *J Clin Pathol* (1987) **40**:335–41.

Linder HH, The anatomy of the fasciae of the neck with particular reference to the spread and treatment of intra-oral infections (Ludwig's) that have progressed into adjacent fascial spaces, *Ann Surg* (1986) **204**:705–14.

Rapoport Y, Himelfarb MZ, Zikk D et al, Cervical necrotizing fasciitis of odontogenic origin, *Oral Surg Oral Med Oral Pathol* (1991) **72**:15–18.

Suss SJ, Middleton DB, Cellulitis and related skin conditions, *Am Fam Physician* (1987) **36:**126–36.

Tharakaram S, Keczkes K, Necrotizing fasciitis – a report of five patients, *Int J Dermatol* (1988) **27:**585–8.

Umbert IJ, Winkelmann RK, Oliver GF et al, Necrotizing fasciitis: a clinical, microbiologic and histopathologic study of 14 patients, *J Am Acad Dermatol* (1989) **20:**774–81.

Weisengreen HH, Ludwig's angina: historical review and reflections, *Ear Nose Throat J* (1986) **65:**21–4.

243   Baden E, Caverivière P, Carbonnel S, Sinus histiocytosis with massive lymphodenopathy (Destombes–Rosai–Dorfman syndrome) occurring as a single enlarged submandibular lymph node: a light and immunohistochemical study with review of the literature, *Oral Surg Oral Med Oral Pathol* (1987) **64:**320–6.

Blinder D, Ramon Y, Hendler S et al, Idiopathic submandibular abscesses in children, *Int J Oral Maxillofac Surg* (1986) **15:**292–5.

Ioachim HL, Lymphadenitides. In: Ioachim HL, ed. *Lymph Node Biopsy* (J B Lippincott: Philadelphia, 1982) 35-96.

Manders SM, Lucky AW, Perioral dermatitis in childhood, *J Am Acad Dermatol* (1992) **27:**688–92.

Unger PD, Rappaport KM, Strauchen JA, Necrotizing lymphadenitis: Kikuchi's disease, *Arch Path Lab Med* (1987) **111:**1031–5.

Zelickson BD, Roenigk RK, Actinic cheilitis, *Cancer* (1990) **65:**1307–11.

244   Aine L, Maki M, Reunala T, Coeliac-type dental enamel defects in patients with dermatitis herpetiformis, *Acta Derm Venereol (Stockh)* (1992) **72:**25–7.

Chan LS, Regezi JA, Cooper KD, Oral manifestations of linear IgA disease, *J Am Acad Dermatol* (1990) **22:**362–5.

Chorzelski TP, Jablonska S, Maciejowska E, Linear IgA bullous dermatosis of adults, *Clin Dermatol* (1991) **9:**383–92.

Economopoulou P, Laskaris G, Dermatitis herpetiformis: oral lesions as an early manifestation, *Oral Surg Oral Med Oral Pathol* (1986) **62:**77–80.

Jablonska S, Chorzelski TP, Rosinska D et al, Linear IgA bullous dermatosis of childhood (chronic bullous dermatosis of childhood), *Clin Dermatol* (1991) **9:**393–401.

Katz SI, Blistering skin diseases: new insights, *N Engl J Med* (1985) **313** (Edit):1657–8.

Porter SR, Bain SE, Scully C, Linear IgA disease manifesting as recalcitrant desquamative gingivitis, *Oral Surg Oral Med Oral Pathol* (1992) **74:**179–82.

Scully C, Midda M, Eveson JW, Adult linear immunoglobulin A disease manifesting as desquamative gingivitis, *Oral Surg Oral Med Oral Pathol* (1990) **70:**450–3.

Wiesenfeld D, Martin A, Scully C et al, Oral manifestations in linear IgA disease, *Br Dent J* (1982) **153:**389–99.

245   Edwards S, Wojnarowska F, Armstrong LM, Chronic bullous disease of childhood with oral mucosal scarring, *Clin Exp Dermatol* (1991) **16:**41–3.

Hietanen J, Clinical and cytological features of oral pemphigus, *Acta Odontol Scand* (1982) **40:**403–14.

Ho VC, Stein HB, Ongley RA, Penicillamine-induced pemphigus, *J Rheumatol* (1985) **114:**583–6.

Kirtschig G, Wojnarowska F, Autoimmune blistering diseases: an up-date of diagnostic methods and investigations, *Clin Exp Dermatol* (1994) **19:**97–112.

Lamey P-J, Rees TD, Binnie WH et al, Oral presentation of pemphigus vulgaris and its response to systemic steroid therapy, *Oral Surg Oral Med Oral Pathol* (1992) **74**:54–7.

Singer KH, Hashimoto K, Jensen PJ et al, Pathogenesis of autoimmunity in pemphigus, *Ann Rev Immunol* (1985) **3**:87–108.

Yancey KM, The diagnosis and biology of bullous diseases, *Arch Dermatol* (1994) **130**:983-7.

246   Acosta E, Gilkes JJ, Ivanyi L, Relationship between serum autoantibody titres and the clinical activity of pemphigus, *Oral Surg Oral Med Oral Pathol* (1985) **60**:611–14.

Ahmed AR, Blose DA, Pemphigus vegetans: Neumann type and Hallopeau type, *Int J Dermatol* (1984) **23**:135–41.

Borradori L, Saada V, Tybojad M et al, Oral intraepidermal IgA pustulosis and Crohn's disease, *Br J Dermatol* (1992) **126**:383-6.

Camisa C, Helm TN, Paraneoplastic pemphigus is a distinct neoplasia-induced autoimmune disease, *Arch Dermatol* (1993) **129**:883–6.

Helm TN, Camisa C, Valenzuela R et al, Paraneoplastic pemphigus. A distinct autoimmune vesiculobullous disorder associated with neoplasia, *Oral Surg Oral Med Oral Pathol* (1993) **75**:209–13.

Laskaris GC, Sklavounov A, Stratigos J, Bullous pemphigoid, cicatricial pemphigoid and pemphigus vulgaris: a comparative clinical survey of 278 cases, *Oral Surg Oral Med Oral Pathol* (1982) **54**:656–62.

Liu AY, Valenzuela R, Helm TN et al, Indirect immunofluorescence on rat bladder transitional epithelium: a test with high specificity for paraneoplastic pemphigus, *J Am Acad Dermatol* (1993) **28**:696–9.

Paterson AJ, Lamey PJ, Lewis MA et al, Pemphigus vulgaris precipitated by glibenclamide therapy, *J Oral Pathol Med* (1993) **22**:92–5.

Premalatha S, Jayakumar S, Yesudian P et al, Cerebriform tongue: a clinical sign in pemphigus vegetans, *Br J Dermatol* (1981) **104**:587–91.

Stevens SR, Griffiths CE, Anhalt GJ et al, Paraneoplastic pemphigus presenting as a lichen planus pemphigoides-like eruption, *Arch Dermatol* (1993) **129**:866–9.

247   Antonelli JR, Bachiman R, Scherer W, Mucous membrane pemphigoid: a disease of the elderly, *Special Care in Dentistry* (1991) **11**:143–7.

Firth NA, Rich AM, Radden BG et al, Direct immunofluorescence of oral mucosal biopsies: a comparison of fresh-frozen tissue and formalin-fixed, paraffin-embedded tissue, *J Oral Pathol Med* (1992) **21**:358–63.

Liu HN, Rogers RS, Clinical variants of pemphigoid, *Int J Dermatol* (1986) **25**:17–27.

Manton SM, Scully C, Mucous membrane pemphigoid – an elusive diagnosis, *Oral Surg Oral Med Oral Pathol* (1988) **66**:37–40.

Matthews RW, Pinkney RCN, Scully C, The management of intransigent desquamative gingivitis with dapsone, *Ann Dent* (1989) **48**:41–3.

Peng T, Wisengard RJ, Levine MJ, Gingival basement membrane antigens in desquamative lesions of the gingiva, *Oral Surg Oral Med Oral Pathol* (1986) **61**:584–9.

Silverman S, Gorsky M, Lozada-Nur F et al, Oral mucous membrane pemphigoid, *Oral Surg Oral Med Oral Pathol* (1986) **61**:233–7.

Vincent SD, Lilly GE, Baker KA, Clinical, historic, and therapeutic features of cicatricial pemphigoid, *Oral Surg Oral Med Oral Pathol* (1993) **76:**453–9.

248 Edwards S, Wilkinson JD, Wojnarowska F, Angina bullosa haemorrhagica – a report of three cases and review of the literature, *Clin Exp Dermatol* (1990) **15:**422–4.

Grattan CEH, Small D, Kennedy CTC et al, Oral herpes simplex infection in bullous pemphigoid, *Oral Surg Oral Med Oral Pathol* (1986) **61:**40–3.

Stephenson P, Lamey P-J, Scully C et al, Angina bullosa haemorrhagica: clinical and laboratory features in 30 patients, *Oral Surg Oral Med Oral Pathol* (1987) **63:**560–5.

Stephenson P, Scully C, Prime SS et al, Angina bullosa haemorrhagica: lesional immunostaining and haematological findings, *Br J Oral Maxillofac Surg* (1987) **25:**488–91.

249 Gebel K, Hornstein OP, Drug-induced erythema multiforme: results of a long-term retrospective study, *Dermatologica* (1984) **168:**35–40.

Lozada-Nur F, Gorsky M, Silverman S, Oral erythema multiforme: clinical observations and treatment of 95 patients, *Oral Surg Oral Med Oral Pathol* (1989) **67:**36–40.

Nesbit SP, Gobetti JP, Multiple occurrences of oral erythema multiforme after secondary herpes simplex: report of case and review of the literature, *J Am Dent Assoc* (1986) **112:**348–52.

250 Araujo OE, Flowers FP, Stevens–Johnson syndrome, *J Emerg Med* (1984) **2:**129–35.

Ting HC, Stevens–Johnson syndrome: a review of 34 cases: *Int J Dermatol* (1985) **24:**587–91.

251 Handlers JP, Abrams AM, Aberk AM, Squamous cell carcinoma of the lip developing in discoid lupus erythematosus, *Oral Surg Oral Med Oral Pathol* (1985) **60:**382–6.

Karjalainen TK, Tomich CE, A histopathologic study of oral mucosal lupus erythematosus, *Oral Surg Oral Med Oral Pathol* (1989) **67:**547–54.

Schiodt M, Oral manifestations of lupus erythematosus, *Int J Oral Surg* (1984) **13:**101–47.

252 Bowden JR, Scully C, Eveson JW et al, Multiple myeloma and bullous lichenoid lesions: an unusual association, *Oral Surg Oral Med Oral Pathol* (1990) **70:**587–9.

Scully C, Elkom M, Lichen planus: review and update on pathogenesis, *J Oral Pathol* (1985) **14:**431–58.

Scully C, Prime SS, Matthews JP et al, Mucosal diseases of uncertain etiology: oral lichen planus: cellular immunological changes in epithelium and lamina propria. In: Mackenzie IC, Squier CA, Dabelsteen E, eds, *Oral Mucosal Diseases: Biology, Etiology and Therapy* (Laegeforeningens Forlag: Copenhagen, 1987) 78–84.

253 Barnard NA, Scully C, Eveson JW et al, Oral cancer development in patients with oral lichen planus, *Oral Pathol Med* (1993) **22:**421–4.

De Jong WFB, Albrecht M, Banoczy J et al, Epithelial dysplasia in oral lichen planus, *Int J Oral Surg* (1984) **13:**221–5.

Hietanen J, Pihlman K, Linder E et al, No evidence of hypersensitivity to dental restorative materials in oral lichen planus, *Scand J Dent Res* (1987) **95:**320–7.

Holmstrup P, The controversy of a premalignant potential of oral lichen planus is over, *Oral Surg Oral Med Oral Pathol* (1992) **73:**704–6.

Holmstrup P, Thorn JJ, Rindum J et al, Malignant development of lichen planus-affected oral mucosa, *J Oral Pathol Med* (1988) **17**:219–25.

Laine J, Kalimo K, Forssell H et al, Resolution of oral lichenoid lesions in patients allergic to mercury compounds, *Br J Dermatol* (1992) **126**:10–15.

Marder MZ, Deesen KC, Transformation of oral lichen planus to squamous cell carcinoma, *J Am Dent Assoc* (1982) **105**:55–60.

Murti PR, Daftary DK, Bhonsle RB et al, Malignant potential of oral lichen planus: observations in 722 patients from India, *J Oral Pathol* (1986) **15**:71–7.

Sigurgeirsson B, Lindelöf B, Lichen planus and malignancy. An epidemiologic study of 2071 patients and a review of the literature, *Arch Dermatol* (1991) **127**:1684–8.

Voute ABE, de Jong WFB, Schulten EAJM et al, Possible premalignant character of oral lichen planus: the Amsterdam experience, *J Oral Pathol Med* (1992) **21**:326–9.

254 Church LF Jr, Schosser RH, Chronic ulcerative stomatitis associated with stratified epithelial specific antinuclear antibodies, *Oral Surg Oral Med Oral Pathol* (1992) **73**:579–82.

Eversole LR, Ringer M, The role of dental restorative metals in the pathogenesis of oral lichen planus, *Oral Surg Oral Med Oral Pathol* (1984) **57**:383–7.

Finne K, Goranson K, Winckler L, Oral lichen planus and contact allergy to mercury, *Int J Oral Surg* (1982) **11**:236–9.

James J, Ferguson MM, Forsyth A et al, Oral lichenoid reactions related to mercury sensitivity, *Br J Oral Maxillofac Surg* (1987) **25**:474–80.

Markitzui A, Katz J, Pisanty S, Lichenoid lesions of oral mucosa associated with ketoconazole, *Mykosen* (1986) **29**:317–22.

Wiesenfeld D, Scully C, Macfadyen EE, Multiple lichenoid drug reactions in a patient with Ferguson-Smith disease, *Oral Surg Oral Med Oral Pathol* (1982) **54**:527–9.

256 Mostofi RS, Hayden NP, Soltani K, Oral malignant acanthosis nigricans, *Oral Surg Oral Med Oral Pathol* (1983) **56**:372–4.

Sedano H, Gorlin RJ, Acanthosis nigricans, *Oral Surg Oral Med Oral Pathol* (1987) **63**:462–7.

257 MacLeod RI, Soames JV, Lichen sclerosis et atrophicus of the oral mucosa, *Br J Oral Maxillofac Surg* (1991) **39**:64–5.

Marren P, Millard P, Chia Y et al, Mucosal lichen sclerosus/lichen planus overlap syndromes, *Br J Dermatol* (1994) **131**:118–23.

Schulten EA, Starink TM, van der Waal I, Lichen sclerosus et atrophicus involving the oral mucosa: report of two cases, *J Oral Pathol Med* (1993) **22**:374–7.

Scully C, Eveson JW, Pigmented purpuric stomatitis, *Oral Surg Oral Med Oral Pathol* (1992) **74**:780–2.

Chapter 15

260 Jonsson R, Heyden G, Westberg NG et al, Oral lesions in systemic lupus erythematosus: a clinical histopathological and immunopathological study, *J Rheumatol* (1984) **11**:38–42.

Mutlu S, Richards A, Maddison P et al, Gingival and periodontal health in systemic lupus erythematosus, *Community Dent Oral Epidemiol* (1993) **21**:158–61.

Pisetsky DS, Systemic lupus erythematosus, *Med Clin North Am* (1986) **70**:337–53.

354

Schiodt M, Oral manifestations of lupus erythematosus, *Int J Oral Surg* (1984) **13**:101–47.

261 Black CM, Welsh KI, Maddison PJ et al, HLA antigens, autoantibodies and clinical subsets in scleroderma, *Br J Rheumatol* (1984) **23**:267–71.

Eversole LR, Jacobson PL, Stone CE, Oral and gingival changes in systemic sclerosis (scleroderma), *J Periodontol* (1984) **55**:175–8.

Furst DE, Clements PJ, Saab M et al, Clinical and serological comparison of 17 chronic progressive systemic sclerosis (PSS) and 17 CREST syndrome patients matched for sex, age and disease duration, *Ann Rheum Dis* (1984) **43**:794–801.

Grassi W, Core P, Carlino G et al, Labial capillary microscopy in systemic sclerosis, *Ann Rheum Dis* (1993) **52**:564–9.

Hopper FE, Giles AD, Orofacial changes in systemic sclerosis: report of a case of resorption of mandibular angles and zygomatic arches, *Br J Oral Surg* (1982) **20**:129–34.

Livingstone JZ, Scott TE, Wigley FM et al, Systemic sclerosis (scleroderma): clinical, genetic and serologic subsets, *J Rheumatol* (1987) **14**:512–18.

Nagy G, Kovacs J, Zeher M et al, Analysis of the oral manifestations of systemic sclerosis, *Oral Surg Oral Med Oral Pathol* (1994) **77**:141–6.

262 Isaacson PG, Extranodal lymphomas: the MALT concept, *Verh Dtsch Ges Pathol* (1992) **76**:14–23.

Scully C, Sjögren's syndrome: clinical and laboratory features, immunopathogenesis and management, *Oral Surg Oral Med Oral Pathol* (1986) **62**:510–23.

Scully C, Oral parameters in the diagnosis of Sjögren's syndrome, *Clin Exp Rheumatol* (1989) **7**:113–18.

Scully C, Orofacial manifestations in the rheumatic disorders, *Dental Update* (1989) **16**:240–6.

Scully C, Diseases of the salivary glands, *Br Dent J* (1992) **172**:358–9.

Skopouli FN, Drosos AA, Papaioannou T et al, Preliminary diagnostic criteria for Sjögren's syndrome, *Scand J Rheumatol* (1986) **61**(suppl):22–5.

St Clair EW, New developments in Sjögren's syndrome, *Curr Opin Rheumatol* (1993) **5**:604–12.

263 Condemi JJ, The autoimmune diseases, *JAMA* (1987) **258**:2920-9.

Cunningham JD Jr, Lowry LD, Head and neck manifestations of dermatomyositis–polymyositis, *Otolaryngol Head Neck Surg* (1985) **93**:673–7.

264 Alfaro-Giner A, Penarrocha-Diago M, Bagan-Sebastian JV, Orofacial manifestations of mixed connective tissue disease with an uncommon serologic evolution, *Oral Surg Oral Med Oral Pathol* (1992) **73**:441–4.

Fox RI, Michelson PE, Howell FV, Ocular and oral problems in arthritis, *Postgrad Med* (1985) **78**:87–93.

Gibson J, Lamey PJ, Zoma A et al, Tongue atrophy in mixed connective tissue disease, *Oral Surg Oral Med Oral Pathol* (1991) **71**:294–6.

Krane SM, Simon LS, Rheumatoid arthritis: clinical features and pathogenetic mechanisms, *Med Clin North Am* (1986) **70**:263–84.

Porter SR, Malamos D, Scully C, Mouth–skin interface: 2. Connective tissue and metabolic disorders, *Update* (1986) **33**:94–6.

265 Armstrong RD, Fernandes L, Gibson T et al, Felty's syndrome presenting without arthritis, *BMJ* (1983) **287:**1620.

Barrett AW, Griffiths MJ, Scully C, Osteoarthrosis, the temporomandibular joint and Eagle's syndrome, *Oral Surg Oral Med Oral Pathol* (1993) **75:**273–5.

Breedveld FC, Factors affecting the incidence of infections in Felty's syndrome, *Arch Intern Med* (1987) **147:**915–20.

Goupille P, Fouquet B, Goga D et al, The temporomandibular joint in rheumatoid arthritis: correlations between clinical and tomographic features, *J Dent* (1993) **21:**141–6.

Kononen M, Wolf J, Kilpinen E et al, Radiographic signs in the temporo-mandibular and hand joints in patients with psoriatic arthritis, *Acta Odontol Scand* (1991) **49:**191–6.

Larheim TA, Storhaug K, Tveito L, Temporomandibular joint involvement and dental occlusion in a group of adults with rheumatoid arthritis, *Acta Odont Scand* (1983) **41:**301–9.

Ogden GR, Complete resorption of the mandibular condyles in rheumatoid arthritis, *Br Dent J* (1986) **160:**95–7.

Sienknecht CW, Urowitz MB, Pruzanski W et al, Felty's syndrome: clinical and serological analysis of 34 cases, *Ann Rheum Dis* (1977) **36:**500–7.

Wilson AW, Brown JS, Ord RA, Psori-atic arthropathy of the temporo-mandibular joint, *Oral Surg Oral Med Oral Pathol* (1990) **70:**555–8.

266 Cawson RA, Scully C, Temporo-mandibular joint disorders, *Medicine International* (1986) **2:**1149–51.

Feinmann C, Harris M, Psychogenic facial pain, *Br Dent J* (1984) **156:**165–8, 205–8.

Moss RA, Garrett JC, Temporomandibu-lar joint dysfunction syndrome and myofascial pain dysfunction syndrome, *J Oral Rehabil* (1984) **11:**3–28.

Porter SR, Scully C, Temporomandibular joint disorders, *Medicine International* (1990) **76:**3170–1.

Yusuf H, Rothwell PS, Temporo-mandibular pain–dysfunction in patients suffering from atypical facial pain, *Br Dent J* (1986) **161:**208–12.

267 Singer FR, Paget's disease of bone – a slow virus infection? *Calcif Tissue Int* (1980) **31:**185–7.

Smith BJ, Eveson JW, Paget's disease of bone with particular reference to dentistry, *J Oral Pathol* (1981) **10:**233–47.

268 Katz JO, Underhill TE, Multilocular radiolucencies, *Dent Clin North Am* (1994) **38:**63–81.

Strickberger SA, Schulman SP, Hutchins GM, Association of Paget's disease of bone with calcific aortic valve disease, *Am J Med* (1987) **82:**953–6.

Waldron CA, Fibro-osseous lesions of the jaws, *J Oral Maxillofac Surg* (1993) **51:**828–35.

Zajac AJ, Phillips PE, Paget's disease of bone: clinical features and treatment, *Clin Exp Rheumatol* (1985) **3:**75–88.

269 Forman D, Leiblich S, Berger J et al, Unusual treatment of an aggressive polyostotic fibrous dysplasia with a 3-year follow-up, *Oral Surg Oral Med Oral Pathol* (1990) **70:**150–4.

Lello GE, Sparrow OC, Craniofacial polyostotic fibrous dysplasia, *J Maxillofac Surg* (1985) **13:**267–72.

Mizuno A, Kuroyanagi-Nakajima M, Akiyama Y et al, Facial fibrous dysplasia: report of a case, *Oral Surg Oral Med Oral Pathol* (1991) **72**:284–8.

Pierce AM, Wilson DF, Goss AN, Inherited craniofacial fibrous dysplasia, *Oral Surg Oral Med Oral Pathol* (1985) **60**:403–9.

270 Feuillan PP, McCune–Albright syndrome, *Curr Therap Endocrinol Metabol* (1994) **5**:205–9.

Triantafillidou K, Antoniades K, Karakosis D et al, McCune–Albright syndrome. Report of a case, *Oral Surg Oral Med Oral Pathol* (1993) **75**:571–4.

271 Faircloth WJ Jr, Edwards RC, Farhood VW, Cherubism involving a mother and daughter: case reports and review of the literature, *J Oral Maxillofac Surg* (1991) **49**:535–42.

Ireland AJ, Eveson JW, Cherubism: a report of a case with an unusual post-extraction complication, *Br Dent J* (1988) **164**:116–17.

Levine B, Skope L, Parker R, Cherubism in a patient with Noonan syndrome: report of a case, *J Oral Maxillofac Surg* (1991) **49**:1014-18.

Zachariades N, Papanicolaou S, Xypolyta A, Cherubism, *Int J Oral Surg* (1985) **14**:138–45.

Chapter 16

274 Anonymous, Cystic hygroma, *Lancet* (1990) **335**:511–12.

Chandler JR, Mitchell B, Branchial cleft, cysts, sinuses and fistulae, *Otolaryngol Clin North Am* (1981) **1**:175–85.

Emery PJ, Cystic hygroma of the head and neck: a review of 37 cases, *J Laryngol Otol* (1984) **98**:613–19.

Goldberg R, Motzkin B, Marion R et al, Velo-cardio-facial syndrome: a review of 120 patients, *Am J Med Genet* (1993) **45**:313–19.

Ingoldby CJ, Unusual presentation of branchial cysts: a trap for the unwary, *Ann R Coll Surg Engl* (1985) **67**:175–6.

Marcone M, Suprenant P, Branchial arch cyst, case report and review of the literature, *Oral Health* (1985) **75**:29–33.

Osborne TE, Haller JA, Levin LS et al, Submandibular cystic hygroma resembling a plunging ranula in a neonate: review and report of a case, *Oral Surg Oral Med Oral Pathol* (1991) **71**:16–20.

Shidara K, Uruma T, Yasuoka Y et al, Two cases of nasopharyngeal branchial cyst, *J Laryngol Otol* (1993) **107**:453–5.

275 Jones MC, Facial clefting. Etiology and developmental pathogenesis, *Clin Plast Surg* (1993) **20**:599–606.

Leck I, The geographical distribution of neural tube defects and oral clefts, *Br Med Bull* (1984) **40**:390–5.

Melnick M, Cleft lip (+/- cleft palate) etiology: a search for solutions, *Am J Med Genet* (1992) **42**:10–14.

Wada T, Mizokawa N, Miyazaki T et al, Maxillary dental arch growth in different types of cleft palate, *Cleft Palate J* (1984) **21**:180–92.

Shprintzen RJ, Morphologic significance of bifid uvula, *Pediatrics* (1985) **75**:553–61.

Transactions of the 75th Annual World Dental Conference: Belgrade, September 1985, Symposium on cleft palate, *Int Dent J* (1986) **36**:115–45.

276 Brooks JK, Leonard CO, Coccaro PJ Jr, Opitz (BBB/G) syndrome: oral manifestations, *Am J Med Genet* (1992) **43**:595–601.

Cheney ML, Familial incidence of lip pits, *Am J Otolaryngol* (1986) **7**:311–13.

Daley TD, Intraoral sebaceous hyperplasia. Diagnostic criteria, *Oral Surg Oral Med Oral Pathol* (1993) **75**:343–7.

Fernando C, Tongue tie, *Med J Aust* (1991) **155**:724.

Kern I, Tongue tie, *Med J Aust* (1991) **155**:33–4.

Monk BE, Fordyce spots responding to isotretinoin therapy, *Br J Dermatol* (1993) **129**:355.

Ohishi M, Yamamoto K, Higuchi Y, Congenital dermoid fistula of the lower lip, *Oral Surg Oral Med Oral Pathol* (1991) **71**:203–5.

Rintala AE, Ranta R, Lower lip sinuses, epidemiology, microforms and transverse sulci, *Br J Plastic Surg* (1981) **34**:25–30.

Vilppula AH, Yli-Kertlula UL, Terha PE et al, Sebaceous glands in the buccal mucosa in patients with rheumatic disorders, *Scand J Rheumatol* (1983) **12**:337–42.

277 Buchholz F, Schubert C, Lehmann-Willenbrock E, White sponge naevus of the vulva, *Int J Gynaecol Obstet* (1985) **23**:505–7.

Ciola B, Ramey CA, White sponge naevus of the oral mucosa, *J Conn State Dent Assoc* (1976) **51**:122–6.

Frithiof L, Banoczy J, White sponge naevus (leukoedema exfoliativum mucosae oris): ultrastructural observations, *Oral Surg Oral Med Oral Pathol* (1976) **41**:607–22.

McDonagh AJ, Gawkrodger DJ, Walker AE, White sponge naevus successfully treated with topical tetracycline, *Clin Exp Dermatol* (1990) **15**:152–3.

Nichols GE, Cooper PH, Underwood PB Jr et al, White sponge nevus, *Obst Gynecol* (1990) **76**:545–8.

Wright S, Levy IS, White sponge naevus and ocular coloboma, *Arch Dis Child* (1991) **66**:514–16.

278 Gupta SK, Sharma OP, Malhotra S et al, Cleido-cranial dysostosis – skeletal abnormalities, *Australas Radiol* (1992) **36**:238–42.

Hall BD, Syndromes and situations associated with congenital clavicular hypoplasia or agenesis, *Prog Clin Biol Res* (1982) **164**:279–88.

Ilic D, Cleidocranial dysplasia, *Proc Eur Prosthodontic Assoc* (1980) **4**:101–4.

Tan KL, Tan LK, Cleidocranial dysostosis in infancy, *Pediatr Radiol* (1981) **11**:114–16.

279 Migliorisi JA, Blenkinsopp PT, Oral surgical management of cleidocranial dysostosis, *Br J Oral Surg* (1980) **18**:212–20.

Monasky D, Winkler S, Icenhower JB et al, Cleidocranial dysostosis: two case reports, *NY State Dent J* (1983) **49**:236–8.

Trimble LD, West RA, McNeill RW, Cleidocranial dysplasia (comprehensive treatment of the dentofacial deformities), *J Am Dent Assoc* (1982) **105**:661–6.

280 Cohen MM Jr, Kreiborg S, An updated pediatric perspective on the Apert syndrome, *Am J Dis Child* (1993) **147**:989–93.

Cohen MM Jr, Kreiborg S, Skeletal abnormalities in the Apert syndrome, *Am J Med Genet* (1993) **47**:624–32.

Ferraro NF, Dental, orthodontic and oral/maxillofacial evaluation and treatment in Apert syndrome, *Clin Plast Surg* (1991) **18**:291–307.

Kreiborg S, Crouzon syndrome: a clinical and roentgeno-cephalometric study, *Scand J Plast Reconstr Surg* (1981) **18** (Suppl):1–198.

Rubenstein SE, Divecha V, Maskell A, Crouzon syndrome, *NY State Dent J* (1982) **48:**620–2.

Singh M, Craniosynostosis: Crouzon disease and Apert's syndrome, *Indian J Pediatr* (1983) **20:**608–12.

281 Caouette-Laberge L, Bayet B, Larocque Y, The Pierre Robin sequence: review of 125 cases and evolution of treatment modalities, *Plast Reconstr Surg* (1994) **93:**934–42.

Christian CL, Lachman RS, Aylsworth AS et al, Radiological findings in Hallermann–-Streiff syndrome: report of five cases and a review of the literature, *Am J Med Genet* (1991) **41:**508–14.

Cohen MM Jr, Hallermann–Streiff syndrome: a review, *Am J Med Genet* (1991) **41:**488–99.

Honda E, Inoue T, Domon M et al, Dental radiographic signs characteristic to Hallermann–Streiff syndrome, *Oral Surg Oral Med Oral Pathol* (1990) **70:**121–5.

Kolar JC, Farkas LG, Munro IR, Surface morphology in Treacher Collin's syndrome: an anthropometric study, *Cleft Palate J* (1985) **22:**266–74.

Ohishi M, Murakami E, Haita T et al, Hallermann–Streiff syndrome and its oral complications, *ASDC J Dent Child* (1986) **53:**32–7.

Raulo Y, Tessier P, Mandibulo-facial dysostosis: analysis, principles of surgery, *Scand J Plast Reconstr Surg* (1981) **15:**251–6.

Rintala A, Ranta R, Stegers T, On the pathogenesis of cleft palate in the Pierre Robin syndrome, *Scand J Plast Reconstr Surg* (1984) **18:**237–40.

Sarkar P, Chamyal PC, Kalra SK et al, Treacher Collins' syndrome, *J Indian Med Assoc* (1980) **75:**221–2.

Slootweg PJ, Huber J, Dentoalveolar abnormalities in oculomandibulodyscephaly (Hallermann–Streiff syndrome), *J Oral Pathol* (1984) **13:**147–54.

282 Byers PH, Steiner RD, Osteogenesis imperfecta, *Annu Rev Med* (1992) **43:**269–82.

Hollister DW, Molecular basis of osteogenesis imperfecta, *Curr Probl Dermatol* (1987) **17:**76–94.

Jones AC, Baughman RA, Multiple idiopathic mandibular bone cysts in a patient with osteogenesis imperfecta, *Oral Surg Oral Med Oral Pathol* (1993) **75:**333–7.

Lachman RS, Tiller GE, Graham JM Jr et al, Collagen, genes and the skeletal dysplasias on the edge of a new era: a review and update, *Eur J Radiol* (1992) **14:**1–10.

Mundlos S, Spranger J, Genetic disorders of connective tissues, *Curr Opin Rheumatol* (1991) **3:**832–7.

Pope FM, Nicholls AC, Molecular abnormalities of collagen in human disease, *Arch Dis Child* (1987) **62:**523–8.

Prockop DJ, Kivirikko KI, Heritable diseases of collagen, *N Engl J Med* (1984) **311:**376–86.

Schwartz S, Tsipouras P, Oral findings in osteogenesis imperfecta, *Oral Surg Oral Med Oral Pathol* (1984) **57:**161–7.

Smith R, ed. *The Brittle Bone Syndrome: Osteogenesis Imperfecta* (Butterworths: London 1983).

283 Droz-Desprez D, Azou C, Bordigoni P et al, Infantile osteopetrosis: a case report on dental findings, *J Oral Pathol Med* (1992) **21:**422–5.

Juniper RP, Caffey's disease, *Br J Oral Surg* (1982) **20:**281–7.

Mintz SM, Martone CH, Anavi Y, Avoiding problems in patients with craniotubular bone disorders, *J Am Dent Assoc* (1993) **124**:116-18.

Turnpenny PD, Davidson R, Stockdale EJ et al, Severe prenatal infantile cortical hyperostosis (Caffey's disease), *Clin Dysmorphol* (1993) **2**:81–6.

284 Gorlin RJ, Focal palmoplantar and marginal gingival hyperkeratosis – a syndrome, *Birth Defects* (1976) **12**:239–42.

Laskaris G, Vareltzidis A, Avgerinou G, Focal palmoplantar and oral mucosa hyperkeratosis syndrome: a report concerning five members of a family, *Oral Surg Oral Med Oral Pathol* (1980) **50**:250–3.

Lucker GPH, Van der Kerkhof PCM, Steijlen PM, The hereditary palmoplantar keratoses: an updated review and classification, *Br J Dermatol* (1994) **131**:1–14.

Martin MD, Nusbacher C, The patient with ichthyosis, *Oral Surg Oral Med Oral Pathol* (1985) **59**:581–4.

Williams ML, Ichthyosis: mechanisms of disease, *Pediatr Dermatol* (1992) **9**:365–8.

285 Burge SM, Wilkinson JD, Darier–White disease: a review of the clinical features in 163 patients, *J Amer Acad Dermatol* (1992) **27**:40–50.

Clarke A, Hypohidrotic ectodermal dysplasia, *J Med Genet* (1987) **24**:659–63.

Clarke A, Phillips DIM, Brown R et al, Clinical aspects of X-linked hypohidrotic ectodermal dysplasia, *Arch Dis Child* (1987) **62**:989–96.

Crawford PJM, Aldred MJ, Clarke A, Clinical and radiographic dental findings in X-linked hypohidrotic ectodermal dysplasia, *J Med Genet* (1991) **28**:181–5.

Freire-Maia N, Pinheiro M, *Ectodermal Dysplasia: a Clinical and Genetic Study* (Alan R Liss: New York, 1984)

Guckes AD, Brahim JS, McCarthy GR et al, Using endosseous dental implants for patients with ectodermal dysplasia, *J Am Dent Assoc* (1991) **122**:59–62.

Macleod RI, Munro CS, The incidence and distribution of oral lesions in patients with Darier's disease, *Br Dent J* (1991) **171**:133–6.

286 Ainsworth SR, Aulicino PL, A survey of patients with Ehlers–Danlos syndrome, *Clin Orthop* (1993) **286**:250–6.

Bond PJ, Friend GW, Meridith MW, Ehlers–Danlos syndrome identified from periodontal findings: case report, *Pediatr Dent* (1993) **15**:212–13.

Dyne KM, Vitellaro-Zuccarello L, Bacchella L et al, Ehlers–Danlos syndrome type VIII: biochemical, stereological and immunocytochemical studies on dermis from a child with clinical signs of Ehlers–Danlos syndrome and a family history of premature loss of permanent teeth, *Br J Dermatol* (1993) **128**:458–63.

Fridrich KL, Fridrich HH, Kempf KK et al, Dental implications in Ehlers–Danlos syndrome. A case report, *Oral Surg Oral Med Oral Pathol* (1990) **69**:431–5.

Gosney MBE, Unusual presentation of a case of Ehlers–Danlos syndrome, *Br Dent J* (1987) **163**:54–6.

Hartsfield JK Jr, Kousseff BG, Phenotypic overlap of Ehlers–Danlos syndrome types IV and VIII, *Am J Med Genet* (1990) **37**:465–70.

Sacks H, Zelig D, Schabes G, Recurrent temporomandibular joint subluxation and facial ecchymosis leading to diagnosis of Ehlers–Danlos syndrome: report of surgical management and review of the literature, *J Oral Maxillofac Surg* (1990) **48**:641–7.

Wright JT, Comprehensive dental care and general anaesthetic management of hereditary epidermolysis bullosa, *Oral Surg Oral Med Oral Pathol* (1990) **70**:573–8.

Wright JT, Fine J-D, Johnson LB, Oral soft tissues in hereditary epidermolysis bullosa, *Oral Surg Oral Med Oral Pathol* (1991) **71**:440–6.

Wright JT, Fine JD, Johnson L, Hereditary epidermolysis bullosa: oral manifestations and dental management, *Pediatr Dent* (1993) **15**:242–8.

287 Briggaman RA, Gammon WR, Woodley DT, Epidermolysis bullosa acquisita of the immunopathological type (dermolytic pemphigoid), *J Invest Dermatol* (1985) **85** (Suppl):795–845.

Eady RAJ, Tidman MJ, Heagerty AHM et al, Approaches to the study of epidermolysis bullosa, *Curr Probl Dermatol* (1987) **17**:127–41.

Fine JD, Bauer EA, Briggaman RA et al, Revised clinical and laboratory criteria for subtypes of inherited epidermolysis bullosa, *J Am Acad Dermatol* (1991) **24**:119–35.

288 Burgess MC, Incontinentia pigmenti: six cases of Bloch–Sulzberger syndrome, *Br Dent J* (1982) **152**:195–6.

Hersh SP, Pachyonychia congenita. Manifestations for the otolaryngologist, *Arch Otolaryngol Head Neck Surg* (1990) **116**:732–4.

Himelhoch DA, Scott BJ, Orsen RA, Dental defects in incontinentia pigmenti, *Pediatr Dent* (1987) **9**:236–9.

Milam PE, Griffin TJ, Shapiro RD, A dentofacial deformity associated with incontinentia pigmenti: report of a case, *Oral Surg Oral Med Oral Pathol* (1990) **70**:420–4.

Vogt J, Matheson J, Incontinentia pigmenti (Bloch–Sulzberger syndrome). A case report, *Oral Surg Oral Med Oral Pathol* (1991) **71**:454–6.

289 Devlin MF, Barrie R, Ward-Booth RP, Cowden's disease: a rare but important manifestation of oral papillomatosis, *Br J Oral Maxillofac Surg* (1992) **30**:335–6.

Rosenberg-Gertzman CB, Clark M, Gaston G, Multiple hamartoma and neoplasia syndrome (Cowden's syndrome), *Oral Surg Oral Med Oral Pathol* (1980) **49**:314–16.

Swart JGN, Lekkas C, Allard RHB, Oral manifestations in Cowden's syndrome, *Oral Surg Oral Med Oral Pathol* (1985) **59**:264–8.

Takenoshita Y, Kubo S, Takeuchi T et al, Oral and facial lesions in Cowden's disease: report of two cases and a review of the literature, *J Oral Maxillofac Surg* (1993) **51**:682–7.

290 Scully C, Down's syndrome. In: Chamberlain EV, ed. *Contemporary Obstetrics and Gynaecology* (Northwood Publications: London 1977) 231–9.

Scully C, Down's syndrome. In: Crown S, ed. *Practical Psychiatry* (Northwood Publications: London 1981) 208.

Stabholz A, Mann J, Sela M et al, Caries experience, periodontal treatment needs, salivary pH, and *Streptococcus mutans* counts in a preadolescent Down's syndrome population, *Special Care in Dentistry* (1991) **11**:203–8.

291 Modeer T, Barr M, Dahllof G, Periodontal disease in children with Down's syndrome, *Scand J Dent Res* (1990) **98**:228–34.

Reuland-Bosma W, van Dijk J, Periodontal disease in Down's syndrome: a review, *J Clin Periodontol* (1986) **13**:64–73.

Scully C, Down's syndrome: aspects of dental care, *J Dent* (1976) **4**:167–74.

Yavuzyilmaz E, Ersoy F, Sanal O et al, Neutrophil chemotaxis and periodontal status in Down's syndrome patients, *J Nihon Univ Sch Dent* (1993) **35**:91–5.

292 Caballero LR, Robles JLD, Caballero CR et al, Tooth pits: an early sign of tuberous sclerosis, *Acta Derm Venereol (Stockh)* (1987) **67**:457–9.

Fryer AE, Chalmers A, Connor JM et al, Evidence that the gene for tuberous sclerosis is on chromosome 9, *Lancet* (1987) **i**:659–61.

Scully C, Orofacial manifestations in tuberous sclerosis, *Oral Surg Oral Med Oral Pathol* (1977) **44**:706–16.

Scully C, Oral mucosal lesions in association with epilepsy and cutaneous lesions: Pringle–Bourneville syndrome, *Int J Oral Surg* (1981) **10**:68–72.

Smith D, Porter SR, Scully C, Gingival and other oral manifestations in tuberous sclerosis, *Periodontal Clinical Investigations* (1993) **15**:13–18.

Thomas D, Rapley J, Strathman R et al, Tuberous sclerosis with gingival overgrowth, *J Periodontol* (1992) **63**:713–17.

293 Geist JR, Gander DL, Stefanac SJ, Oral manifestations of neurofibromatosis types I and II, *Oral Surg Oral Med Oral Pathol* (1992) **73**:376–82.

Leading article, Neurofibromatosis, *Lancet* (1987) **i**:663–4.

Neville BW, Hann J, Narang R et al, Oral neurofibrosarcoma associated with neurofibromatosis type I, *Oral Surg Oral Med Oral Pathol* (1991) **72**:456–61.

Scully C, Orofacial manifestations of the neurodermatoses, *J Dent Child* (1980) **47**:255–60.

294 Kuster W, Happle R, Neurocutaneous disorders in children, *Curr Opin Pediatr* (1993) **5**:436-40.

MacIntyre DR, Hislop SWG, Ross JW et al, The basal cell naevus syndrome, *Dental Update* (1985) **12**:630–5.

Reese V, Frieden IJ, Paller AS et al, Association of facial hemangiomas with Dandy–Walker and other posterior fossa malformations, *J Pediatr* (1993) **122**:379–84.

Uram M, Zubillaga C, The cutaneous manifestations of Sturge–Weber syndrome, *J Clin Neuro Ophthalmol* (1982) **2**:245–8.

295 Evans DG, Farndon PA, Burnell LD et al, The incidence of Gorlin syndrome in 173 consecutive cases of medulloblastoma, *Br J Cancer* (1991) **64**:959–61.

Gorlin RJ, Nevoid basal-cell carcinoma syndrome, *Medicine* (1987) **66**:98–113.

Howell JB, Nevoid basal cell carcinoma syndrome: profile of genetic and environmental factors in oncogenesis, *J Am Acad Dermatol* (1984) **11**:98–104.

296 Biesbrock AR, Aguirre A, Multiple focal pigmented lesions in the maxillary tuberosity and hard palate: a unique display of intraoral junctional nevi, *J Periodontol* (1992) **63**:718–21.

Buchner A, Hansen LS, Pigmented nevi of the oral mucosa, *Oral Surg Oral Med Oral Pathol* (1980) **49**:55–62.

Giardiello FM, Welsh SB, Hamilton SR et al, Increased risk of cancer in the Peutz–Jeghers syndrome, *N Engl J Med* (1987) **316**:1511–14.

Rodu B, Martinez MG, Peutz–Jeghers syndrome and cancer, *Oral Surg Oral Med Oral Pathol* (1984) **58**:584–8.

362

Wilson DM, Pitts WC, Hintz RL et al, Testicular tumors with Peutz–Jeghers syndrome, *Cancer* (1986) **57:**2238–40.

297 Barrett AW, Griffiths MJ, Scully C, The de Lange syndrome in association with a bleeding tendency: oral surgical implications, *Int J Oral Maxillofac Surg* (1993) **22:**171–2.

Gorlin RJ, Pindborg JJ, Cohen MM, *Syndromes of the Head and Neck*, 2nd edn (McGraw-Hill: New York, 1976) 253–5.

Scully C, The de Lange syndrome, *J Oral Med* (1980) **35:**32–4.

298 Boraz RA, Cri-du-chat syndrome: dental considerations and report of case, *Special Care in Dentistry* (1990) **10:**13–15.

Lin AE, Doshi N, Flom L et al, Beemer–Langer syndrome with manifestations of an orofaciodigital syndrome, *Am J Med Genet* (1991) **39:**247–51.

Pearn J, Gage J, Genetics and oral health, *Aust Dent J* (1987) **32:**1–10.

Scully C, Davison MF, Orofacial manifestations of the cri-du-chat (5p-) syndrome, *J Dent* (1980) **7:**313–20.

Singh KS, Trisomy 13 (Patau's syndrome): a rare case of survival into adulthood, *J Ment Defic Res* (1990) **34:**91–3.

299 Verloes A, Ayme S, Gambarelli D et al, Holoprosencephaly–polydactyly ('pseudotrisomy 13') syndrome: a syndrome with features of hydrocephalus and Smith–Lemli–Opitz syndromes. A collaborative multicentre study, *J Med Genet* (1991) **28:**297–303.

300 Bakaeen G, Scully C, Hereditary gingival fibromatosis in a family with the Zimmermann–Laband syndrome, *J Oral Pathol Med* (1991) **20:**457–9.

Chadwick B, Hunter B, Hunter L et al, Laband syndrome, *Oral Surg Oral Med Oral Pathol* (1994) **78:**57–63.

301 Gazit E, The stomatognathic system in myotonic dystrophy, *Eur J Orthodont* (1987) **9:**160–4.

Thayer HH, Genshaw J, Oral manifestations of myotonic muscular dystrophy, *J Am Dent Assoc* (1966) **72:**1405–11.

Chapter 17

304 Evans CRH, Oral ulceration after contact with the houseplant *Dieffenbachia*, *Br Dent J* (1987) **162:**467–8.

Gatot A, Arbelle J, Leiberman A et al, Effects of sodium hypochlorite on soft tissues after its inadvertent injection beyond the root apex, *J Endodontics* (1991) **17:**573–4.

Linebaugh ML, Koka S, Oral electrical burns: etiology, histopathology and prosthodontic treatment, *J Prosthodontics* (1993) **2:**136–41.

Touyz LZG, Hille JJ, A fruit mouthwash chemical burn, *Oral Surg Oral Med Oral Pathol* (1984) **58:**290–2.

305 Daley TD, Wysocki GP, Day C, Clinical and pharmacological correlations in cyclosporin-induced gingival hyperplasia, *Oral Surg Oral Med Oral Pathol* (1986) **62:**417–21.

Dongari A, McDonnell HT, Langlais RP, Drug-induced gingival overgrowth, *Oral Surg Oral Med Oral Pathol* (1993) **76:**543–8.

Glenert U, Drug stomatitis due to gold therapy: a clinical and histologic study, *Oral Surg Oral Med Oral Pathol* (1984) **58:**52–6.

Hassell TM, Epilepsy and the oral manifestations of phenytoin therapy. In: Myers HM, ed. *Monographs in Oral Science* (Karger: Basel 1981) 9.

Hassell TM, Hefti AF, Drug-induced gingival overgrowth: old problem, new problem, *Crit Rev Oral Biol Med* (1991) **2**:103–37.

Seymour RA, Calcium channel blockers and gingival overgrowth, *Br Dent J* (1991) **170**:376–9.

Seymour RA, Heasman PA, *Drugs, disease and the periodontium* (Oxford University Press: Oxford 1992) 1–201. Seymour RA, Jacobs DJ, Cyclosporin and the gingival tissues, *J Clin Periodontol* (1992) **19**:1–11.

Shaftic AA, Widdup LL, Abate MA et al, Nifedipine-induced gingival hyperplasia, *Drug Intell Clin Pharm* (1986) **20**:602–5.

Slavin J, Taylor J, Cyclosporin, nifedipine and gingival hyperplasia, *Lancet* (1987) **ii**:739.

Stinnett E, Rodu B, Grizzle WE, New developments in understanding phenytoin-induced gingival hyperplasia, *J Am Dent Assoc* (1987) **114**:814–16.

Varga E, Tyldesley WR, Carcinoma arising in cyclosporin-induced gingival hyperplasia, *Br Dent J* (1991) **171**:26–7.

306 Diamond JP, Chanda A, Williams C et al, Tranexamic acid-related ligneous conjunctivitis with gingival and peritoneal lesions, *Br J Ophthalmol* (1991) **75**:753–4.

308 Thomas D, Buchanan N, Teratogenic effects of anticonvulsants, *J Pediatr* (1981) **99**:163–70.

Winter RM, Donnai D, Burn J et al, Fetal valproate syndrome: is there a recognisable phenotype? *J Med Genet* (1987) **24**:692–5.

309 Dummett CO, Pertinent considerations in oral pigmentations, *Br Dent J* (1985) **158**:9–12.

Wollina U, Funfstuck V, Chloroquine-induced isolated palatal hyperpigmentation, *Deutsche Zeitschrift fur Mund-, Kiefer-, und Gesichts-Chirurgie* (1990) **14**:104–5.

310 Rogers SN, Vale JA, Oral manifestations of poisoning, *Br Dent J* (1993) **174**:141–3.

311 Buchner A, Hansen LS, Amalgam pigmentation (amalgam tattoo) of the oral mucosa: a clinicopathological study of 268 cases, *Oral Surg Oral Med Oral Pathol* (1980) **49**:139–47.

Dayan D, Buchner A, Moscona D et al, Pigmentation of the oral mucosa after root filling with AH-26: a light and electron microscopic study, *Clin Prevent Dent* (1983) **5**:25–9.

Owens BM, Johnson WW, Schuman NJ, Oral amalgam pigmentations (tattoos): a retrospective study, *Quintessence Int* (1992) **23**:805–10.

Owens BM, Schuman NJ, Johnson WW, Oral amalgam tattoos: a diagnostic study, *Compendium* (1993) **14**:210, 212, 214.

Peters E, Gardner DG, A method of distinguishing between amalgam and graphite in tissue, *Oral Surg Oral Med Oral Pathol* (1986) **62**:73–6.

Rahman A, Foreign bodies in the maxillary antrum, *Br Dent J* (1982) **153**:308.

312 Lee SM, Lee SH, Generalized argyria after habitual use of AgNO3, *J Dermatol* (1994) **21**:50–3.

Tunnessen WW, McMahon KJ, Basser M, Acrodynia: exposure to mercury from fluorescent light bulbs, *Pediatrics* (1987) **79**:786–9.

313 Aragon SB, Dalwick MF, Buckley S, Pneumomediastinum and subcutaneous emphysema during third molar extraction under general anaesthesia, *J Oral Maxillofac Surg* (1986) **44**:141–4.

Belfiglio EJ, Fox LJ, Extensive subcutaneous emphysema crossing the midline after extraction: report of case, *J Am Dent Assoc* (1986) **112**:646–8.

Chuong R, Boland TJ, Piper MA, Pneumomediastinum and subcutaneous emphysema associated with temporomandibular joint surgery, *Oral Surg Oral Med Oral Pathol* (1992) **74**:2–6.

Rossiter JL, Hendrix RA, Iatrogenic subcutaneous cervicofacial and mediastinal emphysema, *J Otolaryngol* (1991) **20**:315–19.

314 Anderson JA, Adkinson NF, Allergic reactions to drugs and biological agents, *JAMA* (1987) **258**:2891–9.

Atkinson JC, Frank MM, Oral manifestations and dental management of patients with hereditary angioedema, *J Oral Pathol Med* (1991) **20**:139–42.

Brickman C, Tsokos G, Balow J et al, Immunoregulatory diseases associated with hereditary angioedema, *J Allergy Clin Immunol* (1986) **77**:749–57, 758–67.

Candelaria LM, Huttula CS, Angioedema associated with angiotensin-converting enzyme inhibitors, *J Oral Maxillofac Surg* (1991) **49**:1237–9.

Clemmensen O, Hjarth N, Perioral contact urticaria from sorbic acid and benzoic acid in a salad dressing, *Contact Dermatitis* (1982) **8**:1–6.

Dyer PD, Late-onset angioedema after interruption of angiotensin converting enzyme inhibitor therapy, *J Allergy Clin Immunol* (1994) **93**:947–8.

Ley SJ, Williams RC, A family with hereditary angioedema and multiple immunologic disorder, *Am J Med* (1987) **82**:1046–51.

McCarthy NR, Diagnosis and management of hereditary angioedema, *Br J Oral Maxillofac Surg* (1985) **23**:123–7.

Peacock ME, Brennan WA, Strong SL et al, Angioedema as a complication in periodontal surgery: report of a case, *J Periodontol* (1991) **62**:643–5.

Zeitoun IM, Dhanrajani PJ, Angioneurotic edema mimicking Ludwig's angina: a case report, *J Oral Maxillofac Surg* (1993) **51**:601–3.

315 Amphlett J, Colwell WC, Edentulous vestibuloplasty using the palatal graft technique, *J Prosthet Dent* (1982) **48**:8–14.

Ehrl PA, Oro-antral communication, *Int J Oral Surg* (1980) **9**:351–8.

Pogrel MA, Intraoral dermis grafting – has it any advantages? *Oral Surg Oral Med Oral Pathol* (1985) **60**:598–603.

316 Carl W, Oral complications in cancer patients, *Am Fam Physician* (1983) **27**:161–70.

Fleming TJ, Oral tissue changes of radiation-oncology and their management, *Dent Clin North Am* (1990) **34**:223–37.

Jacob RF, Management of xerostomia in the irradiated patient, *Clin Plast Surg* (1993) **20**:507–16.

Maguire A, Murray JJ, Craft AW et al, Radiological features of the long-term effects from treatment of malignant disease in childhood, *Br Dent J* (1987) **162**:99–102.

Rothwell BR, Prevention and treatment of the orofacial complications of radiotherapy, *J Am Dent Assoc* (1987) **114**:316–22.

317 Haddock A, Porter SR, Scully C, Submandibular gustatory sweating, *Oral Surg Oral Med Oral Pathol* (1994) **77**:317.

May JS, McGuirt WF, Frey's syndrome: treatment with topical glycopyrrolate, *Head & Neck* (1989) **11**:85–9.

Mealey BL, Bilateral gustatory sweating as a sign of diabetic neuropathy, *Oral Surg Oral Med Oral Pathol* (1994) **77**:113–15.

318 Scully C, Chen M, Tongue piercing (oral body art), *Br J Oral Maxillofac Surg* (1994) **32**:37–8.

INDEX